TRAUMA SURGERY

This B

I

The KEY TOPICS Series

Advisors:

T.M. Craft *Department of Anaesthesia and Intensive Care, Royal United Hospital, Bath, UK*
C.S. Garrard *Intensive Therapy Unit, John Radcliffe Hospital, Oxford, UK*
P.M. Upton *Department of Anaesthetics, Royal Cornwall Hospital, Treliske, Truro, UK*

Anaesthesia, Second Edition
Obstetrics and Gynaecology, Second Edition
Accident and Emergency Medicine
Paediatrics, Second Edition
Orthopaedic Surgery
Otolaryngology
Ophthalmology
Psychiatry
General Surgery
Renal Medicine
Trauma
Chronic Pain
Oral and Maxillofacial Surgery
Oncology
Cardiovascular Medicine
Neurology
Neonatology
Gastroenterology
Thoracic Surgery
Respiratory Medicine
Orthopaedic Trauma Surgery

Forthcoming titles include:

Critical Care
Accident and Emergency Medicine, Second Edition

KEY TOPICS IN
ORTHOPAEDIC
TRAUMA SURGERY

G.S. KEENE
FRCS Orth
Consultant Trauma and Orthopaedic Surgeon,
Addenbrooke's Hospital, Cambridge, UK

A.H.N. ROBINSON
FRCS Orth
Consultant Trauma and Orthopaedic Surgeon,
Addenbrooke's Hospital, Cambridge, UK

M.G. BOWDITCH
FRCS Orth
Specialist Registrar in Trauma and Orthopaedic Surgery,
Addenbrooke's Hospital, Cambridge, UK

D.J. EDWARDS
FRCS Orth
Consultant Trauma and Orthopaedic Surgeon,
Addenbrooke's Hospital, Cambridge, UK

Consultant Editor

A.C. ROSS
MB FRCS
Consultant Orthopaedic Surgeon, Royal United Hospital and
Royal National Hospital for Rheumatic Diseases, Bath, UK

βIOS
SCIENTIFIC
PUBLISHERS

A CIP catalogue record for this book is available from the British Library.

ISBN 1 85996 291 2

BIOS Scientific Publishers Ltd
9 Newtec Place, Magdalen Road, Oxford OX4 1RE, UK
Tel. +44 (0)1865 726286. Fax +44 (0)1865 246823
World Wide Web home page: http://www.bios.co.uk/

Important Note from the Publisher
The information contained within this book was obtained by BIOS Scientific Publishers Ltd from sources believed by us to be reliable. However, while every effort has been made to ensure its accuracy, no responsibility for loss or injury whatsoever occasioned to any person acting or refraining from action as a result of information contained herein can be accepted by the authors or publishers.

The reader should remember that medicine is a constantly evolving science and while the authors and publishers have ensured that all dosages, applications and practices are based on current indications, there may be specific practices which differ between communities. You should always follow the guidelines laid down by the manufacturers of specific products and the relevant authorities in the country in which you are practising.

Production Editor: Jonathan Gunning.
Typeset by Footnote Graphics, Warminster, UK.
Printed by TJ International Ltd, Padstow, UK.

CONTENTS

ABBREVIATIONS

3D	three dimensional
AAOS	American Academy of Orthopaedic Surgeons
ACJ	acromioclavicular joint
ACL	anterior cruciate ligament
ADH	antidiuretic hormone
ADL	activities of daily living
AFO	ankle foot orthosis
AIDS	acquired immune deficiency syndrome
AIS	Abbreviated Injury Scale
ALARA	as low as reasonably achievable
ALIF	anterior lumbar interbody fusion
ALRUD	acute longitudinal radio-ulnar dissociation
AMBRI	atraumatic multidirectional bilateral rehabilitation and rarely inferior capsular shift
AO	Arbeitsgemeinschaft für Osteosynthesefragen
AP	antero-posterior
APACHE	Acute Physiology and Chronic Health Evaluation
APC	antero-posterior compression
ARDS	adult respiratory distress syndrome
ASIF	Association for the Study of Internal Fixation
ATLS	Advanced Trauma Life Support
AVN	avascular necrosis
BMP	bone morphogenic protein
BP	blood pressure
C5	5th cervical
C6	6th cervical
C8	8th cervical
CCL	coracoclavicular ligament
cm	centimetre
CM	combined mechanism
CMCJ	carpo-metacarpal joint
CO	cervical orthosis
CPP	cerebral perfusion pressure
CRP	C-reactive protein
CSF	cerebrospinal fluid
CT	computerized tomogram
CTO	cervicothoracic orthosis
Da	Dalton
DCP	dynamic compression plate
DCS	dynamic condylar screw
DIC	disseminated intravascular coagulation
DIPJ	distal interphalangeal joint
DISI	dorsal intercalated segment instability
DNA	deoxyribonucleic acid

DRUJ	distal radio-ulnar joint
DVLA	Driver and Vehicle Licensing Authority
DVT	deep venous thrombosis
ECG	electrocardiogram
ECRB	extensor carpi radialis brevis
ECU	extensor carpi ulnaris
EDC	extensor digitorum communis
EGF	epidermal growth factor
EMG	electromyelogram
EPL	extensor pollicis longus
ESR	erythrocyte sedimentation rate
EUA	examination under anaesthetic
FCR	flexor carpi radialis
FCU	flexor carpi ulnaris
FDP	flexor digitorum profundus
FDS	flexor digitorum superficialis
FES	fat embolism syndrome
FFA	free fatty acid
FGF	fibroblast growth factor
FPL	flexor pollicis longus
GCS	Glasgow Coma Scale
Gy	Gray
HGV	heavy goods vehicle
HIV	human immunodeficiency virus
HO	heterotopic ossification
HRT	hormone replacement therapy
im	intramuscular
ICP	intracranial pressure
ICU	intensive care unit
IGF	insulin-like growth factor
IM	intramedullary
ISS	Injury Severity Score
iv	intravenous
IVP	intravenous pyelogram
K-wire	Kirschner wire
KAFO	knee ankle foot orthosis
kg	kilogram
l	litre
lb/in^2	pounds per square inch
lb	pound
LC	lateral compression
LC-DCP	low contact dynamic compression plate
LCL	lateral collateral ligament
LD	lethal dose
LMN	lower motor neurone
LSO	lumbo-sacral orthosis
MCL	medial collateral ligament

MCPJ	metacarpo-phalangeal joint
MSC	mesenchymal stem cells
MESS	Mangled Extremity Severity Score
mm	millimetre
mmHg	millimetres of mercury
MO	myositis ossificans
MPa	megapascal
MRI	magnetic resonance imaging
MSC	mesenchymal stem cells
MTOS	Major Trauma Outcome Study
MTPJ	metatarso-phalangeal joint
MUA	manipulation under anaesthetic
N	Newton
NAI	non-accidental injury
NCS	nerve conduction studies
NG	nasogastric
NHS	National Health Service (United Kingdom)
NISSA	nerve injury, ischaemia, soft tissue contamination, skeletal, shock and age score
Nm^{-2}	Newtons per square metre
NSAID	non-steroidal anti-inflammatory drug
OI	osteogenesis imperfecta
ORIF	open reduction and internal fixation
OS	osteogenic sarcoma
PA	postero-anterior
PaO_2	partial pressure of oxygen – arterial
PASG	pneumatic anti-shock garment
PCL	posterior cruciate ligament
$PaCO_2$	partial pressure of carbon dioxide – arterial
PDGF	platelet-derived growth factor
PDS	poly-p-dioxanone
PGA	polyglycolic acid
PHBA	poly-β-hydroxybutyric acid
PHSS	Peterborough Hip Scoring System
PIPJ	proximal interphalangeal joint
PLA	polylactic acid
PLIF	posterior lumbar interbody fusion
PR	per rectum
PTH	parathyroid hormone
ROM	range of movement
RTA	road traffic accident
RTS	Revised Trauma Score
SCIWORA	spinal cord injury without radiological abnormality
SCJ	sternoclavicular joint
sec	second
SF-36	Short Form-36
S–H	Salter–Harris

SI	sacroiliac
SIRS	systemic inflammatory response syndrome
SOMI	sterno-occipito-mandibular immobilizer
SUFE	slipped upper femoral epiphysis
Sv	sievert
T1	1st thoracic
TER	total elbow replacement
TFCC	triangular fibrocartilage complex
TGF	transforming growth factor
THR	total hip replacement
TKR	total knee replacement
TLO	thoraco-lumbar orthosis
TLSO	thoraco-lumbo-sacral orthosis
TPN	total parenteral nutrition
TS	Trauma Score
TSR	total shoulder replacement
TUBS	traumatic unilateral Bankart lesion in which surgery is often indicated
UCL	ulnar collateral ligament
UK	United Kingdom
UMN	upper motor neurone
VISI	volar intercalated segment instability
VS	vertical shear
WAD	whiplash-associated disorders
w_t	tissue weighting factors
μm	micrometre

PREFACE

Orthopaedic trauma surgery is a specialist field in its own right. A high standard of knowledge is required by Specialist Registrars for the daily care of trauma patients and for the Fellowship Examination – the 'FRCS Orth'. This book has been written for specialist registrars in trauma and orthopaedic surgery, and other specialists involved in trauma care. The book will be of value to allied professionals, nurses, physiotherapists and lawyers.

The principles of non-operative and operative fracture management have been covered concisely. The common treatment principles are discussed, but there is not room for long management algorithms or discussion of every treatment option. The text is dogmatic and attempts to steer a safe course through controversial areas of trauma care. From our own experience, the principles of basic science are the hardest to grasp and the most difficult to research from other sources; we have therefore attempted to address this issue.

We acknowledge that such texts as *Rockwood and Green's Fractures in Adults*, or *Skeletal Trauma* by Browner and colleagues are vastly more comprehensive. Our book is not intended as a substitute for these texts, but rather as a practical and manageable clinical guide and revision aid, concentrating on the key topics faced by orthopaedic trauma surgeons. The book complements *Key Topics in Orthopaedic Surgery* with minimal crossover in content.

We thank Mr Alistair Ross FRCS for reviewing the manuscript and thank all those at BIOS Scientific Publishers who have waited for delivery of the manuscript. Most importantly, we cannot acknowledge highly enough the training we ourselves have received over the years from our senior colleagues in Cambridge and indeed throughout East Anglia, who have given us the inspiration to write this book.

G.S. Keene
A.H.N Robinson
M.G. Bowditch
D.J. Edwards

ACHILLES TENDON RUPTURE

Rupture of the Achilles tendon classically occurs in the middle-aged, often sedentary male, during sudden ankle dorsiflexion, excessive strain during the heel-off phase of gait, or following direct trauma. The mean age of presentation is 35 years and 60% of ruptures occur during recreational sport. Fifteen to twenty per cent occur during non-sporting everyday activities. Acute rupture may be seen in the amateur or professional athlete.

The pathological process leading to sudden rupture is poorly understood. Rupture typically occurs 3–6 cm above the insertion site. This is an area of relatively poor blood supply, aggravated by decreased perfusion during stretching, contraction and advancing age. In addition, there are changes to the cross-linking of collagen fibres and degenerative changes with age. There is a correlation between Achilles tendon rupture and blood group O. Some 5–15% of patients report a history of pain in the tendon for several months before presentation. These factors in combination appear responsible for sudden rupture.

Diagnosis

A history of sudden pain or an audible snap is the classic presentation, followed by difficulty walking. On examination there is a visible and palpable defect in the tendon (masked by swelling in late presentation) and weakness of plantarflexion. There may be some active plantarflexion due to plantaris, flexor hallucis longus and tibialis posterior function. Simmonds' test is positive – with the patient prone, or kneeling on a chair, squeezing the calf does not produce passive plantarflexion.

Where the clinical findings are circumspect, the diagnosis can be confirmed by ultrasound or magnetic resonance imaging (MRI), although this is seldom required.

Management

The relative merits of conservative and surgical management remain controversial.

1. Non-operative treatment is favoured by many, to reduce the risk of surgical complications. With early presentation, less than 48 hours, the tendon ends can often be felt to oppose on passive plantarflexion. A cast in equinnus should be applied and changed at 4 and 6 weeks to bring the foot up to a more neutral position, before removing the cast at 8 weeks. There are conflicting reports as to whether the cast should be above or below the knee, and when weight-bearing should begin. A below-knee cast is considered acceptable and protected weight-bearing considered safe after 6 weeks, but should continue for 4 or more weeks after cast removal. Re-rupture rates are higher following conservative treatment, with greater tendon elongation and weaker plantarflexion.

2. Surgical repair is favoured in the athlete, as the re-rupture rate is lower. Through a short postero-medial incision, the tendon ends should be identified, approximated, and the paratenon closed. Lateral incisions can damage the sural nerve and midline incisions are prone to adhesions and subsequent irritation in footwear. A tourniquet is seldom required. A similar regimen of plaster treatment is required, with weight-bearing at around 4 weeks. The re-rupture rate is lower and rehabilitation more rapid, although an overall complication rate of around 10% is reported.

Various percutaneous methods have been advocated, but these seem to confer little advantage, with a significant potential for sural nerve damage.

3. *Late repair* of neglected tendon ruptures is difficult, because the proximal tendon migrates as contracture develops in the calf muscle. If direct repair cannot be achieved, options for reconstruction include:

- Interposition reconstruction with strips of fascia lata.
- V–Y gastrocplasty, or advancement of the central fascia from the gastroc-soleus complex.
- Flexor digitorum longus, flexor hallucis longus, peroneus brevis, or plantaris interposition transfer.

Rehabilitation

Physiotherapy should begin after removal of the cast. Protected weight-bearing should continue for 4 weeks and a 2 cm heel raise is used for 6 weeks. Calf muscle strength is greater following surgical repair, with a calf strength greater than 85% of normal, compared to 75% for conservative treatment. Jogging should not be commenced for 4 months after the rupture and more vigorous sport gradually introduced after 6 months. It is advisable to avoid badminton, the most common causative sport, and other sports demanding repetitive forced plantarflexion, for 12 months.

Better results, strength and range of movement, with faster recovery and return to sport, are reported for surgical repair using a mobile cast or brace, allowing early active plantarflexion and restricted dorsiflexion. This is because immobilization in a cast leads to calf muscle atrophy, fibro-fatty connective tissue matures into adhesions, and scar tissue bridges the tendon and paratenon. Finally, early movement improves the blood supply and promotes healing.

Complications

The complications of surgery must be balanced against the effects on rehabilitation and return to sport.

1. *Re-rupture* is seen in 1.5% (range 0–7%) of surgically repaired and 13% (range 4–50%) of conservatively treated ruptures.

2. *Tendon elongation and muscle weakness* are greater following conservative treatment in most reports, although some workers have found no loss of strength with conservative management.

3. *Deep infection, superficial infection, fistula and skin necrosis* each have an incidence of 1–2% following surgical repair, increasing the overall complications of operative treatment compared to non-operative treatment.

Further reading

Cetti R, Christensen S-E, Ejsted R *et al*. Operative versus non-operative treatment of Achilles tendon rupture. *American Journal of Sports Medicine*, 1993; 21: 791–799.

Cetti R, Henriksen LO, Jacobsen KS. A new treatment of ruptured Achilles tendons. *Clinical Orthopaedics*, 1994; 308: 155–165.

Related topic of interest

Hand – tendon injuries, p. 93

AMPUTATION AND REPLANTATION

This chapter considers amputation and replantation. Should the severely mangled limb be salvaged and should an already amputated limb be replanted?

Amputation

Traumatic amputation accounts for 11% of all amputations, and in the under 50s the figure approaches 50%. The decision to amputate is difficult. The limb must be considered both in the context of the patient's acute condition and long-term health. Economic, social and psychological factors should be assessed, ideally involving the patient in the decision-making process. Independent orthopaedic and plastic surgical opinions on the feasibility of limb salvage are helpful. Prognostic factors include:

1. *Local factors.* The following are linked to a poor outcome:

- Vascular injury, especially if the warm ischaemia time exceeds 6 hours.
- Gustilo IIIc injury, in which the amputation rate is 40–88%.
- Infrapopliteal vascular injury of all three vessels – these have amputation rates around 100%.
- Neurological injury – the restoration of protective sensation is critical to successful outcome.
- Soft tissue crush injury – as opposed to sharp cutting injury.
- Loss of bone length in the lower limb.
- Compartment syndrome.
- Pre-existing limb disease – atherosclerosis.

2. *Systemic factors.* The following are linked to a poor outcome:

- Age.
- Smoking.
- Pre-existing conditions – diabetes mellitus.
- Associated polytrauma. The Hanover group advocate amputation in Gustilo III fractures, when the Injury Severity Score (ISS) exceeds 40. This reduces the risk from systemic release of breakdown products, reducing the threat to renal and pulmonary function, therefore putting life before limb.
- Systemic hypotension.

3. *Absolute and relative indications.* Lange suggested the following indications for amputation in Gustilo IIIc tibial injuries:

(a) Absolute
- Warm ischaemia time exceeding 6 hours.
- Complete posterior tibial nerve disruption.

(b) Relative
- Associated polytrauma.
- Severe ipsilateral foot trauma.
- Fracture with major soft tissue injury and bony reconstruction anticipated.

4. *Scoring systems.* To aid the decision-making process, various scoring systems have been devised, the Mangled Extremity Severity Score (MESS) being the most

commonly used (*Table 1*). This score was developed retrospectively by assessing the outcome in patients with Gustilo IIIc tibial fractures. A score of >7 was predictive of amputation in 100% of cases. Subsequent studies have been less convincing, with a reported sensitivity of 22% and specificity of 53%. Interobserver variability is a problem.

The MESS has been modified to the NISSA (nerve injury, ischaemia, soft tissue contamination, skeletal, shock and age score). Despite the usefulness of scores, no method is fail-safe and clinical judgement remains paramount.

5.   Other indications for amputation. Entrapment of the patient by the limb and attempting to prevent the development of 'crush' syndrome.

6.   Late indications for amputation. These are an infected or functionless limb.

7.   Prognosis. The outcome after reconstruction can be good, but late amputation rates of 12–61% are reported. In the amputation group, the best results reported in young patients demonstrated 96% return to work with a prosthesis. Only 16% considered themselves disabled at 2-year follow-up.

Replantation

'Replantation' is the reattachment of a part that has been completely separated, as opposed to 'revascularization' of a partially amputated limb or digit. Generally, revascularization is easier and more successful, as some of the venous and lymphatic drainage remains in continuity.

Table 1. The Mangled Extremity Severity Score (MESS)

Factor	Points
A–Energy	
Low energy (closed fracture, stab, low-velocity gunshot)	1
Medium energy (open, multiple fractures, dislocation)	2
High energy (close-range gunshot, high-velocity gunshot, crush)	3
Massive crush (contamination, avulsion of soft tissues)	4
B–Limb ischaemia	
Diminished pulse, no ischaemia	1*
No pulse, paraesthesiae, slow capillary refill	2*
No pulse, cool, paralysed, anaesthetic, no capillary refill	3*
C–Shock	
Stable BP	0
Hypotensive, responds to i.v. fluids	1
Persistent systolic BP <90 mmHg	2
D–Age	
<30 years	0
30–50 years	1
>50 years	2

*Double score if ischaemia time is >6 hours.

1. Indications. The ideal part for replantation should have been sharply severed at a single level. There should be a short warm ischaemia time: <6 hours if muscle is present and <12 hours with digits. These figures are doubled for cold ischaemia. Replantation requires prolonged operating times and is inappropriate in the poly-traumatized patient or those in poor general health. Replantation is most important in the upper limb. Lower limb replants are less common as the initial mechanism of injury tends to make the limb less suitable for replantation, and good function can be achieved with modern lower limb orthoses. An attempt at replantation should usually be made in children, whatever the injury.

2. Transport. The amputated part is either transported wrapped in a swab moistened with isotonic saline, or immersed in isotonic saline within a plastic bag. The swab is then placed on, or the bag in, ice. Care must be taken to avoid frostbite by direct contact with ice.

3. Surgery. The surgical technique includes achieving bone stability, tendon repair, and microsurgical nerve, arterial and venous anastomoses. If the amputated part contains muscle, arterial circulation should be re-established as early as possible, possibly using a temporary shunt. It may be necessary to shorten the bones to prevent tension in the repaired soft tissues.

4. Prognosis. Replantation survival exceeding 80% is achievable. The best results are with replantation of the thumb, finger distal to the flexor digitorum superficialis (FDS) insertion, wrist and forearm. The expected range of movement is approximately 50% of normal. Cold insensitivity lasts 2 years. With proximal and lower limb replantation, recovery takes 3–5 years.

Further reading

Helfet DL, Howey T, Sanders R *et al.* Limb salvage versus amputation: preliminary results of the mangled extremity severity score. *Clinical Orthopaedics and Related Research*, 1990; **256**: 80–86.

Nugent IM, Ivory JP, Ross AC. Amputation and prosthetics. In: *Key Topics in Orthopaedic Surgery*. Oxford: BIOS Scientific Publishers Ltd, 1995; 15–17.

Rosenberg GA, Patterson BM. Limb salvage versus amputation for severe fractures of the tibia. *Orthopaedics*, 1998; **21**: 343–349.

Sanders R, Swiontowski M, Nunley J *et al.* The management of fractures with soft-tissue disruptions. *Journal of Bone and Joint Surgery*, 1993; **75A**: 778–788.

Related topics of interest

Hand – neurovascular and soft tissue injuries, p. 85; Principles of soft tissue management, p. 223

ANKLE FRACTURES

Ankle fractures are the commonest lower limb fractures. The prevalence and age of presentation are increasing.

Mechanism and classifications

Mechanisms of injury include both high-energy injuries (e.g. road traffic accidents (RTA), falls from a height and sports injuries), and low-energy injuries (e.g. falls, twists or slips). The most common age groups are young sportsmen and late-middle-age obese females.

Three classifications are popular:

- Simple descriptive (Henderson, 1932).
- Lauge–Hansen, 1950.
- Weber, 1972 (expanded by AO, 1979).

1. Descriptive classification. This is based on the number of malleoli involved (bi/tri-malleolar) and the displacement.

2. Lauge–Hansen classification. This is based on the position of the foot (supinated or pronated) and the direction of the deforming force (abduction, adduction or external rotation) at the time of injury. Ninety five per cent of fractures are classified into one of five groups, with up to four stages of injury severity and damaged structures for each group (*Figure 1*). While not easily remembered, these fracture patterns are invaluable for closed reduction techniques.

- Supination – adduction.
  - I. Transverse distal fibula fracture or lateral ligament rupture.
  - II. Vertical medial malleolus fracture.
- Supination – external rotation (of talus in mortice).
  - I. Anterior talo-fibular ligament rupture +/– avulsion fracture of antero-lateral tibia (Tillaux).
  - II. Spiral/oblique fibula fracture (anterior distal) at syndesmosis.
  - III. Posterior malleolus fracture or posterior tibio-fibular ligament rupture.
  - IV. Low medial malleolus fracture or ligament rupture.
- Pronation – abduction.
  - I. Transverse medial malleolus fracture or medial ligament rupture.
  - II. Syndesmosis disruption.
  - III. Short transverse or oblique fibula fracture above joint.
- Pronation – external rotation.
  - I. Transverse medial malleolus fracture or medial ligament rupture.
  - II. Anterior tibio-fibular ligament rupture +/– avulsion fracture.
  - III. Oblique fibula fracture (antero-superior) at/above syndesmosis (proximal fibula = Maisonneuve fracture).
  - IV. Posterior malleolus fracture or posterior tibio-fibular ligament rupture.
- Pronation – axial compression (pilon).

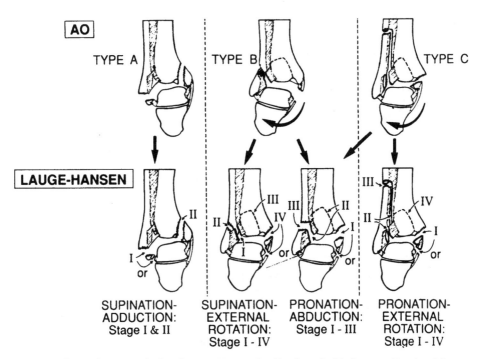

Figure 1. The AO (Danis–Weber) and Lauge–Hansen classification of ankle fractures. Reprinted from Sangeorzan BJ and Hansen ST (1990) *Orthopaedic Knowledge Update III*, p. 615. With permission from American Academy of Orthopaedic Surgeons.

3. *Weber classification.* This is based on the level of the fibula fracture relative to the syndesmosis (*Figure 1*). More proximal type C fractures are less stable. The three types are:

A. Below.
B. At the level.
C. Above.

Clinical assessment

Acute presentation with pain, swelling and inability to weight-bear is typical, but some 'stable' fractures present late. Examination to determine the extent of injury and stability is essential. Ligamentous injury is detected clinically by location of tenderness and swelling. Stress testing is rarely possible acutely. Skin viability must be assessed and immediate reduction of a fracture/dislocation performed if the skin is ischaemic.

Imaging

AP, lateral and mortise (internal rotation 15°) radiographs are usually adequate. Assessment includes the measurement of:

- Medial and superior joint space (4 mm, or <1 mm difference).
- Talar tilt (angle between tibial articular surface and superior talus on mortise view) <5°.

- Talocrural angle (angle between distal tibia articular surface and malleoli) 8–15°.
- Tibio-fibular overlap should be >1 mm on all views.

Talar shift is important – 1 mm of lateral talar shift reduces the area of joint contact by 40%.

Initial management

After appropriate resuscitation, the management objectives for the limb are:

- Protection of the soft tissue envelope.
- Correction of gross deformity.
- Initial stabilization.
- Detailed assessment of fracture stability.

Open wounds require debridement, lavage, antibiotics and delayed closure or reconstruction. Closed injuries require attention to the soft tissues to reduce skin tension and minimize swelling – high elevation for 5 to 7 days and possibly cryo-cooling may be necessary before surgery.

Definitive management

The objectives are:

- Anatomical reduction of the articular surface.
- Bone union.
- Non-infected, viable soft tissue envelope.
- Early movement and restoration of function.

Fractures should be assessed for stability and further displacement.

1. _Undisplaced fractures_ of lateral malleolus alone, without talar shift, are usually stable and managed non-operatively with cast immobilization for 6 weeks. Partial weight-bearing is allowed after 2 weeks, if subsequent X-rays demonstrate no displacement.

2. _Undisplaced, but potentially unstable fractures_ involving both malleoli (fractures or ligament) may be managed non-operatively with cast immobilization, but require close clinical and radiological monitoring for at least 3 weeks. Weight-bearing can then be introduced. There is evidence of a better outcome with surgical stabilization if facilities do not allow close follow-up. Five to ten per cent of medial malleolar fractures fail to unite and merit late radiological assessment.

3. _Displaced isolated lateral malleolar fractures_ do not require anatomical reduction of the fibula and are managed non-operatively in a cast, with early weight-bearing.

4. _Displaced isolated medial malleolar fractures_ are uncommon pronation injuries and require anatomical reduction. Often periosteum is trapped in the fracture and open reduction and internal fixation (ORIF) is required with two cancellous lag screws or a tension band wire. Left untreated non-union may result.

5. _Displaced bimalleolar or trimalleolar fractures_ are generally unstable and require operative treatment. Closed reduction and cast immobilization can be used if close follow-up is maintained, as redisplacement is common when swelling resolves. Closed treatment is most suitable for those with higher complication rates – poor skin, elderly, diabetics, rheumatoids, alcoholics and the immuno-compromised. ORIF prevents redisplacement, allowing early weight-bearing, early mobilization and less frequent follow-up.

Surgical fixation

1. **Fibular fractures** are the key to restoration of joint congruity and are addressed first. Oblique fibula fractures are stabilized with lag screws and a lateral neutralization plate. A posterior anti-glide plate is recommended in porotic bone. Transverse fractures are stabilized with a dynamic compression plate.

2. **Medial malleolar fractures** are fixed with lag screws or a tension band wire.

3. **Posterior malleolar fractures** should be stabilized with lag screws if ≥25% of the articular surface is involved.

4. **Diastasis of the syndesmosis** follows pronation injuries. The indications for fixation of Weber type C fractures are controversial.

- If a medial fracture is adequately stabilized, talar shift will not occur. If the medial ligament is ruptured, joint stability by ligament repair is not adequate and a diastasis screw is required.
- Studies suggest residual diastasis is likely despite fibular fixation, if the fibular fracture is ≥4.5 cm above the joint, but not if ≤3 cm. Between 3 and 4.5 cm is a 'grey' area. The intra-operative 'hook' test is a good method to identify significant dynamic diastasis.
- Proximal fibular fractures are not usually fixed and a diastasis screw is used.

5. **Syndesmosis stabilization** is by direct open repair, or 'closed' reduction and temporary stabilization with a screw. The screw should be 4.5 mm fully threaded, non-lagged, crossing three cortices just proximal to the syndesmosis and inserted with the ankle in neutral. Non-weight-bearing is maintained for 6–8 weeks and the screw may be removed under local anaesthetic or left *in situ*.

Complications

(a) Early: non-operative
- Inadequate reduction.
- Redisplacement.

(b) Early: operative
- Delayed wound-healing.
- Wound infection.
- Osteomyelitis.
- Sural nerve injury or neuroma.

(c) Late
- Mal/non-union, diastasis.
- Joint pain, stiffness, instability.
- Joint degeneration occurs despite optimal management and is related to cartilage damage at the time of injury.
- Late arthrodesis rates are <5%.

Further reading

Michelson JD. Fractures about the ankle. *Journal of Bone and Joint Surgery*, 1996; **77A**: 142–152.

Vander Griend R, Michelson JD, Bone LB. Fractures of the ankle and distal part of the tibia. *Journal of Bone and Joint Surgery*, 1996; **78A**: 1772–1783.

Related topic of interest

Tibial pilon fractures, p. 284

BIOMATERIALS – BONE

Bone consists of the mineral calcium hydroxyapatite $[Ca_{10}(PO_4)_6(OH)_2]$, collagen and glycosaminoglycans which bind collagen. Hydroxyapatite is strong in compression, whereas collagen gives bone flexibility and tensile strength. The weakest area is the cement line between osteons. Bone is $3\times$ as light, $10\times$ as flexible, but has approximately the same tensile strength as cast iron. Any material deforms under load, yet to act as a skeleton the deformations must be small. Bone tested in the laboratory is dead, but the data obtained are important and form the basis of the stress/strain curve – the formal expression of strength and stiffness.

Stress/strain curves

1. Stress. This is the intensity of a force, expressed as force per unit area (Nm^{-2} or Pascal).

2. Strain. Linear strain is defined as the deformation, or change in length of an object, as a result of loading. Angular (shear) strain is the rotational equivalent. Strain is a proportion and has no units.

3. Stress (Y axis) plotted against strain (X axis) (Figure 1). The resulting curve consists of two lines, with an almost vertical element and an almost horizontal element. The vertical element is the elastic portion where deformation is temporary, and if the deforming force is removed, the structure returns to its original length (like an elastic band). In this elastic range stress is proportional to strain and the stress/strain ratio is known as *Young's modulus of elasticity – 'E'.* The horizontal element is the plastic portion where increasing the stress on the subject leads to permanent deformity. The point of change from vertical to horizontal is known as the *yield point* or *proportional limit.*

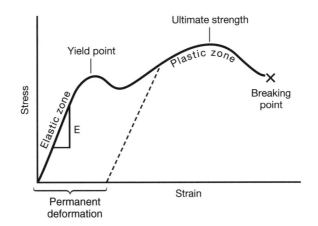

Figure 1. The stress–strain curve. E = Young's modulus. The area under the curve is the energy stored.

4. Ultimate strength. Stress/strain curves are plotted by testing material to destruction. The point at which the material fractures, at the end of the plastic portion of the curve, is the ultimate strength. The area under the curve is the total energy stored – this is released at the time of fracture.

5. Materials are either brittle or ductile. Brittle materials have no plasticity and ultimate failure occurs at, or soon after, the yield point (e.g. glass). Ductile materials are plastic and deform greatly before ultimate failure (e.g. metal).

The properties of bone

Fractures occur when a bone is stressed beyond its ultimate strength. This point will be affected by patient-related (intrinsic) and extrinsic factors.

Intrinsic factors

1. Bone density. The compressive and tensile strength of bone is proportional to the density. The porosity of cortical bone is 3–30%. Cancellous bone can have a porosity of >90%. Cancellous bone has a lower ultimate strength, is 10% as stiff, but 500% as ductile as cortical bone.

2. Patient age. Bone is more ductile in the young, leading to the characteristic greenstick and plastic deformation types of failure. With increasing age, as well as osteoporosis, bone becomes more brittle. The modulus of elasticity reduces by 1.5% per annum. In the elderly, bone may be osteoporotic – cortical bone is resorbed endosteally, widening the intramedullary canal. The bony trabeculae of cancellous bone become thinner. The resultant reduction in bone density weakens the bone and the ultimate strength reduces by 5–7% per decade.

3. Bone geometry
- The longer a bone, the greater the potential bending moment.
- The larger the cross-sectional area, the greater the stress to failure.
- The area moment of inertia measures the amount of bone in a cross-section and the distance from the neutral axis. The more bone further from the axis, the stronger and stiffer the bone. In a cylinder the relationship is to the power four.

4. Wolff's law (1892). This states that bone is laid down in response to stress and resorbed where stress is absent. Consequently there can be *localized* areas of reduced density (after plate removal due to stress shielding) or *systemic reduction* after prolonged recumbency.

5. Stress raisers. A cortical defect occupying 20% of the diameter, caused for example by a tumour or screw removal, can reduce the strength of a bone by up to 60%. Screw defects heal over in 8 weeks.

6. Muscle function. Muscle protects bone. An example is the skier's 'boot top' fracture of the tibia – contraction of the triceps surae, resisting ankle flexion, compresses the posterior tibial cortex. As bone is weaker in tension than in compression, the fracture starts anteriorly.

Extrinsic factors

1. ***The magnitude of the force.*** Bone has a considerable margin of safety between the forces experienced in daily activity and those required to cause a fracture. The greater the area under the stress/strain curve, the more energy will be released at the time of fracture; thus osteoporotic fractures are not associated with as much soft tissue damage as fractures of denser bone.

2. ***The rate of stress application to the bone.*** Bone exhibits viscoelasticity – the ultimate strength increases when loaded at a faster rate. Thus with a fast rate of loading, bone stores more energy before failure and this excess energy is released at failure.

3. ***The direction of application of stress.*** Bone does not have the same strength if loaded in different directions – a property known as anisotropicity. Bone is less strong and less stiff when stressed from side to side, than from end to end. In general, bone is strongest and stiffest in the direction in which it is loaded *in vivo* (longitudinally for a long bone). Even when tested in the same direction, bone is strongest in compression, weakest in tension, with shear being intermediate.

4. ***Fatigue failure.*** In common with most materials, bone fails at lower stresses when repeatedly stressed. A fracture typically occurs after a few repetitions of a high load, or many repetitions of a lower load. The ability of bone to repair micro-fractures protects it from this phenomenon.

Fracture patterns

There are three principal stress planes: tension, compression and shear. Individually or in combination these determine the plane of fracture.

- Tension: transverse fracture.
- Compression: oblique fracture.
- Bending: a bent bone has tension and compression sides. The tension side fractures first, transversely. The fracture propagates across to the compression side, creating a butterfly fragment.
- Torsion: spiral.
- Comminution is a function of the energy stored in the bone at the time of fracture.

Stress fractures

For a stress fracture, the rate of microfracture exceeds the rate of repair and there are two principal theories as to the cause:

- A stress fracture follows fatigue from repetitive stress.
- There is defective muscle activity and the absence of protective muscle function predisposes to fracture.

Further reading

Hipp JA, Hayes WC. Biomechanics of fractures. In: Browner BD, Jupiter JB, Levine AM, Trafton PG, eds. *Skeletal Trauma*. Philadelphia: WB Saunders, 1998; 97–130.

Nordin M, Frankel VH. Biomechanics of bone. In: *Basic Biomechanics of the Musculoskeletal System*, 2nd Edn. Philadelphia: Lea and Febiger, 1989; 3–29.

Related topics of interest

Biomaterials – implants in trauma, p. 15; Biomechanics of fracture implants and implant removal, p. 19; Bone structure, p. 34

BIOMATERIALS – IMPLANTS IN TRAUMA

Implants have traditionally been made of metal, but recently bioresorbable implants have been introduced. The 'ideal' implant should fulfil the following criteria:

- Biocompatibility – inert, non-immunogenic, non-toxic, non-carcinogenic.
- Strength – sufficient tensile, compressive and torsional strength, stiffness and fatigue resistance, for early resumption of function.
- Workability – easy to manufacture and implant.
- Corrosion free.
- Inexpensive.
- No affect on subsequent radiological imaging.
- Avoidance of prominence, sparing the need for removal.

Metal implants

Types of metal implant

Stainless steel and titanium are the principal metals used in trauma. Cobalt–chromium is used for joint replacement implants.

1. **Stainless steel,** as 316L stainless steel, is a chromium (13–15.5%) and nickel (17–19%) alloy, low (L) in carbon (0.03%). Nickel provides corrosion resistance and stabilizes the crystalline structure, while chromium provides an oxidized surface, reducing corrosion.

2. **Titanium** is used in one of four pure forms, or as an alloy. Adding oxygen, making the implant stronger and more brittle, modifies the form. Type 4 has the highest oxygen content. Titanium superalloys (e.g. Ti-6Al-4V) are also used.

3. **Cobalt–chromium** alloys (e.g. cobalt–chromium–molybdenum, vitallium) are used in replacement implants, but seldom in trauma devices.

Processing

Changing the atomic and crystalline structure of the metal during processing can alter the properties of metals:

- Casting – liquid metal is poured into a mould.
- Wrought – cast metal is modified by rolling or extruding.
- Forging – metal is heated and then subjected to a force, increasing strength and hardness, but decreasing ductility.
- Cold working – metal is repeatedly loaded with loads greater than the yield point.
- Annealing – metal is heated and cooled to toughen it.
- Passivation – creates an oxide covering over the surface of a metal, generally by placing the implant in nitric acid, improving biocompatibility and reducing corrosion. In 316L stainless steel, chromium and nickel form an oxide coat that reforms in air when scratched.

Table 1 quantifies some of the alterations in properties achieved by processing metals.

Table 1. Comparison of yield and tensile strength in different materials

Metal	Yield strength (MPa)	Ultimate tensile strength (MPa)
Cortical bone	130	150
316L SS hot-forged	250	600
316L SS cold-worked	690	860
316L SS cold-forged	1200	1350
Titanium	485	550
Ti-6Al-4V	795	860

L, low.
SS, stainless steel.

Properties

*1. **Corrosion*** can be caused by electrochemical currents which arise when two dissimilar metals are in contact – known as *galvanic corrosion*. However, currents can also arise between two areas of the same metal, due to variations in tension, leading to *crevice corrosion*. Areas of high-stress gradients lead to stress corrosion and micromovement abrading two surfaces leads to *fretting corrosion*.

*2. **Fatigue failure*** is the result of cyclical or repetitive loading below the ultimate stress, causing a fracture. A fracture occurs after a few repetitions of a high load, or many repetitions of a lower load. The *endurance limit* is the stress at which the material under load will not have failed after 10 million cycles. It is considered that failure will never occur after this many cycles and assumed that orthopaedic implants are stressed 2 million cycles per year. The endurance limit is 900 MPa for cold-forged 316L stainless steel and 520 MPa for Ti-6Al-4V.

*3. **Creep*** is the progressive deformation of a material over time, under constant load.

Choice of materials

316L stainless steel is commonly used and is cheap, with adequate ductility, yield and ultimate strength. A small number of people are hypersensitive to nickel and chromium. Steel is not perfect and for this reason titanium is used in some situations. The advantages of titanium are:

- Less fatigable after large numbers of cycles.
- Greater modulus of elasticity, 6× that of bone (cf 12× for steel), and there is less stress shielding with titanium implants.
- More biocompatible, forming a direct interface with the bone, promoting bony ingrowth.
- Less interference with MRI or CT.
- Less interference with radiotherapy, for example following pathological fractures.

The disadvantages of titanium are:

- Expense.
- Sensitivity to stress risers (scratches).

- Pure titanium has a low tensile strength, making it less suitable for use in the lower limb.

Bioresorbable implants

Types of bioresorbable implants

Organic molecules can be polymerized and formed into filaments, rods and screws. The production process is complex and closely regulated. The principal bioresorbable polymers are:

- Polyglycolic acid (PGA).
- Polylactic acid (PLA).
- Poly-p-dioxanone (PDS).
- Poly-β-hydroxybutyric acid (PHBA).

*1. **Bioresorbable implants*** are low in strength, but this can be increased using reinforcing techniques, such as sintering under pressure. The reinforced products are prefixed with the letters 'SR'. Sterilization is by irradiation or ethylene oxide.

*2. **Non-reinforced implants*** have a tensile strength of 30–70 MPa, increasing to 450 MPa for SR-PLA (cf *Table 1*).

*3. **Degradation is by hydrolysis,*** until the molecular weight is reduced to 5000 Da, when a foreign body reaction supersedes. Complete loss of strength of the implant occurs between 1 month (SR-PGA), and 1 year (SR-PLA) depending on the polymer. Complete resorption takes between 3 months (SR-PGA) and 6 years (SR-PLA).

*4. **The use of bioresorbable implants is controversial***

Advantages are:

- No removal of hardware, with cost and morbidity savings.
- Less stress shielding and weakening of bone.
- Absence of metal toxicity.

The disadvantages are:

- The initial implant is expensive, with a finite shelf-life.
- The strength of the implant is low.
- Foreign body reactions occur, with reports of osteolysis, sinus formation and implant extrusion.
- Synovitis has been reported with PLA and PGA.

Clinical experience

Bioresorbable implants have been used in paediatric, hip, ankle, elbow and wrist fractures. Initial reports of 15% redisplacement and 8% sinus formation after the fixation of ankle fractures with PGA rods have lead to scepticism. Lower rates of sinus formation are seen with PLA, which resorbs more slowly.

In summary, until the mechanical properties can be improved, it will not be possible to use these implants for fixation and allow early mobilization with weight-bearing.

Further reading

Blasier RD, Bucholz R, Cole W *et al.* Bioresorbable implants: applications in orthopedic surgery. *Instructional Course Lectures*, 1997; **46**: 531–546.

Disegi J, Wyss H. Implant materials for fracture fixation: a clinical perspective. *Orthopaedics*, 1989; **12**: 75–79.

Related topics of interest

Biomaterials – bone, p. 11; Biomechanics of fracture implants and implant removal, p. 19

BIOMECHANICS OF FRACTURE IMPLANTS AND IMPLANT REMOVAL

The aim of surgical intervention is to anatomically reduce and stabilize the fracture securely, while causing the least possible interference with healing. In the laboratory, structural rigidity (or stiffness) is tested by recording the axial, bending (flexural) and torsion stiffness of the implant applied to an osteotomized bone.

Wires

1. ***Cerclage wires*** of <1 mm diameter do not interfere with cortical blood supply, although broader bands (e.g. Parham bands) do. Wires can be used to produce interfragmentary compression. A surgical knot gives the maximum compression, although for practical purposes a twist may be better. Commercially available systems, such as the Dall–Miles system (Howmedica Inc, Rutherford, NJ) are stronger still, but expensive. They are used to secure fractures, plates and allografts, when the femoral cortex is 'blocked' by an intramedullary implant.

2. ***Tension band wiring*** is commonly performed. The most frequent application is the olecranon; other suitable sites are the patella, medial malleolus and femoral greater trochanter. The principle used is that an unyielding band or wire on the tension side of a bone converts tension to compression. The compression is dynamic, optimal compression only being achieved with functional activity.

Drills

The cutting edge of a drill is at the tip and the helical flutes remove the bone debris. Optimum drill speed is low: 750–1250 rpm. The most common cause of drill breakage is bending, and use of a drill sleeve can help to avoid this.

Screws

Screws have a core (inner solid centre) and an outer diameter. The pitch is the distance between threads.

1. ***Screws break*** in two ways. Either by excess torque during insertion, or by bending. After implantation, bending occurs secondary to a loose plate. The bending and shear strength is determined by the core diameter.

2. ***Pullout strength*** is proportional to the area of thread in contact with bone – increased either by increasing the outer diameter, or reducing the pitch. Over the first 6 weeks following insertion, the pullout strength increases to 150% of that at insertion.

3. ***Self-tapping screws*** manufactured with cutting flutes to cut a thread are controversial. The advantages are:

- Reduced operative time.
- Impaction of bone around the thread during insertion, increasing hold.

The disadvantages are:

- The cutting flutes reduce the area of thread. Pullout strength is reduced by 10% if the threads are not advanced through the distal cortex.
- Insertion requires increased torque.
- There is a mild increase in temperature as the screw is inserted.
- Reinsertion may be compromised by the screw cutting a new path, although there are studies showing no reduction in pullout strength with 12 re-insertions.

4. *Cancellous screws* do not have flutes, but gain a better hold when the cancellous bone is not tapped.

5. *Cannulated screws* have a larger core diameter to accommodate the guide wire, reducing the pullout strength by 20%.

Plates

The strength of a plate is defined by the equation BH^3 (B = width; H = height or thickness). Thus, increasing the thickness of a plate increases the rigidity to the power three. Plate failure is usually due to fatigue and is more likely if there is a gap after fixation.

Plates can be used for a number of different functions:

- Neutralization – protecting a lag screw from torsional, shear and bending forces.
- Compression – achieved by:
(i) Placing a lag screw through the plate.
(ii) The eccentric screw hole of a dynamic compression plate (DCP), producing up to 600N of compression. Two holes can be compressed, as there is the potential for 1.8 mm of glide.
(iii) The external tensioning device.
(iv) Pre-bending the plate 1–2 mm off the bone at the fracture site.
(v) Placing the plate on the tension side of the bone.
(vi) Compression hip screws, buttress and antiglide plates can also be used in compression.
- The LC-DCP (low contact-DCP) has been designed with certain proposed advantages over the DCP. It is made of type 4 titanium, and is cut away on the undersurface, with scalloping between the screw holes. This allows:
(i) A modulus of elasticity closer to bone.
(ii) Improved biocompatibility.
(iii) Decreased interference with periosteal blood supply (the contact area is 50% that of a DCP).
(iv) The stiffness between screw holes is approximately that at a screw hole.
(v) Improved fatigue life.
(vi) Wider angle of screw insertion.
(vii) Compressibility from either end of the screw hole, with advantages for the fixation of segmental fractures.

Intramedullary nails

The original Küntscher nails were slotted with a 'V'. Later the cloverleaf cross-section was introduced. The cloverleaf cross-section increased the stiffness of the nail and the slot allowed better interference fit with the cortex. The unlocked nail relies on interference fit with the cortex to provide torsional stability. The axial and torsional stability of unlocked nails is poor.

1. ***Improving torsional stability***. Methods are:

- Reaming. Flexible reaming (speed two-thirds that of a drill) allows the insertion of a larger nail with a better interference fit, but damages the endosteal blood supply.
- The use of fins or flutes on the nail
- Interlocking the nail with screws, providing torsional and axial stability.

2. ***Slots in nails are controversial.*** Slots reduce the torsional stiffness, but have little effect on bending stiffness. Theoretical advantages of the slot are that it allows some flexibility to promote callus formation, and reduces risk of fracture during insertion. Increasing the diameter of the nail increases the stiffness according to the fourth power of its radius. Some small, unreamed nails are not cannulated and are not inserted over a guide wire. The small diameter dictates the need for a solid cross-section.

3. ***Working length.*** This is the distance over which the nail is unsupported by bone. The distance may be <1 mm with a transverse fracture, but several centimeters with a comminuted fracture. In torsion, stiffness is inversely proportional to the working length, and in bending it is inversely proportional to the square of the working length.

Implant removal

The complication rates following metalware removal vary from 3 to >40%. The principal problems are neurovascular damage and refracture. The removal of forearm plates is the most frequently associated with problems. Refracture is caused by two principal phenomena:

1. ***Removing a screw*** leaves a stress riser in the bone. If the size of the hole is significantly greater than 20–30% of the diameter of the bone, the weakness rises exponentially. Thus 3.5 mm screws are recommended in the forearm.

2. ***Bone under a plate demineralizes,*** either by stress protection or bone necrosis caused by the plate occluding the periosteal blood supply. The AO group favour the latter, and recommend removal of forearm plates at >18 months, by which time the blood supply is re-established. This theory is favoured as the refracture rate drops with later plate removal.

Further reading

Mazzoca AD, Caputo AE, Browner BD *et al.* Principles of internal fixation. In: Browner BD, Jupiter JB, Levine AM, Trafton PG, eds. *Skeletal Trauma.* Philadelphia: WB Saunders, 1998; 287–348.

Müller ME, Allgöwer M, Schneider R, Willenegger H, eds. *Manual of Internal Fixation*, 3rd Edn. Berlin: Springer-Verlag, 1991; 4–95.

Related topics of interest

Biomaterials – implants in trauma, p. 15; Principles of operative fracture management, p. 220

BIRTH INJURIES

The incidence of birth injuries in the Western World is <2 per 1000 live births and decreasing with advances in obstetric care. Injuries are associated with breech presentation, shoulder dystocia and birth weight over 4 kg. Injuries are also seen in premature and very small neonates. The two most common injuries are fractures of the clavicle and brachial plexus lesions.

Specific injuries

1. Fractures of the clavicle are the most common birth injury, accounting for 40% of the total. Particular risk factors include high birth weight and shoulder dystocia. The fracture – usually in the middle third – is recognized by pain on handling and pseudoparalysis of the limb. Five per cent are associated with a brachial plexus injury and neonates should be reassessed to exclude a neurological deficit at 2 weeks. Parental reassurance, cautious handling and occasionally support for the arm in a sling is the only treatment required.

2. Brachial plexus injuries (obstetric palsies) are seen in 0.8 per 1000 live births following traction on the arm or head, and comprise around 40% of all birth injuries. There may be an associated fracture of the clavicle in 10–15% of cases. The diagnosis is either obvious after birth with a flail limb, or made by a high index of suspicion following a difficult delivery. Shoulder X-rays should be obtained to exclude a fracture. Three types of palsy are recognized:

- *Erb's palsy* affects the upper trunk and occurs when the head is abducted from the shoulders during delivery, stretching the C5/6 nerve root. The arm lies in a position of internal rotation, with the forearm in pronation. There is no active shoulder abduction or elbow flexion, but there is active flexion of the digits. Erb's palsy carries the best prognosis with spontaneous recovery in 90% of cases.
- *Klumpke's palsy* affects the lower trunk and more commonly follows breech presentation, with severe abduction of the arms or extension of the neck during delivery. There may be a Horner's sign, which is a bad prognostic factor. Bilateral injuries are reported.
- *Total plexus palsy* is occasionally seen, often with a Horner's sign, and has a very poor prognosis as spontaneous recovery is rare.

Within a few days of birth, the pattern of injury becomes more obvious. The principle of treatment is to maintain passive movement and close observation for signs of recovery, as 80–90% recover spontaneously. Early recovery of biceps and deltoid function, within a couple of months, are good prognostic signs. Physiotherapy should be maintained to prevent contractures. Absent biceps function at 3 months is the primary indication for surgical exploration. Reconstruction by nerve grafting or neurotization is usually required as end to end repair is rarely feasible. The outcome is proportional to the extent of the lesion.

3. Fractures of the humerus are generally transverse, middle-third fractures. The humerus is treated by support for about 2 weeks – shortening and angulation of up to 50° rapidly correct. There are occasional instances of separation of the physis from the metaphysis in the humerus and rare reports of dislocations around the elbow.

4.   Fractures of the femur are again most commonly middle third and transverse. Treatment is by cautious vertical gallows traction, or strapping the lower limb to the chest with the hip and knee flexed, or in a hip spica. The proximal fragment tends to stay in flexion, if the injury followed an extended breech presentation, and should therefore be treated with the hip flexed. Angular malunion remodels well. Fracture separation of the proximal or distal physis is rare.

5.   Cervical injuries occasionally follow breech presentation and where the neonate survives, cause cord injury. Damage to the cord can sometimes be confused or attributed to a neuromuscular condition.

Late reconstruction of the neglected obstetric palsy

The untreated brachial plexus palsy results in deformity and loss of function due to paralysis and contracture.

- The shoulder assumes a position of internal rotation and a progressive contracture of subscapularis may need to be released to restore external rotation. Isolated weakness of abduction and external rotation may be addressed by transfer of latissimus dorsi and teres major. A rotation humeral osteotomy may be required.
- Hand deformities are often severe and results of surgery are poor in the neglected palsy. Wrist-drop can sometimes be improved by transfer of flexor carpi ulnaris (FCU) to extensor carpi radialis brevis (ECRB), although tenodesis in extension improves the grasp more reliably.

Further reading

Gilbert A, Brockman R, Carlioz H. Surgical treatment of brachial plexus birth palsy. *Clinical Orthopaedics*, 1991; **264**: 39–47.
Lamb DW. *The Paralysed Hand*. Edinburgh: Churchill Livingston, 1993.

Related topic of interest

Shoulder – brachial plexus injuries, p. 243

BONE DEFECTS, TRANSPORT AND LATE RECONSTRUCTION

Reconstituting bone defects by transport of bone was developed by Ilizarov in Russia in the 1960s, capitalizing on the production of callus with distraction. The technique has been widely developed to address established non-union, infected non-union and for the primary management of some complex fractures. In trauma situations, defects of 3–12 cm can be reconstructed by bone transport. Defects of 7–10 cm have a 95% healing rate after transport and docking.

Principles and techniques

Extensive counselling of the patient and family is essential before surgery. Careful pre-operative planning is mandatory.

The three phases of treatment are:

- Latency.
- Distraction.
- Consolidation.

Deformities can be corrected in a single or multiple planes, restoring the mechanical axis. Construction of the frame generally requires four-point fixation to maintain a mechanical advantage for segment lengthening and correction of angular deformity.

Hypertrophic non-unions are vascular, with a dense collagen interface, and bone formation follows primary distraction. Hypotrophic non-unions are avascular, with non-reactive bone ends, so compression is initially required before distraction. Ilizarov demonstrated marked hypervascularity of the bone and limb after corticotomy and distraction, which is essential to the principle of bone transport.

1. *Open or closed corticotomy* in the metaphysis is performed and bone transported to bridge the defect, after application of a frame. New bone is formed by the gradual distraction of vascular bone surfaces. Progenitor cells from the medullary canal on both sides of the corticotomy and distraction sites are responsible for new bone formation. Bone forms in this process of distraction osteogenesis by pure intramembranous ossification in uniform zones, after a latency period of 3–5 days, before distraction is started.

The corticotomy must be 'low-energy', with a series of drill holes and an osteotome, preserving the blood supply and preferably the periosteal tube. The corticotomy should ideally be in metaphyseal, rather than diaphyseal, bone, as the blood supply is more favourable.

2. *Distraction osteogenesis* is a gradual process. At the site of distraction, type I collagen is formed centrally, giving a radiolucent central band. Osteoblasts secrete osteoid matrix into the collagen as mineralization continues. Longitudinal columns of bone are formed, parallel to the distraction force, which become interconnected transversely.

3. **Transformation osteogenesis** is the conversion into bone of non-osseous interposition materials at the docking site. On some occasions the docking site must be opened and the bone ends freshened.

Technical considerations

1. **Distraction** proceeds at 0.5–1 mm/day in adults, in four increments, and at 1–2 mm/day in children. The distraction rate is a balance between the rate of distraction osteogenesis with an adequate blood supply and premature consolidation. The effect on the soft tissues must also be considered.

2. **Consolidation** is required after distraction osteogenesis, once length has been restored before the frame is removed. The consolidation time is 5× the distraction time in adults and 2× in children. The total duration of treatment, or *healing index,* is 1 month/cm in children and 2–3 month/cm in adults.

3. **During distraction osteogenesis** the blood supply is derived from the periosteal and not the osteal surface, so distraction over an intramedullary device is possible. However, this is seldom required.

4. **Circular or ring frames** provide greater stiffness and stability than monolateral frames, which impart an eccentric load to the bone by their inherent cantilever design. Circular frames are the most versatile, allowing greater control and correction of alignment. Wires under tension and half pins can be used. During lengthening, the tibia has a tendency to go into flexion and valgus. The stiffness and stability of a frame depends upon:

- Diameter of the wires.
- Tension in the wires.
- Number and angular relationship of wires.
- Number of rings.
- Spacing between rings.

5. **Bifocal treatment** is most frequently applied, transporting a single bone block.

6. **Multifocal treatment** is the transport of bone in two directions, which allows more rapid closure of an intercalary gap, or treatment of a wider gap.

7. **To reduce the healing time** the docking site can be grafted, or an intramedullary nail inserted.

8. **Complications,** to which this technique is frequently prone, include:

- Neurological injury.
- Inadequate soft tissue cover.
- Joint subluxation.
- Joint stiffness.
- Loss of alignment.
- Pin-tract infections.
- Delayed consolidation.
- Non-union.

Further reading

Aronson J. Limb-lengthening, skeletal reconstruction and bone transport with the Ilizarov method. *Journal of Bone and Joint Surgery*, 1997; **79A**: 1243–1258.

Ilizarov GA. *The Transosseus Osteosynthesis: Theoretical and Clinical Aspects of the Regeneration and Growth of Tissue*. New York: Springer, 1992.

Pederson WC, Sanders WE. Management of bone loss. In: Rockwood CA, Green DP, Bucholz RW, Heckman JD, eds. *Fractures in Adults*, 4th Edn. Philadelphia: Lippincott-Raven, 1996; 360–366.

Related topics of interest

Bone grafting, p. 28; Bone healing, p. 31; Non-union – infected, p. 150; Non-union and delayed union, p. 153

BONE GRAFTING

Bone graft is used to assist new bone formation and hence bone healing, and to replace bone lost through trauma or a chronic process. Graft takes the form of autograft, with or without a blood supply, allograft or xenograft. Autograft is most commonly used and the incorporation process should be understood.

The mechanism of graft incorporation, enveloping graft bone with viable new bone, depends upon revascularization by the host, but the precise bio-histological process is ill understood. However, the incorporation of bone graft has very similar features to fracture healing. Osteoblasts play a vital role and lay down bone mineral in an identical manner to that seen in fracture healing. The fundamental requirement is a good blood supply for vascular ingrowth.

Types of graft

- Autograft – non-vascularized, cancellous or cortical, morsellized, block or bulk.
- Autograft – vascularized, cortical strut.
- Allograft – cancellous or cortical, morsellized or strut.
- Xenograft (experimental/research tool).
- Bone substitutes.

Graft incorporation

1. When autograft is harvested, the blood supply is sacrificed; however, some osteogenic cells survive transplantation and promote new bone formation. In addition, the autograft induces bone formation and may stimulate surrounding tissues to undergo metaplasia into bone. The autograft acts as an *osteoconductor*, providing a template or scaffold, for host osteoblasts and osteoclasts to function, leading to *osteoinduction*, with new bone formation and incorporation of the autograft.

2. After bone grafting, a good blood supply delivers a haematoma rich in nutrients, platelet-derived growth factors (PDGF), lymphocytes, plasma cells, osteoblasts and polynuclear cells. An inflammatory response is established. As granulation tissue develops with an ingrowth of capillary buds, reticular cells and macrophages follow. Interleukin 1 and 6, bone morphogenic protein (BMP) and insulin-like growth factors (IGF) are secreted, stimulating osteoblast and osteoclast activity. Osteogenic cells arise from the differentiation of primitive mesenchymal cells, originating from the host and possibly the graft.

3. Cancellous and cortical bone have different structures. Once the inflammatory response is established, granulation tissue has formed and osteogenic cells have become active (which takes about 3 weeks), there follows a different incorporation process for the two tissue types.

4. Small cancellous autograft bone chips are revascularized in 4–6 weeks. Primitive mesenchymal cells differentiate into osteoblasts, covering the surface of dead autograft trabeculae and depositing osteoid. This becomes annealed to the core of grafted bone, which it eventually covers. At this stage, 4–6 weeks after grafting, the bone becomes more radiodense and the graft strengthens. Over the next few weeks and months, osteoclasts resorb the entrapped core of grafted bone, haemopoetic marrow elements become established, mature lamellar bone is formed and normal radiodensity returns.

5. **Cortical bone revascularization** is a much slower process and even after several years may not be complete. Initially there is a resorptive phase, as capillary cutter cones grow into pre-existing Haversian canals from the periphery. Vigorous osteoclast activity develops, which leads to loss of mechanical strength and reduced radiodensity. Structural weakening of 40% occurs in the first 2–6 months, but normal strength is regained over the next year or more, as osteoblastic activity follows resorption. The process of resorption and replacement, after vessel ingrowth and vascularization from the graft bed, is described as 'creeping substitution'.

6. **Defects up to 6 cm are suitable for cancellous autografting.** Larger defects should be filled with cortical bone, but incorporation takes much longer and may never be complete.

7. **Papineau grafting may be used in cases of an exposed, infected non-union.** The exposed surface is allowed to granulate and then autograft chips are applied. Once these are covered by granulation tissue, epithelialization may grow in from the surrounding skin, or a split skin graft is applied. This is an elementary, safe, but very slow technique.

Autogenous graft harvesting

1. **The iliac crest is an ideal donor site,** anterior or posterior. Large cortico-cancellous graft blocks can be harvested from the inner or outer table. Chips of cancellous graft are taken after elevating the cortex. Tube saws prevent the need for a wide and potentially painful surgical exposure if only small volumes of graft are required.

2. **To promote osteogenic cell survival,** graft should not be left exposed to the air before implantation, but stored in chilled blood or a saline soaked swab.

Vascularized autografts

Autograft on a vascularized pedicle or as a free graft is suitable for larger bone defects. Microsurgical transfer of rib, iliac crest, radius or preferably fibula may be used. In the leg, the fibula may be transferred to create a tibio-fibular synostosis in established tibial non-union. Vascularized grafts lose some of their osteogenic potential, but healing and union are similar to the process of fracture healing, without creeping substitution.

Allografts

1. **Morsellized cancellous chips,** cortical struts, or in some cases massive structural allografts are used to reconstruct defects, although seldom indicated in trauma surgery. The osteogenic potential of allograft is substantially inferior to autograft, leading to slower revascularization and incorporation by creeping substitution. The risk of infection in the post-trauma setting with a bone defect is substantial.

2. *Union* is initially by callus formation and partial bridging at the margins of the host–allograft interface, with some rounding off of the allograft strut. There is bone resorption and associated loss of strength, followed by gradual revascularization, creeping substitution and incorporation. With cortical allograft, this is a slow process over many years and seldom complete.

Xenograft

Bone harvested from other animals is used only for experimental purposes. The development of bovine spongiform encephalitis and Creutzfeld–Jakob disease may prohibit the future use of xenografts.

Ceramics and bone substitutes

Tricalcium phosphate and hydroxyapatite have a pore size of 100–400 μm, which is effective for bone ingrowth by osteoconduction, in the presence of marrow cells. These substitutes may be effective for filling metaphyseal bone defects, but the rate of ingrowth and remodelling are slow and the biomechanical properties are poor.

Further reading

Friedlander GE. Bone grafting. In: Dee R, Hurst LC, Gruber MA, Kottmeier SA, eds. *Principles of Orthopaedic Practice*, 2nd Edn. New York: McGraw-Hill, 1997; 79–85.
Pederson WC, Sanders WE. Management of bone loss. In: Rockwood CA, Green DP, Bucholz RW, Heckman JD, eds. *Fractures in Adults*, 4th Edn. Philadelphia: Lippincott-Raven, 1996; 360–366.

Related topics of interest

Bone defects, transport and late reconstruction, p. 25; Bone healing, p. 31

BONE HEALING

Fracture healing is a specialized form of tissue healing and similar to other histopathological repair processes. An understanding of normal bone formation and structure is essential. Bone consists of mesenchymal cells embedded in a mineralized extracellular matrix for strength and stiffness, with type I collagen predominating. The periosteum, with an inner cambium or vascular layer and outer fibrous layer, plays a vital role in fracture healing.

The process of fracture healing is similar to the process occurring at an active growth plate. Woven (immature) bone formed within callus after a fracture, with rapid turnover and irregular mineralization giving it a blurred radiographic appearance, is replaced by lamellar (mature) bone. Fracture healing consists of three distinct phases: inflammation, repair and remodelling. The formation of callus, in response to fracture movement, is a vital part of healing called indirect healing and is followed by a process of remodelling. Rigid internal fixation interferes with this natural process, leading to direct or primary healing without abundant callus formation.

Phases of fracture healing

1. Acute inflammation. This is the first phase of healing in response to haematoma formation at a fracture site. The haematoma provides a source of haematopoietic cells secreting growth factors (cytokines) to promote healing. A classical inflammatory response secondary to mediators is evoked, leading to vascular ingrowth and cell proliferation, with an influx of polymorphonuclear leucocytes, macrophages and lymphocytes. Exudate and necrotic tissue are removed by demolition. From osteogenic precursors, pluripotent mesenchymal stem cells (MSC), osteoblasts and fibroblasts proliferate, producing a new matrix.

2. Repair process. The process starts with organization of the haematoma into granulation tissue and a change of environment from slightly acidic (the acidic tide), to neutral and subsequently slightly alkaline (the alkaline tide), promoting alkaline phosphatase activity. Periosteal vessels are stimulated by angiogenic fibroblast growth factors to produce capillary buds. Osteoclasts, derived from monocytes and monocytic progenitors, resorb non-viable bone, possibly under stimulus from prostaglandins. Proliferation of the MSCs leads to formation of a matrix of fibrous tissue and cartilage. After mineralization this forms woven bone, described as fracture callus. Hard callus is formed at the periphery by intramembranous bone formation, and soft callus is formed in the central region, with a higher cartilage content, by endochondral ossification. Eventually a mass of callus bridges the fracture margins and clinical union has occurred.

Initially the matrix consists of types I, III and V collagen, glucosaminoglycans, proteoglycans and other non-collagenous proteins acting as enzymes, growth factors and mediators. Some of this collagen is converted to types II and IX collagen and then type I collagen predominates during osteogenesis, mineralization and remodelling.

Local oxygen tension, pH, electrical charge and numerous growth factor mediators (cytokines) which are non-collagenous proteins, mostly released from platelets and cells, promote the repair process of cartilage and bone formation. These factor mediators include fibroblast growth factor (FGF), platelet-derived growth factor (PDGF) and the progression factor transforming growth factor beta (TGF-β). These mediators and others, such as IGF-I, IGF-II and epidermal growth factor (EGF) encourage mitoses. BMP and TGF-β stimulate the differentiation of MSCs into the specialist cells required for bone healing.

When the fracture margins are stable and anatomically aligned, either by impaction at the time of a fracture or secondary to rigid internal fixation, direct bone healing occurs, without abundant fracture callus formation and replacement, in a manner similar to remodelling or natural turnover of bone. With cortical contact, octeoclasts arranged in cutting cones or heads cross the fracture margins, followed by osteoblasts, forming lamellar bone with new haversian systems. Defects up to 200 μm can be crossed in this manner, known as *contact healing*.

Larger gaps, of 200 to 1000 μm are first filled with woven bone and then lamellar bone in a different orientation to the original lamellar bone, before remodelling. This bridging of small gaps is known as *gap healing*.

As well as demonstrating a change in pH, the fracture site is marginally electronegative which promotes fracture healing and hence electrical stimulation may be used to promote fracture healing.

3. Remodelling phase. This starts during the repair phase and sees the conversion of woven bone to lamellar bone, with restoration of the normal matrix. The process may take several months or years, and is demonstrated radiographically by the cortical and trabecular patterns returning to normal. The bone returns to its normal shape by responding to loading and stress – Wolff's Law.

4. Fracture union. Commonly assessed clinically and radiographically. The stiffness of a healing fracture can be measured accurately to define the point of union. This is more accurate than clinical assessment, but at present only a research tool.

5. Delayed and non-union. This occurs when the healing process is slow or fails. Union may fail with minimal callus formation, hypotrophic non-union, or with abundant callus formation, hypertrophic non-union. A non-union bridged by fibrocartilage is a pseudarthrosis.

Injury and patient variables may delay fracture healing. Injury variables include soft tissue damage from high-energy or open fractures, soft tissue interposition, infection, bone disease and poor local blood supply. Patient variables include age, comorbidity, corticosteroids, malnutrition and smoking. Fracture healing is also altered by the presence or absence of surgical stabilization.

Further reading

Pan WT, Einhorn TA. The biochemistry of fracture healing. *Current Orthopaedics*, 1992; **6**: 207–213.

Walter JB, Talbot IC. Healing of specialised tissues. In: Walter JB, Israel MS (eds.) *General Pathology*. New York: Churchill Livingstone, 1996; 181–186.

Wozney JM, Rosen V. Bone morphogenic protein and bone morphogenic protein gene family in bone formation and repair. *Clinical Orthopaedics and Related Research*, 1998; **346**: 26–37.

Related topics of interest

Bone grafting, p. 28; Bone structure, p. 34; Non-union and delayed union, p. 153

BONE STRUCTURE

There are two types of bone – mature or *lamellar* bone and immature or *woven* bone. Both types consist of cells, and a partly organic, partly mineral extracellular matrix of collagen fibres embedded in a ground substance providing strength and stiffness. Periosteum is the dense layer of fibro-connective tissue covering bone. It is thicker in children.

Bone provides skeletal support and protection for the soft tissues, mechanical advantage for muscles and a centre for mineral metabolism.

The majority of bone is formed from mesenchymal tissues by mineralization of a cartilage model, *endochondral ossification*, but some is formed by direct mineralization of mesenchymal layers without a cartilage model, *intramembranous ossification*. Unmineralized bone is known as osteoid.

Bone

Lamellar bone is an organized, regular, stress-orientated structure which may be cortical or cancellous. Woven bone has a high cell turnover and content, a less organized structure and higher water content, making it weaker and more deformable than lamellar bone. Woven bone is formed first in the embryonic skeleton, and following a fracture, before being replaced by organized lamellar bone. Bone remodels and changes shape according to load and stress – *Wolff's law*.

1. Cortical or compact bone has tightly packed haversian systems, or osteons, with a central haversian canal for nerves and vessels. The slow turnover of cortical bone occurs at the cement line, where osteoblasts and osteoclasts are active, which is the margin of the osteon.

2. Cancellous or trabecular bone undergoes faster turnover and is less dense. By weight, only 20% of the skeleton is cancellous bone, which is more elastic than cortical bone with a smaller Young's modulus.

Cells

There are four cell types in bone:

1. Osteoblasts, derived from undifferentiated mesenchymal cells or stromal cells, synthesize and secrete bone matrix. Osteoblasts have similar characteristics to fibroblasts.

2. Osteocytes, the most common cell line, control the microenvironment, and the concentration of calcium and phosphate in bone matrix. Osteocytes are derived from osteoblasts trapped in the matrix, communicating with each other by long cytoplasmic processes, called canaliculi. Osteocytes are stimulated by calcitonin and inhibited by parathyroid hormone (PTH).

3. Osteoclasts, derived from circulating monocyte progenitors and therefore stem cells, are multinucleate giant cells responsible for resorbing bone under stimulation by PTH, vitamin D, prostaglandins, thyroid hormone and glucocorticoids. They are inhibited by calcitonin. Resorption occurs at the cell surface by the enzymatic activity of tartrate-resistant acid phosphatase and carbonic anhydrase.

4. *Osteoprogenitor cells* line the Haversian canals and periosteum, before being stimulated to differentiate into osteoblasts and other cells.

Matrix

Organic and mineral components form non-cellular bone, called the matrix.

1. *The organic* component consists of type I collagen for tensile strength, proteoglycans for compressive strength, glycoproteins and phospholipids. The collagen is a triple helix of tropocollagen. Tensile strength is increased by cross-linking. Forty per cent of the matrix is made up by the organic component, which itself is 90% type I collagen.

2. *The inorganic* component is mineral, mostly poorly crystalline calcium hydroxyapatite, which mineralizes bone and provides compressive strength. A small amount of the inorganic component is osteocalcium phosphate.

Periosteum

Bone is covered by periosteum, a fibro-connective tissue, with an inner cambium and outer fibrous layer. The cambium layer is vascular and osteogenic, producing cortical bone. The outer layer is fibrous and continuous with joint capsules. Periosteum plays an important role in fracture healing.

Bone formation

The formation of bone is mostly by mineralization of a cartilage model, endochondral ossification and sometimes directly by intramembranous ossification.

1. *Endochondral ossification* is the principal system of bone formation and growth. Initially a cartilaginous model, derived from mesenchymal tissue condensation, is formed. Vascular invasion, with osteoprogenitor cells differentiating into osteoblasts, leads to the formation of a primary centre of ossification. The epiphysis is a secondary centre at the bone ends, leaving an area between for longitudinal growth – the physis.

The physis consists of three zones for chondrocyte growth and transformation:

- The **reserve zone** is where resting cells store products required for subsequent maturation. This zone is on the epiphyseal side of the physis. Gaucher's disease affects this zone.
- The **proliferative zone** is an area of cell proliferation and matrix formation, with longitudinal growth as the chondrocytes become organized or stacked in an area of high oxygen tension and high proteoglycan concentration. Achondroplasia is a defect in this zone.
- The **hypertrophic zone** has three areas of *maturation*, *degeneration* and *provisional calcification*. In this zone, cells first accumulate calcium as they increase in size and then die, releasing calcium for mineralization. Osteoblasts are active in this zone, with calcification of the cartilage, promoted by low oxygen tension and low proteoglycan. Mucopolysaccharide diseases affect the zone, with chondrocyte degeneration, and in rickets there is reduced provisional calcification. Physeal fractures occur through the zone of provisional calcification.

2. _Intramembranous ossification_ is a process of bone formation without a cartilage precursor during embryonic life, and in some areas during fracture healing. Mesenchymal cells aggregate into layers or membranes, followed by osteoblast invasion and bone formation.

Hormonal control

The micro-environment of bone formation is under hormonal control, probably by hundreds of polypeptides, and knowledge of this control is expanding rapidly. This hormonal control is especially relevant to fracture healing. The principal agent is BMP, a member of the TGF-β superfamily. There are several types of BMP responsible for formation of bone, cartilage and connective tissue, the hallmark being the induction of endochondral bone formation, by the differentiation of cells into cartilage and bone phenotypes. This also involves other factors including TGF-β, IGF and FGF.

In the clinical setting, additional BMP may help stimulate new bone formation to bridge defects, which integrates well with host bone.

Further reading

Fawcett DW, Jensh RP. Bone. In: _Bloom and Fawcett: Concise Histology._ New York: Chapman and Hall, 1997; 69–79.

Revell PA. Bone structure. In: Hughes SPF, McCarthy I, eds. _Sciences Basic to Orthopaedics._ London: WB Saunders, 1998; 1–14.

Schiller AL. Bones and joints. In: Rubin E, Farber JL, eds. _Pathology._ Philadelphia: Lippincott-Raven, 1988; 1304–1315.

Wozney JM, Rosen V. Bone morphogenic protein and bone morphogenic protein gene family in bone formation and repair. _Clinical Orthopaedics and Related Research_, 1998; **346**: 26–37.

Related topics of interest

Bone grafting, p. 28; Bone healing, p. 31

CLASSIFICATION OF FRACTURES

There are almost as many fracture classifications as orthopaedic surgeons. The classification of fractures by eponyms has made documentation and comparison of fractures, to determine the epidemiology, management and outcome, difficult. This problem has been addressed by AO/ASIF, who have successfully introduced a complex alphanumeric classification for long bone fractures, but the classification does not comprehensively cover pelvic, spinal and some other fractures.

Fracture classifications

1. AO classification. This is alphanumeric, ascribing a code specific to every fracture with increasing complexity, which identifies the anatomical location (*Figure 1*), type, group and subgroup of the fracture.

Fracture location is identified by the first two numbers. The first number refers to the bone involved: 1, humerus; 2, radius and ulna; 3, femur; 4, tibia and fibula; 5, spine; 6, pelvis; 7, wrist and hand; 8, foot. The second number refers to the bone segment: 1, proximal metaphyseal; 2, diaphyseal; 3, distal metaphyseal. The metaphyseal/diaphyseal junction is a point equivalent to the width of the metaphysis, such that the metaphyseal segment forms a square. The two exceptions are the proximal femur, where the proximal segment is above a line through the lower border of the lesser trochanter, and the ankle, where malleolar fractures are segment 44.

Fracture type is identified by the letter A, B or C. Metaphyseal fractures are: A,

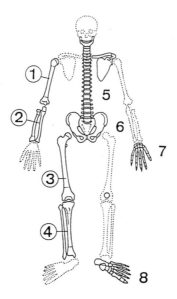

Figure 1. The 'AO' man, showing the numbering of different bones. Reprinted from Müller ME, Allgöwer M, Schneider R, Willenegger H, *Manual of Internal Fixation*, 3rd Edn, p. 121, fig. 3, 1991. ©Springer-Verlag.

extra-articular; B, partial intra-articular with a simple split; C, complex intra-articular. Diaphyseal fractures are: A, simple two-fragment; B, wedge with a butterfly fragment; C, multifragmentary.

The last two digits of the code identify the group and subgroup, referring to increasing complexity, with three groups for each fracture type and three subgroups for each group. Hence for each segment there are nine groups and 27 subgroups. These are not possible to memorize!

A recent classification for pelvic, acetabular, spinal, foot and hand fractures has been introduced, largely based on eponymous classifications.

The AO classification is not exhaustive, and for some fractures eponyms remain popular and universally accepted as detailed below.

2. The Salter–Harris (SH) classification of physeal fractures is based on the prognosis of the injury. Type I, a transverse fracture through the physis; type II, a fracture through the physis, with a small fragment of metaphysis; type III, an intra-articular fracture crossing the epiphysis and out through the physis; type IV, an oblique intra-articular fracture through the epiphysis and physis into the metaphysis; type V, a crush injury of the physis. Rang expanded this to include a perichondral ring injury as type VI.

Types V and VI are difficult to diagnose and may not be apparent until complications become evident.

3. The Frykman classification of distal radial fractures is an eight-part classification, I to VIII. Odd numbers have an intact ulnar styloid and even numbers an ulnar styloid fracture. Types I and II are extra-articular; types III and IV extend into the radio-carpal joint; types V and VI into the radio-ulnar joint; types VII and VIII involve both the radio-carpal and radio-ulnar joint.

4. The Milch classification refers to medial and lateral condylar fractures of the humerus, with type I passing through the capitellum or medial condyle, fracturing off the condyle, leaving the trochlear ridge intact. Type II fractures pass close to the trochlear sulcus and by including the trochlear ridge allow elbow joint subluxation.

5. The Neer four-part classification of proximal humeral fracture/dislocations depends on the number of displaced segments, defining displacement as >1 cm or >45°. The proximal humerus is considered in four segments: the articular head, lesser tuberosity, greater tuberosity and shaft. Fractures may be 1 (undisplaced), 2, 3 or 4-part, with anterior or posterior dislocation. Head splitting articular fractures are usually 3 or 4-part.

6. The Tile classification of pelvic fractures is: A, stable; B, rotationally unstable, but vertically stable; C, rotationally and vertically unstable.

7. The Letournel and Judet classification of acetabular fractures has five elemental and five associated, or more complex, configurations. The elemental patterns include: posterior wall, posterior column, anterior wall, anterior column and transverse. The associated patterns include: T-shaped, posterior column and wall, transverse and posterior wall, anterior wall or column with posterior hemitransverse and finally, both column fractures.

8. The Thompson and Epstein classification for posterior hip dislocation includes five configurations: type I with no associated fracture or small fragments; type II with a large single posterior rim fracture; type III with a comminuted rim fracture; type IV with an acetabular floor fracture; type V with a femoral head fracture.

9. The Pipkin classification of femoral head fractures includes: type I with a caudad head fragment below the fovea centralis; type II with a cephalad fracture above or including the fovea centralis; type III with a femoral head and neck fracture; type IV with an associated acetabular rim fracture.

10. The Garden classification of femoral neck fractures has four stages, depending on the degree of displacement seen on AP X-ray. Garden I fractures are incomplete or impacted into valgus; Garden II fractures are complete with minimal or no displacement; Garden III fractures are displaced with angulation of the trabecular lines; and Garden IV fractures are grossly displaced, with the trabecular lines of the head and acetabulum lying parallel.

11. The Pauwel classification of subcapital femoral neck fractures is based on the angle of the fracture line.

12. The Schatzker classification of tibial plateau fractures includes six fracture types: type 1, vertical shear; type 2, vertical shear and compression; type 3, local compression; type 4, medial condyle fracture (considered a fracture/dislocation of the knee); type 5, bicondylar; type 6, tibial plateau and segmental fracture.

13. The Danis–Weber classification of ankle fractures is in three parts, based upon the level of the fibula fracture and hence stability of the ankle joint. Weber A is a supination injury, with a fracture of the lower fibula, below the joint line, with a stable mortice. Weber B passes through the level of the joint line, with a spiral fracture of the fibula, allowing the mortice to displace, but with an intact syndesmosis. Weber C has a more proximal fracture of the fibula with disruption of the syndesmosis.

14. The Lauge–Hansen classification of ankle fractures is based upon the position of the foot at the time of the injury, pronation or supination, and the deforming force, adduction, abduction or rotation, and hence upon the mechanism of injury. The injury patterns are supination–adduction, supination–external rotation, pronation–abduction, pronation–external rotation and pronation–dorsiflexion. Each pattern has several stages.

15. The Hawkins and Canale classification of talar neck fractures includes: type I, minimally displaced vertical fracture; type II, subtalar joint subluxation or dislocation; type III, talar body dislocation from the ankle and subtalar joint; rarely type IV, talar head and body dislocation.

Soft tissue injury classifications

1. The Gustilo and Anderson classification divides open fractures into: type I, puncture wound <1 cm with minimal soft tissue damage; type II, wound >1 cm, with moderate tissue damage; type III, extensive tissue devitalization. Gustilo,

Mendosa and Williams expanded the original classification into: type IIIA, large wound, typically >10 cm, and extensive muscle damage but adequate skin cover; type IIIB, extensive periosteal stripping, with skin damage requiring a reconstructive procedure to close the defect; type IIIC, associated vascular injury requiring repair.

The mechanism of injury, degree of contamination and soft tissue damage are crucial to the classification, not the length of visible skin wound. By definition, high energy, segmental or contaminated fractures are type IIIA, wounds requiring a skin graft or flap are type IIIB and high velocity missile wounds type IIIB or IIIC.

2. The AO classification categorizes skin, muscle–tendon and neurovascular damage separately. Skin wounds are: IO1, from inside out; IO2, <5 cm skin breakage from outside; IO3, >5 cm skin breakage; IO4, considerable skin damage, contusion and loss; IO5, degloving. Muscle–tendon and neurovascular damage are graded from MT1 to MT5 and NV1 to NV5, respectively.

Further reading

Müller ME, Allgöwer M, Schneider R, Willenegger H. *Manual of Internal Fixation*, 3rd Edn. Berlin: Springer-Verlag, 1991; 118–156 (Appendix A).

Related topic of interest

Spinal fracture classification, p. 262

COMPARTMENT SYNDROME

Compartment syndrome is increased soft tissue pressure within an enclosed soft tissue compartment of the extremity, leading to devastating muscle necrosis, contracture, functional impairment and nerve damage. Elevated compartment pressures which compromise the microcirculation usually follow fractures, most commonly of the tibia, and soft tissue crush injuries. Compartment syndrome may be a consequence of burns, gunshot wounds, surgery, prolonged use of a tourniquet or pneumatic anti-shock garment (PASG), and occasionally as a chronic exercise-induced phenomenon.

Diagnosis

In a conscious patient, pain is the earliest feature of elevated compartment pressure. Paraesthesiae, pallor, paralysis and pulselessness are indicative of elevated pressure, but the latter three signs appear late and are not early features. The most reliable sign is significant pain on passive stretching of an involved muscle group, for example flexion or extension of the great toe, or extension of the fingers. Beware the patient requiring excessive analgesia. In the paralysed and intoxicated, the diagnosis is more difficult and an indication for compartment pressure monitoring.

Clinical suspicion is usually enough to warrant surgical exploration. Compartment pressures can be measured with an indwelling catheter device and this is especially useful for the paralysed. Normal pressure in a fascial compartment is around 0 mmHg. Pressures within 20–30 mmHg of the diastolic blood pressure, or an absolute value >40 mmHg, require surgical decompression by fasciotomy. Some units monitor calf pressures in all patients with tibial shaft fractures and all ventilated polytrauma victims. For chronic exercise-induced symptoms, a thallium or other isotope scan may confirm the diagnosis.

Management

Surgical decompression within 4 hours of the onset of the symptoms is the aim of treatment. Where findings are equivocal, the limb should be elevated and reassessed a couple of hours later. However, if the diagnosis is suspected, an unnecessary surgical decompression is uncommon and preferable to compartment ischaemia.

*1. **The leg*** is the most common site for compartment syndrome, following a closed tibial shaft fracture, but elevated pressure may follow open fractures and IM nailing. The four compartments in the leg (anterior, lateral, posterior and deep posterior) must all be released. The anterior compartment is the most frequently involved.

The anterior and lateral compartments are decompressed through a long, 15–20 cm, antero-lateral incision between the fibula and crest of the tibia. The posterior compartments are decompressed through a long medial incision, 2 cm behind the posterior border of the tibia. The fascia is released longitudinally, preserving neurovascular structures – the superficial peroneal nerve is most at risk. In the past, a single lateral incision has been advocated, excising a portion of fibula to achieve decompression of all compartments. This approach does not allow adequate exposure and surgical release. Concern about the cosmetic outcome should not compromise the surgical decompression, as even the skin is a potential constricting structure. The fascial and skin incisions are left open and the wound inspected under anaesthesia two days later. At this stage, it may be possible to close part of the skin wound, but usually a split-skin graft is required at 7–10 days. Techniques to appose the skin edges by tension from elastic bands, or other elastic devices to improve the cosmetic outcome, should be used with caution and the skin wound must *never* be closed under tension.

2. *The forearm* may develop compartment syndrome following trauma or surgery, especially when the deep fascia has been closed. A supracondylar fracture of the distal humerus may also be associated with compartment syndrome, when the circulation has been interrupted. Classically the volar compartments are affected. The forearm is decompressed through a longitudinal volar incision, zig-zagged across the wrist into the palm, to include release of the carpal tunnel. It is uncommon to need to release the dorsal compartments through a second dorsal approach. The same approach to wound care is required.

3. *The hand and foot* may develop compartment syndrome, following fractures and crush injuries. While these are uncommon, the diagnosis should not be over-looked and the relevant compartments decompressed.

4. *Full thickness burns* cause constriction of the skin, which may be circum-ferential and cause elevated compartment pressure. The eschar should be released with a longitudinal incision. A full thickness burn results in anaesthetic skin, so this can be performed in the resuscitation room, if the situation is urgent.

5. *The thigh* is an occasional site for compartment syndrome, following direct trauma, spontaneous haemorrhage and rarely closed IM nailing. Decompression is performed through a direct lateral approach.

6. *Iatrogenic causes* include tight bandages or plasters, prolonged use of a tourniquet or PASG and fluid extravasation during knee arthroscopy. Treatment is the same and where the diagnosis is suspected, the compartment should be released. Plasters and bandages should be split, opened down to the skin and the limb reassessed.

Late sequelae

Fibrosis of necrotic muscle occurs when surgical decompression has been unsuc-cessful, too late, or the diagnosis overlooked. Fibrosis leads to contracture and ineffective muscle function. There may be a mild contracture, for example with clawing of the toes, or a florid Volkmann's ischaemic contracture. Tendon transfers may occasionally be indicated to improve function.

Related topics of interest

ELBOW DISLOCATION

Dislocation of the elbow is second only in frequency to dislocation of the shoulder. Simple dislocation carries a good prognosis. There are two theories for the mechanism of injury: firstly hyperextension causing the olecranon to impinge in the olecranon fossa 'levering' out the joint, and secondly axial loading of the slightly flexed joint causing dislocation.

Classification

Elbow dislocation is classified according to the direction of forearm displacement. Posterior dislocation is commonest, with anterior, medial and lateral being rarer. Divergent dislocation, where the radius and ulna dissociate to either side of the humerus may occur, either antero-posterior with the radius anterior and the ulna posterior, or medio-lateral. Ulnar and radial dislocation may occur in isolation.

Clinical presentation

1. Typically acute and if delayed beyond 7 days constitutes a 'neglected' case, seldom reducible by closed means.

2. Clinically the equilateral triangle formed by the olecranon, medial and lateral epicondyles is disrupted, differentiating dislocation from supracondylar fracture.

3. Careful neuro-vascular assessment should be documented at presentation and repeated after reduction.

Associated injuries

1. Vascular injury. If arterial injury is suspected, an arteriogram should be obtained after reduction. The presence of distal pulses does not exclude significant arterial injury. Historically, good results have been reported with simple ligation of the brachial artery; however, modern standards of care advocate vascular reconstruction.

2. Neurological injury. The median, ulnar, anterior interosseous and radial nerves can all be injured. The radial is the least often involved and anterior interosseous palsy the most difficult to diagnose, because of the lack of sensory involvement. The median and ulnar nerves can be trapped within the joint during reduction and the development of post-reduction palsy requires surgical exploration. For palsy present before reduction it is customary to wait 3 months, obtain electromyelogram (EMG) studies and if recovery does not occur spontaneously, undertake surgical exploration.

3. Fracture dislocation. The incidence of associated fractures varies from 16% to 62%, reflecting the unreliable detection of osteochondral fragments. Fracture dislocation is associated with a poorer outcome.

4. Medial epicondyle avulsion. Occurs in adults or children and requires early recognition, as retained joint fragments lead to articular surface damage. ORIF is usually required, although success with closed reduction is reported.

5. *Muscular injury.* Avulsion of the triceps is associated with anterior dislocation, possibly with an associated bony fragment. Following reduction of anterior dislocation, triceps function should be assessed and reattachment performed if required.

Treatment

1. *Closed reduction is favoured.* Posterior dislocation can usually be reduced under sedation, by one of two methods. Firstly, extension of the elbow to 'unlock' it, which may predispose to nerve entrapment; or secondly, application of longitudinal forearm traction, with digital pressure over the olecranon. The elbow is immobilized in 100° flexion in a plaster slab for 7–10 days, before commencing mobilization. Physiotherapy may be helpful but is seldom required, and forced passive mobilization should be avoided. In the presence of a significant fracture, for example an unfixed coronoid process fracture, immobilization may be increased to 3 weeks.

2. *Other patterns of dislocation.* These are rare and closed reduction is usually successful.

3. *Indications for open surgery.* These include:

- Open dislocation.
- Significant fracture requiring fixation.
- Entrapped soft tissue, blocking reduction.
- Vascular injury requiring surgery.
- Ligamentous repair (seldom improving the result).
- Irreducible neglected dislocation.

4. *With persistent instability,* despite fixation of fractures, there are three options:

- Ligamentous repair (usually lateral).
- A hinged external fixator, or brace.
- Passing a Steinman pin across the joint – while this prevents dislocation, stiffness, heterotopic ossification and pin breakage may follow.

Complications

1. *Ectopic calcification and heterotopic ossification (HO).* Ectopic ossification is mineralization of normal anatomical structures (such as collateral ligaments) and is usually associated with minimal symptoms. HO is the laying down of heterotopic bone in a previous haematoma, which leads to stiffness. HO occurs more frequently after head injury, burns, massive trauma and prolonged immobilization. The role of ill-timed surgery (after 3 days) and forceful passive mobilization are debated. Treatment is excision once the ossification is mature (trabeculated with a rim), typically around 6–8 months, and should include prophylactic indomethacin for 6 weeks post-operatively.

2. *Chronic instability.* While frank recurrent dislocation is rare, there is increasing awareness of 'elbow instability' as a long-term sequel, with patients complaining of clunking or snapping in the elbow. The critical lesion is damage to the lateral collateral ligament (LCL), specifically the ulnar part.

Prognosis

The prognosis is good in the simple dislocation. Recovery takes 3–6 months and many patients are left with 10–15° flexion contracture.

Paediatrics

The peak age of dislocation is 10–13 years, against 5 years for supracondylar fractures. Intra-articular entrapment of the medial epicondyle must be considered. In common with adults, posterior dislocation is commonest and early active flexion at 5 days is advised to avoid stiffness.

Further reading

Josefsson PO, Johnell O, Gentz CF. Long-term sequelae of simple dislocation of the elbow. *Journal of Bone and Joint Surgery*, 1984; **66A**: 927–930.

Modabber MR, Jupiter JB. Reconstruction for post-traumatic conditions of the elbow joint. *Journal of Bone and Joint Surgery*, 1995; **77A**: 1431–1442.

O'Driscoll SW, Morrey BF, Korinek S *et al.* Elbow subluxation and dislocation: a spectrum of instability. *Clinical Orthopaedics*, 1992; **280**: 186–197.

Related topics of interest

Humeral fractures – distal, p. 107; Radius and ulna – diaphyseal fractures, p. 230; Radius and ulna – fractures around the elbow, p. 236

FEMORAL FRACTURES – DISTAL

Distal or supracondylar femoral fractures are difficult to treat. Sir Reginald Watson-Jones stated in 1957 that 'few injuries present more difficult problems than supracondylar fractures of the femur'.

Epidemiology

Distal femoral fractures represent 7% of all femoral fractures. Fifty per cent are extra-articular supracondylar fractures and 50% have an intra-articular extension. Of the intra-articular group, 80% are intercondylar and 20% involve the condyles. Twenty five per cent of all fractures are open. Associated neurovascular or ligamentous injuries are relatively rare and present in <15% of cases.

There is a bimodal age distribution for supracondylar fractures. A younger, predominantly male, group is affected following high-energy polytrauma. An elderly, predominantly female, osteoporotic group is affected following minimal trauma.

Anatomy and mechanism of injury

The distal femoral metaphysis is a 9 cm transitional zone from the thick cortical region of the shaft to the broad condylar region. There is a thin cortex and a wide cancellous area. There are numerous muscle and ligamentous attachments, which cause deforming forces. Gastrocnemius rotates the distal fragment posteriorly, while the strong adductors cause varus angulation. Intercondylar fractures are splayed open by discordant muscle action.

In most cases, axial loading with a varus or valgus force leads to a distal femoral fracture. In the young this is usually a high-energy injury, typically an RTA, with considerable comminution, displacement and soft tissue trauma. In the elderly with osteoporotic bone, a fall on a flexed knee is the most common mechanism of injury. A long spiral supracondylar fracture is the result, sometimes complicated by a femoral prosthesis above or below the fracture. Rarely, a fracture occurs without obvious trauma in the immobile, as a result of severe osteoporosis.

Fracture classification

Various classifications have been described, from simple extra- and intra-articular classifications, to the detailed AO classification (33-A, 33-B and 33-C, depending on site, intra-articular involvement and extent of comminution).

Non-operative management

Non-operative management of these fractures, in a long leg cast or skeletal traction, has proved difficult. The deforming force of the gastrocnemius muscle attachment causes a hyperextension deformity of the distal segment, making accurate reduction difficult. Reduction can be achieved by 90/90 traction, but this is difficult to maintain over a protracted period and subsequent knee stiffness is a problem. Malunion and non-union are common.

Non-operative management is therefore reserved for the minimally displaced fracture, or the elderly, low-mobility patient, particularly if unfit for anaesthesia.

Conservative treatment in the 1960s was reported to give a satisfactory outcome in 67–84% of cases.

Operative management

Operative management is appropriate for open and most displaced fractures. The aims are anatomical reduction of the articular surface, stable fixation and early mobilization, achieved with minimal disruption to the soft tissue envelope and blood supply to the bone. Several techniques are available and all have an application:

- Plate and screws.
- IM nails – rigid and flexible.
- External fixation – monolateral, circular and hybrid.

As there is a wide range of injury patterns, it is important to appreciate that one particular technique is not applicable to all fractures.

1. Screw fixation alone may be appropriate for partial articular or unicondylar fractures (33-B1-3), followed by early mobilization in a cast brace.

2. Plate fixation takes the form of a blade plate, a dynamic condylar screw (DCS), or a condylar buttress plate, after lag screw fixation of any intercondylar extension. Plate fixation is usually through a lateral approach. Bone grafting is advisable for comminuted fractures, especially in the elderly, or when the comminution is on the medial side.

The disadvantages of this technique include the wide exposure necessary to insert the plate, the extensive soft tissue damage and resultant damage to the blood supply, as well as load sparing, or stress shielding by the plate itself. A DCS is preferable to a blade plate, as it allows more flexibility in plate positioning on the femur.

3. Intramedullary devices inserted in a retrograde fashion are becoming increasingly popular. In the past, Zickel supracondylar nails, Rush pins, and Ender's nails have been used. These are inserted through the epicondylar region and are suitable for distal fractures. Unfortunately there is little control of rotation of the distal fragment.

Newer intramedullary devices, inserted through the roof of the intercondylar notch adjacent to the posterior cruciate ligament (PCL) attachment, have significant advantages. This type of device allows load sharing by virtue of the intramedullary placement, as well as controlling length and rotation by interlocking screw fixation. Supplementary screw fixation to stabilize condylar fractures is possible anterior or posterior to the nail. The advantage of this technique is the relative ease of insertion, together with minimal soft tissue damage. Infection rates are low and union rates approaching 100% have been reported. Implant failure is relatively rare. The lack of periosteal stripping and soft tissue damage allows early knee movement to be regained. These devices, however, do not hold the bone fragments rigidly and therefore cautious mobilization is encouraged with, or without, a cast brace post-operatively.

In the elderly, fixation is often tenuous, and therefore cast brace support and partial or non-weight-bearing is advised for 3 months.

IM nails are ideal for 33-A1 to A3 and C1 and C2 fractures, particularly in the younger group with good bone quality, but are rather unsatisfactory for C3 type fractures where there is significant articular comminution. Open fixation and reconstruction is required.

4. **External fixation** is usually reserved for more severe injuries, 33-C3 type fractures, and open fractures. An anterior bridging fixator is used to stabilize the limb for soft tissue and vascular reconstruction. Minimal open reduction and percutaneous screw or wire fixation may be supported by circular frame stabilization. These techniques minimize soft tissue stripping, yet give adequate fixation for early movement.

Special cases

Some fractures in the elderly may extend down from the tip of a proximal femoral prosthesis. In such cases, fixation can be difficult. Dual plating, cable plating, and modified 'interlock' nailing are the options available. The latter involves engaging the proximal tip within the end of the retrograde nail. Fractures above a total knee replacement may be treated by any of the above methods or revision arthroplasty. If possible, the best technique is an IM nail through the condylar notch, which needs to be a minimum of 12 mm wide.

Complications

1. **Early.** Vascular compromise, infection, malreduction and fixation failure.

2. **Late.** Malunion, non-union (particularly with a fracture above a stiff knee), implant failure and knee stiffness.

Further reading

David SM, Harrow ME, Peindl RD. Comparative biomechanical analysis of supracondylar femur fracture fixation: locked intramedullary nail versus 95-degree angled plate. *Journal of Orthopaedic Trauma*, 1997; **11**; 344–350.

Moed BR. Femur: trauma. In: Kasser JR, ed. *Orthopaedic Knowledge Update 5*. Rosemont, Illinois: American Academy of Orthopaedic Surgeons, 1999; 427–436.

Schatzker J. Fractures of the distal femur revisited. *Clinical Orthopaedics*, 1998; **347**; 43–46.

Related topics of interest

Intramedullary nailing techniques, p. 128; Peri-prosthetic fractures (hip and knee), p. 167; Principles of external fixation, p. 214

FEMORAL FRACTURES – SHAFT

Fractures of the shaft of the femur are relatively common and frequently associated with major trauma. As high-energy injuries, femoral fractures can be life-threatening from open wounds, fat embolism and respiratory compromise. By definition, a shaft fracture is >2.5 cm below the lesser trochanter and >8 cm above the knee joint. Several treatment options are available, each with their own merits and problems.

Classification

Shaft fractures are described by the anatomical site (mid-shaft, junction of upper and middle thirds, etc.) and fracture configuration (transverse, short oblique, multi-fragmentary, etc.). Fractures are often classified by the AO classification (32-A, 32-B or 32-C for the femur), with various subtypes to describe the morphological pattern. The Winquist and Hansen classification from 0 to V is also commonly used.

Associated injuries

Two to five per cent of femoral shaft fractures have associated ipsilateral neck fractures, and hip X-rays are therefore mandatory. Less than 2% have associated condylar fractures. Ipsilateral ligament injuries are reported in 7–49% of fractures, most commonly the anterior cruciate. Meniscal damage is reported in 25–50% of fractures. There is no correlation between ligament and meniscal injuries, but all patients with a haemarthrosis need further assessment. Neurovascular injuries are surprisingly uncommon.

Treatment

1. *Traction* may be used for initial management, or rarely as definitive treatment with balanced skeletal traction in a Thomas splint. A traction force of 10–15 lb is used and the patient's hip and knee are mobilized in bed. When the fracture shows signs of union at 6–8 weeks, the patient is mobilized partially weight-bearing, often in a cast brace. Traction is occasionally advocated where co-morbidity prevents surgical stabilization.

2. *Internal fixation* with an IM nail, inserted by a closed technique with interlocking screws, is the treatment of choice for the majority of femoral shaft fractures, with predictable healing rates. An accurately placed entry point is crucial to successful insertion. The femoral canal should be reamed 1–2 mm greater than the nail diameter. Stability of the knee should be assessed under anaesthetic at the end of the procedure. Infection is seen in less than 1% of cases and non-union is rare even with static interlocking screws. Reconstruction nails, with screws inserted along the femoral neck into the head, are used for ipsilateral femoral neck fractures. Open fractures up to Gustilo–Anderson grade IIIA may be safely treated with intramedullary fixation and appropriate soft tissue management. It may be better to use an external fixator for IIIB and IIIC fractures, or an unreamed nail, although the literature is controversial.

Fixation should be performed within 24 hours of a closed fracture. IM nailing has the advantage of achieving accurate fracture reduction and stabilization, without extensive soft tissue dissection, and early patient mobilization. With rigid fixation and a stable fracture configuration, full weight-bearing is safe at an early stage.

*3. **External fixation** is rarely required for the adult, even with open fractures. Pins with a diameter greater than 5 mm are required for adequate frame stiffness. Knee stiffness may be a major problem due to quadriceps tethering. The long pin tracts are accompanied by infection in 50% of reported cases.

*4. **Dynamic compression plate (DCP) fixation** is seldom indicated. A broad DCP should be employed and with the advent of excellent intramedullary techniques, the only real indication in the adult for DCP fixation is an associated ipsilateral pelvic or acetabular fracture. Early surgical stabilization of a pelvic fracture may be prevented if there is a recent wound around the hip joint.

*5. **Paediatric femoral fractures** are commonly treated by skin or skeletal traction in a Thomas splint to allow fracture union, before mobilization in a suitable cast. For the young infant, and in some centres children up to the age of 10, early immobilization in a hip spica is favoured, obviating the need for prolonged hospital treatment. In the polytraumatized child, plate fixation is indicated, or an external fixator can be used with less disturbance of the soft tissues.

There may be some limb overgrowth, rarely >1 cm, with conservative treatment and hence it is acceptable to allow the fracture to heal with some shortening. Overgrowth is more marked between the ages of 2 and 10 years. IM nailing beyond the age of 12 years, avoiding violation of the distal epiphysis, is considered safe practice.

Complications

- Fat embolus: 1%.
- Infection: 5% after open nailing.
- Infection: <1% after closed nailing.
- Delayed union: 6–9% (defined as 6 months).
- Non-union: 2%.
- Shortening: up to 1.5 cm is compatible with good function.
- External rotation of up to 15° is seen in 20% of patients and well tolerated.

Management of infection and non-union

A deep infection site should be explored and debrided. The IM nail should be removed, the canal reamed up 1 mm, another locked nail inserted and appropriate antibiotics commenced. The fracture will usually heal over 6 months.

Delayed union is uncommon and removal of unbroken locking screws is occasionally required. Established non-union of the femur is rare and should be addressed by exchange IM nailing and occasionally autogenous bone grafting, if the IM bone reamings are thought inadequate.

Further reading

Bucholz RW, Brumback RJ. Fractures of the shaft of the femur. In: Rockwood CA, Green DP, Bucholz RW, Heckman JD, eds. *Rockwood and Green's Fractures in Adults*. Philadelphia: Lippincott-Raven, 1996; 1827–1918.

Wiss DA, Gibson T. Intramedullary nailing of the femur and tibia: indications and techniques. *Current Orthopaedics,* 1994; **8**: 245–254.

Related topics of interest

Femoral fractures – distal, p. 46; Femoral neck fractures – extracapsular, p. 52; Femoral neck fractures – intracapsular, p. 55; Intramedullary implants – reamed and unreamed, p. 125; Intramedullary nailing techniques, p. 128; Polytrauma – management and complications, p. 200

FEMORAL NECK FRACTURES – EXTRACAPSULAR

Extracapsular fractures may be intertrochanteric (between the trochanters) or pertrochanteric (through the trochanters), and are common in the elderly and osteoporotic patient, often following minimal trauma. Extracapsular fractures account for almost 50% of all femoral neck fractures and the proportion is increasing. The mean age of presentation is 80 years, higher than for intracapsular fractures. Eighty per cent occur in women. As the fracture is extracapsular the blood supply to the femoral head is good and the aim of treatment is early surgical stabilization and mobilization. Union rates are high, and late complications of the fracture itself uncommon. However, as the majority of patients are elderly, often with additional medical problems, surgery and bed rest are tolerated poorly, leading to mortality of 33% at 6 months and 38% at 12 months. Mortality is higher than for intracapsular fractures.

Extracapsular fractures occur in younger patients following high-velocity trauma. Subtrochanteric fractures account for the minority of proximal femoral fractures and have a bimodal distribution presenting in young adults and over 65 year olds.

Classification

The AO classification is widely accepted: 31-A1 or 31-A2 for pertrochanteric fractures and 31-A3 for intertrochanteric fractures, with subtypes to describe the morphological pattern. Classification and stability depend upon the degree of comminution and trochanteric involvement. The Boyd and Griffin classification (1949), based on the ease of obtaining and maintaining reduction of the fracture, is often quoted, as is the Evans classification (1949), dividing fractures into stable and unstable groups. Subtrochanteric fractures occur within 2.5 cm of the lesser trochanter.

Radiology

Where the diagnosis is not confirmed by plain AP and lateral X-rays, the hip should be assessed with tomograms, an isotope bone scan, MRI or under the image intensifier. When there is no obvious fracture and pain persists, X-rays should be repeated.

Treatment

The aim of treatment is to achieve early mobilization of the patient, avoiding the attendant complications of prolonged bed rest. Young patients should be treated in the same manner. Rehydration and urgent medical assessment of all patients is vital. Surgery should be performed within 48 hours of the fracture, as confusion, pneumonia, the incidence of pressure sores and the duration of hospital stay all increase significantly after this period if surgery is further delayed.

1. Closed treatment, with skin or skeletal traction for 6–8 weeks will usually achieve sound union and should be reserved for the 2 or 3% of patients where surgery is contraindicated or declined.

Undisplaced fractures can be treated with early mobilization and partial weight-bearing. The fracture should be reassessed regularly with X-rays. Where pain persists, the fracture displaces or the patient is unable to cooperate with mobilization, internal fixation should be performed.

2. *Internal fixation* is the treatment of choice, followed by early mobilization and weight-bearing as tolerated. Careful placement of the patient on the fracture table is essential and an anatomical reduction can often be achieved before opening the fracture.

A variety of devices may be used, but a sliding hip screw-plate system (a dynamic hip screw) is the most popular. Within the femoral neck and head, the sliding screw should lie below the midline on the AP view, centrally on the lateral view and within 10 mm of the subchondral bone, to reduce the possibility of screw cut out. With an anatomical reduction, sliding screw-plate systems are well tolerated. Unstable fractures may require osteotomy or medial displacement of the shaft to enhance stability, as bone continuity along the medial aspect of the upper femur is essential.

Short intramedullary devices may be used, but are less popular. Flexible IM nails, inserted into the femoral neck and head from the condylar region (condylo-cephalic nails) are popular in parts of Europe, with good results.

Subtrochanteric fractures can be treated with a sliding hip screw, but insertion of an intramedullary device by closed means with sound fixation by locking screws into the femoral head is preferable.

3. *Isolated greater and lesser trochanter fractures* are rare and can usually be treated symptomatically.

Additional considerations

Hip fractures consume a large proportion of health care, costing the National Health Service (NHS) £330 million a year, and have a massive impact on society. The incidence of proximal femoral fractures is still rising. The associated morbidity carries major functional, social and financial implications. Preventative measures to reduce the fracture incidence, including hormone replacement therapy (HRT), need further development.

The morbidity following extracapsular fractures is greater than intracapsular fractures and can be measured in the elderly by a variety of means including pain, residential status, use of walking aids and function. The Peterborough Hip Scoring System (PHSS) scores function from 9 to 0 on the ability to perform three functions – shopping, getting out of the house and getting about the house, depending on the level of independence or assistance required. The Mental Test Score can be used to predict mortality, but the PHSS has a superior predictive value.

Complications

- Mortality: 6 months – 33%; 12 months – 38% (3% <60 years, 50% >90 years).
- In-hospital mortality: 15%.
- Delayed union: 1–2%.
- Wound infection: 2–15%.
- Implant failure and screw cut out: 5–16%
- Avascular necrosis: <0.5%.

Further reading

Boyd HB, Griffin LL. Classification and treatment of trochanteric fractures. *Archives of Surgery*, 1949; **58**: 853–866.

Brennan MJ. Intertrochanteric femur fractures. In: Levine AM, ed. *Orthopaedic Knowledge Update Trauma*. Rosemont: American Academy of Orthopaedic Surgeons, 1998; 121–126.

Evans EM. The treatment of trochanteric fractures of the femur. *Journal of Bone and Joint Surgery*, 1949; 31B: 190–203.

Parker MJ, Pryor GA, Thorngren K.-G. *Handbook of Hip Fracture Surgery*. Oxford: Butterworth Heinemann, 1997.

Related topic of interest

Femoral neck fractures – intracapsular, p. 55

FEMORAL NECK FRACTURES – INTRACAPSULAR

Intracapsular fractures are subcapital (at the junction of the head and neck) or transcervical (passing through the neck), and are common in the elderly or osteoporotic patient, often following only a slight injury. Intracapsular fractures account for just under 50% of all femoral neck fractures and the proportion is decreasing. The mean age of presentation is 78 years, lower than for extracapsular fractures. Eighty per cent occur in women. Subcapital fractures are uncommon in the presence of an osteoarthritic hip.

As the fracture is intracapsular, the blood supply to the femoral head is at risk and, especially when displaced, there is a substantial incidence of ovascular necrosis or non-union of the femoral head. With displaced fractures, the risk of avascular necrosis is 20 to 55% and the risk of non-union is 10 to 30%, although it can sometimes be difficult to distinguish the two. Historically, the risk has been considered so great that the majority of displaced subcapital fractures in the elderly have been treated by hemiarthroplasty. Treatment is directed at early mobilization for elderly patients whether following internal fixation or hemiarthroplasty. Surgery and bed confinement are tolerated poorly in the elderly, who often present with co-morbidity, leading to a mortality rate of 24% at 6 months and 29% at 12 months following intracapsular fractures – lower than for extracapsular fractures.

Intracapsular fractures may occur after high-velocity trauma in younger patients and the principle of treatment must be to reduce and stabilize the fracture, accepting a significant risk of failure. Twenty per cent are associated with an ipsilateral femoral shaft fracture. Joint replacement should be considered, but the complication rate following an acute fracture is significantly higher than for total hip replacement (THR) under elective conditions for degenerative disease.

Classification

The Garden classification (1961), based on the degree of displacement on the AP X-ray, is the most popular classification (*Figure 1*). Garden stage I fractures are incomplete or impacted into valgus; Garden II fractures are complete with minimal or no displacement; Garden III fractures are displaced with angulation of the

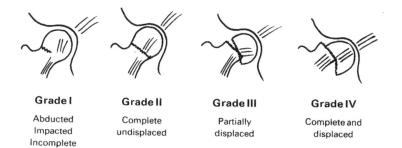

Grade I	Grade II	Grade III	Grade IV
Abducted Impacted Incomplete	Complete undisplaced	Partially displaced	Complete and displaced

Figure 1. Garden classification of subcapital femoral neck fractures. The trabecular lines help in differentiation, particularly between types III and IV. From Keene G, Parker M (1993) The fractured neck of femur – proximal femoral fractures. *Postgraduate Doctor Middle East*, vol. 16, pp. 244–253. Reprinted by permission of PMH Publications.

trabecular lines; and Garden IV fractures are grossly displaced, with the trabecular lines of the head and acetabulum parallel. Stages I and II (20%) have a similar prognosis, as do stages III and IV (80%). The AO classification is also widely accepted: 31-B1, 31-B2 and 31-B3. Pauwel's classification is based on the angle of the fracture line across the femoral neck.

Radiology

Where the diagnosis is not confirmed by plain AP and lateral X-rays, the hip should be assessed with tomograms, an isotope bone scan, MRI, image intensifier, or ultrasound.

Treatment

The aim of treatment is early mobilization, avoiding the attendant complications of bed rest, either by mobilization alone, internal fixation or arthroplasty. Rehydration and urgent medical assessment of all patients is vital. Surgery should be performed within 48 hours of the fracture as confusion, pneumonia, the incidence of pressure sores and the duration of hospital stay all increase significantly with further delay.

1. *Impacted fractures* can be mobilized early when the head is tilted into valgus, weight-bearing as tolerated. However, there is a significant risk of displacement on mobilization, so stabilization of the fracture with three parallel screws is a wise precaution. This can be performed under local anaesthetic if required. Without stabilization, regular radiological review is advisable to assess displacement.

2. *Undisplaced fractures* should be stabilized with three parallel screws or a sliding hip screw with an additional screw to prevent rotation. Where patients are aged over 80 years, there is evidence to suggest a more favourable and predictable outcome with hemiarthroplasty, although the complication rates are higher.

3. *Displaced fractures* are traditionally treated by hemiarthroplasty, with an uncemented Austin Moore type stem, or a cemented stem. The results of late conversion of a hemiarthroplasty to a THR are good. There are no reported benefits of a bipolar prosthesis in patients over 80 years.

There is increasing evidence to suggest that the incidence of avascular necrosis and non-union are not as high as previously perceived, even for displaced fractures. This is a contentious issue and may relate to improved fixation techniques and intra-operative imaging. The current literature suggests more fractures should be reduced and stabilized with parallel screws, rather than performing a hemiarthroplasty. Large randomized controlled trials are needed to assess this further. However, this approach conflicts with reports of a more favourable outcome where hemiarthroplasty is used in patients over 80 years for undisplaced or minimally displaced fractures, rather than internal fixation.

A subcapital fracture can be reduced on the traction table with longitudinal traction and internal rotation, or by the Leadbetter manoeuvre (traction along the line of the femur with the hip and knee flexed at 90°, followed by internal rotation and abduction). The capsule should be incised following internal fixation to release any intracapsular haematoma, which may jeopardize the venous drainage.

4. In younger patients treatment is directed at preserving the femoral head by reduction and fixation within 6 hours of the fracture, accepting that a proportion will develop avascular necrosis requiring further surgery. A good outcome can be expected in 70 to 84% of patients. If a primary THR is performed, the incidence of infection, heterotopic bone formation, early failure and dislocation are all higher than elective situations.

Additional considerations

Hip fractures have a massive impact on society and consume a large proportion of health care resources. The incidence of proximal femoral fractures is rising and costs the NHS around £330 million a year. Although mortality is important, the associated morbidity carries major functional, social and financial implications. Preventative measures to reduce the fracture incidence, including HRT, need further development.

The morbidity following intracapsular fractures is less than in extracapsular fractures and can be measured in the elderly by a variety of means including pain, residential status, use of walking aids and function. The Peterborough Hip Scoring System (PHSS) scores function from 9 to 0 on the ability to perform three functions – shopping, getting out of the house and getting about the house, depending on the level of independence or assistance required. The Mental Test Score can be used to predict mortality, but the PHSS has a superior predictive value.

Complications

- Mortality: 6 months – 24%; 12 months – 29%; following dislocation of hemiarthroplasty – 60–70% at 12 months.
- In-hospital mortality: 15%.
- Infection: 2–20%.
- Non-union: 7–25% in young patients.
- Avascular necrosis: 20–55% ($\propto$ to displacement – 80% in some series).
- Osteoarthritis: 5%.
- Dislocation after THR: 15–30%.

Further reading

Garden RS. Low angle fixation in fractures of the femoral neck. *Journal of Bone and Joint Surgery*, 1961; 43B: 647–663.

Lu-Yao GL, Keller RB, Littenberg B *et al*. Outcomes after displaced fractures of the femoral neck: a meta-analysis of one hundred and six published reports. *Journal of Bone and Joint Surgery*, 1994; 76A: 15–25.

Parker MJ, Myles JW, Anand JK *et al*. Cost benefit analysis of hip fracture treatment. *Journal of Bone and Joint Surgery*, 1992; 74B: 261–264.

Parker MJ, Pryor GA, Thorngren K.-G. *Handbook of Hip Fracture Surgery*. Oxford: Butterworth Heinemann, 1997.

Related topic of interest

Femoral neck fractures – extracapsular, p. 52

FOOT – CALCANEAL FRACTURES

Calcaneal (os calcis) fractures account for 1% of all fractures and 75% of tarsal fractures. They occur most frequently in males of working age and often lead to significant socio-economic problems. The calcaneus has a complex shape, articulating on four surfaces with the talus and cuboid. The calcaneus is important for weight-bearing, lever arm force transmission and foot shape, all of which may be altered by a fracture.

There are two groups of fractures:

1. *Intra-articular fractures* constitute 75% of fractures and follow RTAs and falls from a height (classically a ladder) – both result in axial load. Five to ten per cent are bilateral. Other fractures are commonly associated – 20% have an ipsilateral limb injury, such as tibial plateau or hip fracture, and 10% have a cervical or lumbar spine fracture.

2. *Extra-articular fractures* constitute 25% of calcaneal fractures and follow a twisting injury or low-energy fall, usually resulting in an avulsion type fracture.

Classification

Both intra-articular and extra-articular fractures are classified according to site and displacement.

1. *Extra-articular.* In order of frequency of occurrence, these involve the anterior process (15%), tuberosity, medial process, sustentaculum tali or body.

2. *Intra-articular.* These are initially classified as undisplaced or displaced. This is the basis of the Essex Lopresti (1951) classification using plain X-rays, which distinguishes undisplaced and displaced fractures, sub-dividing displaced fractures into 'central depression' and 'tongue' types. Classifications based on CT appearances described by Sanders, Zwipp, Eastwood and Atkins, are essential for consideration and planning of operative management. These classifications attempt to define the precise nature of the fracture with respect to the number and orientation of fracture lines, degree of displacement and comminution.

Imaging

1. *Plain lateral and axial X-rays* are the most useful views. Occasionally oblique views help identify extra-articular fractures. Bohler's angle, subtended by lines from the highest points on the posterior and anterior processes measured on the lateral X-ray, is normally 25–40°. It is reduced or reversed in intra-articular fractures.

2. *CT scanning,* with multi-planar reformatting, is undertaken to assess intra-articular fractures, if operative reduction and fixation is considered.

Management

1. *Extra-articular.* Most undisplaced fractures are managed by limitation of swelling and immobilization in a short leg cast for 4–6 weeks. Displaced tuberosity fractures, often occurring in the elderly or diabetic with porotic bone, require ORIF.

2. *Intra-articular.* Undisplaced fractures are managed by elevation, ice/cryocuff and early non-weight-bearing mobilization. Partial weight-bearing is started at 6 weeks and full weight-bearing at 12 weeks. The management of displaced intra-articular fractures is more controversial. The principles of management of other displaced intra-articular fractures apply – reduction and early movement. However, this is difficult to achieve and the benefits are questioned. Experience with ORIF has increased considerably over the past 10 years.

The options for treatment are:

- **Non-operative.** As for undisplaced fractures, and most appropriate for the elderly or poor surgical candidate.
- **Closed or percutaneous reduction with or without immobilization.** Results are little different to non-operative treatment, due to poor reduction and immobilization of the joint. Historically, reduction is with the Gissane spike (Essex– Lopresti).
- **ORIF.** This is increasingly the treatment of choice. The aim of surgery is to restore height, alignment and width of the calcaneus, reconstruct neighbouring joints and, with stable fixation, allow early mobilization. Internal fixation is undertaken once swelling has subsided, at 7 to 10 days. Most commonly, the extensile lateral approach is favoured. The sural nerve is preserved and the peroneal tendons reflected 'en masse' to expose the sub-talar joint. The tuberosity and sustentacular fragments are exposed and reduced, followed by the sub-talar joint, before reconstructing the lateral wall. Lag screws and a specially-shaped lateral wall buttress plate are used for internal fixation. Surgery is exacting. Post-operatively, management is similar to the undisplaced with early non-weight-bearing movement.

Complications – non-operative

1. *Foot shape.* A widened heel leads to heel pain, ill-fitting shoes, peroneal tendon impingement and tendinitis.

2. *Articular disruption.* This leads to degenerative change, with subsequent pain and stiffness in the sub-talar joint, especially on rough or uneven ground.

As many as 30–50% of patients walk with pain, require a stick, cannot wear a normal shoe and are unable to return to their previous employment. Twenty five per cent may require late sub-talar fusion.

Complications – operative

1. *Early problems* are wound healing, infection, sural nerve and peroneal tendon injury.

2. *Late problems* are chronic deep infection, implant prominence and failure. Similar long-term problems related to foot shape and sub-talar joint stiffness described above are also encountered. With careful selection and surgical skill, operative complications may be reduced to <5%. Foot shape is improved, but it remains to be shown if the outcome with respect to sub-talar joint function is different.

Further reading

Eastwood DM, Gregg PJ, Atkins RM. Intra-articular fractures of the calcaneum. (Parts I and II). *Journal of Bone and Joint Surgery*, 1993; 75B: 183–195.

Eastwood DM, Phipp L. Intra-articular fractures of the calcaneum: why such controversy? *Injury*, 1997; 28: 247–259.

Stockenhuber N, Wildburger R, Szyszkowitz R. Fractures of the os calcis. *Current Orthopaedics*, 1996; 10: 230–238.

Related topics of interest

Foot – talar fractures, p. 65; Tibial pilon fractures, p. 284

FOOT – METATARSAL AND PHALANGEAL FRACTURES

Metatarsal fractures

Metatarsal fractures are usually the result of a direct blow, although twisting of the forefoot can cause spiral fractures. Fractures at the base of the fifth metatarsal are discussed separately below.

The majority of shaft fractures can be treated non-operatively, with early weight-bearing in a rigid-soled shoe. Internal fixation is rarely indicated, but should be considered in:

- Fractures of the first metatarsal, which are rare. Malunion is poorly tolerated.
- Fractures of the lesser metatarsals, with dorsal or plantar angulation. Medial or lateral angulation is well tolerated. Internal fixation avoids later pressure problems.
- Head fractures.

Fixation is often with a plate in the first ray, and K-wires in the lesser rays. Occasional reduction and fixation is required in the displaced head fracture to maintain a congruent joint. Stiffness is often a long-term problem.

Fractures of the proximal fifth metatarsal

Proximal fifth metatarsal fractures are known as 'Jones' fractures, after Sir Robert Jones, who sustained a fifth metatarsal fracture while dancing. Lawrence and Botte (1993) described three zones of the proximal fifth metatarsal (*Figure 1*).

- Zone I. These are avulsion fractures of the base of the fifth metatarsal, after an inversion injury. The bony fragment is avulsed either by the peroneus brevis, or the lateral cord of the plantar aponeurosis. Treatment is with early protected mobilization (e.g. hard-soled shoe, strapping or cast). Very rarely symptomatic non-union ensues, in which case the fragment is excised and the soft tissues re-attached.
- Zone II. These injuries are similar to type 1 injuries, although healing is slower.
- Zone III. This is the area in which stress fractures occur. There is often a history of pain preceding the acute fracture. Treatment is initially non-weight-bearing in a cast for 6 weeks. If this fails, a percutaneous 4.5 mm semi-threaded cancellous screw is inserted down the medullary canal of the fifth metatarsal. Occasionally it is necessary to open and bone graft the fracture site.

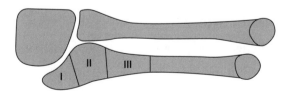

Figure 1. The three fracture zones of the proximal fifth metatarsal.

Turf toe

A hyperextension injury of the first metatarso-phalangeal joint (MTPJ), injuring the plantar capsuloligamentous complex and the cartilage of the first metatarsal head. Treatment is non-operative. Severe injuries sometimes require late repair of the ligaments and debridement of the joint.

Metatarso-phalangeal joint dislocation

Metatarso-phalangeal joint dislocation may affect the hallux, or lesser toes.

1. The hallux. Dislocation of the first MTPJ is rare and associated with high-energy trauma. Most dislocations are dorsal and *simple* (reducible). If stable, the toe is immobilized in a below-knee cast with a toe extension for 4 weeks. If unstable, a K-wire is placed across the reduced joint. *Complex* (irreducible) dislocation occurs when the metatarsal head becomes entrapped on the plantar side of the sesamoid complex. Open reduction through a dorso-lateral, or transverse plantar incision is required. An attempt should be made to repair the sesamoid complex.

2. Lesser toe dislocations. These are usually simple dorso-lateral dislocations and easily reduced by closed means. The toes are then neighbour-strapped for 2 weeks.

Interphalangeal joint dislocation

Interphalangeal joint dislocation is rare. Treatment is with reduction and splinting to the adjacent toe.

Phalangeal fractures

Fractures of the phalanges are due to either a direct blow (an object being dropped from a height onto an unprotected foot) or a stubbing injury.

Simple fractures of the phalangeal shafts can be managed conservatively with strapping. Splinting with tape and immobilization for 2 to 3 weeks is often sufficient.

Displaced intra-articular (condylar) fractures of the interphalangeal joints may require reduction and immobilization with a wire, or occasionally screws. Occasionally formal reduction and fixation is required for patients with severe rotational malalignment.

Further reading

Lawrence SJ, Botte MJ. 'Jones' fractures and related fractures of the proximal fifth metatarsal. *Foot and Ankle*, 1993; **14**: 358–365.
Rodeo SA, O'Brien S, Warren RF *et al.* Turf toe: an analysis of metatarsophalangeal joint sprains in professional football players. *American Journal of Sports Medicine*, 1990; **18**: 280–285.
Shereff MJ. Complex fractures of the metatarsals. *Orthopaedics*, 1990; **13**: 875–882.

Related topics of interest

FOOT – MID-TARSAL FRACTURES

The mid-foot is relatively rigid. The primary articulation is the mid-tarsal or 'Chopart's joint', consisting of the talo-navicular and calcaneo-cuboid joints. The joint is mobile when the calcaneum is pronated, but fixed with the heel supinated. The relative rigidity of this area means that while isolated fractures do occur, the possibility of injury associated with joint sprain, subluxation or dislocation should be considered. Diagnosis of an isolated fracture is only made after exclusion of injuries to other components of the joint complex. Main and Jowett (1975) described five different patterns of injury of the mid-foot associated with instability (see 'Foot – tarsal dislocations', p. 69).

Navicular fractures

Acute navicular fractures can be classified into three types:

- Cortical avulsions (47%).
- Fractures of the tuberosity (24%).
- Fractures of the body (29%).

1. Cortical avulsion fractures occur as a result of an eversion injury and should be treated with a below-knee walking plaster for 4 to 6 weeks. Avulsions of more than 25% of the articular surface should be reduced and fixed with a wire or screw. Persistent displacement of a fragment may give rise to persistent pain requiring fragment excision.

2. Tuberosity fractures occur after eversion of the foot and avulsion of the tibialis posterior tendon or deltoid ligament give rise to the fracture. These fractures are seen in isolation, or in conjunction with compression fractures of the cuboid. The latter is an indicator of injury to the mid-tarsal complex. Treatment of the non-displaced fracture is with a below-knee walking plaster. Occasionally, non-union occurs. In these cases, the fragment is 'shelled out' of the tibialis posterior tendon and the tendon resutured to the bone. Very rarely the acute fracture is displaced >1 cm and acute operative repair is indicated.

3. Navicular body fractures are associated with other injuries, but can occur in isolation. Vertical or longitudinal fractures usually occur in combination with the complex Main and Jowett mid-tarsal injuries. Sangeorzan (1989) described three injury patterns:

- Type 1: fracture in the coronal plane.
- Type 2: the fracture line is dorso-lateral to plantar-medial. The main fragment displaces medially and the forefoot adducts.
- Type 3: a comminuted fracture with lateral displacement of the forefoot.

Treatment is in plaster for the non-displaced fracture. If displaced, type 1 fractures can often be fixed with lag screws. Type 2 and 3 fractures are often comminuted and fixation is difficult. It is permissible to fix fragments to the cuneiforms, but effort should be made to avoid fixing the talo-navicular joint, due to its functional importance.

Cuboid fractures

Fractures of the cuboid can either be avulsion fractures, or compression fractures.

Compression fractures have been described as 'nutcracker fractures'. These are significant because the lateral column of the foot is shortened. These are therefore Main and Jowett lateral stress injuries. Injuries with minimal impaction can be treated with a below-knee walking plaster. Those with severe comminution and lateral column shortening should be opened, reduced, bone-grafted and fixed. This approach gives superior results, avoiding the later need to distract the lateral column and fuse the calcaneal cuboid joint.

Cuneiform fractures

These are rare in isolation and no large series exist. Conservative treatment is favoured.

Stress fractures

Stress fractures of the cuboid and navicular occur, and can usually be treated in a non-weight-bearing cast.

Further reading

Main BJ, Jowett RL. Injuries of the mid-tarsal joint. *Journal of Bone and Joint Surgery*, 1975; **57B**: 89–97.
Sangeorzan BJ, Benirschke SK, Mosca V *et al*. Displaced intra-articular fractures of the tarsal navicular. *Journal of Bone and Joint Surgery*, 1989; **71A**: 1504–1510.

Related topics of interest

Foot – metatarsal and phalangeal fractures, p. 61; Foot – talar fractures, p. 65; Foot – tarsal dislocations, p. 69

FOOT – TALAR FRACTURES

Fractures of the talus are uncommon, but important in view of the complex bony articulations, architecture and vascularity. The talus has a head, neck and body. The head articulates with the navicular, and the body articulates with the ankle mortise and the large posterior calcaneal facet. Over 60% of the talus is covered by articular cartilage. There are no muscle origins or insertions.

The peroneal, anterior and posterior tibial arteries all supply the talus. The lateral part of the body is supplied by the anastomosis between the artery of the tarsal canal and the artery of the tarsal sinus. The medial third of the body is supplied by the deltoid branches of the posterior tibial artery. The head and neck are supplied by branches from the dorsalis pedis and the artery of the tarsal sinus.

Fractures of the talus are subdivided into six anatomical types:

- Neck.
- Body.
- Head.
- Processes.
- Osteochondral.
- Avulsions.

Talar neck fractures

Thirty per cent of talar fractures involve the neck. The term 'aviator's astragalus' has been coined to describe this fracture, as it was most commonly seen after flying accidents, where the foot, resting on the rudder bar, was forcibly dorsiflexed. Dorsiflexion causes impingement of the anterior distal tibia upon the talar neck. Talar neck fractures are often the result of severe trauma and 65% of patients have other fractures.

1. Classification. Hawkins (1970) described three types of talar neck fractures. The very rare type IV was added later by Canale (1978) (*Figure 1*):

- Type I: a vertical, non-displaced fracture.
- Type II: a displaced fracture with subluxation or dislocation of the sub-talar joint.
- Type III: a displaced fracture with dislocation of the body of the talus from both the sub-talar and ankle joints.
- Type IV: fracture of the talar neck associated with dislocation of the talo-navicular joint.

2. Radiographic evaluation. A lateral X-ray of the whole foot and ankle, as well as AP views of the foot and ankle are required. Malleolar fractures are reported in 25% of talar neck fractures.

3. Treatment. Undisplaced fractures should be treated in a below-knee cast for 8 to 12 weeks, at least 6 weeks of which should be non-weight-bearing.

Type II fractures require urgent anatomical reduction. Closed reduction under anaesthesia, followed by casting can be used, but open reduction is often indicated.

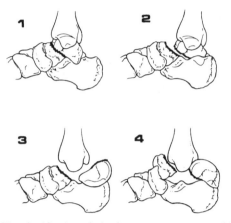

Figure 1. The Hawkins classification of talar fractures. Type IV was added later by Canale. Reproduced from Sangeorzan BJ and Hansen ST (1990) *Orthopaedic Knowledge Update III*, p. 616. With permission from American Academy of Orthopaedic Surgeons.

Three surgical approaches are described: antero-medial, antero-lateral and postero-lateral. The antero-medial and antero-lateral approaches, either individually or combined, allow visualization of the fracture and placement of screws. A postero-lateral approach can be used to internally fix the fracture if closed reduction has been successful. Two small fragment lag screws are the ideal. Post-operatively, the patient is placed in a cast, which should be maintained until fracture union.

Type III fractures are open in 50% of cases. Debridement of the wound is therefore necessary, and open reduction is usually required. A medial malleolar osteotomy, which is said to preserve the blood supply through the deltoid ligament, may be required to aid visualization and reduction.

Type IV fractures are very rare and treated by open reduction and internal fixation.

4. Complications. Good results can be achieved in approximately 70% of type I injuries, although this reduces to approximately 20% of type III injuries. Complications include:

- Skin necrosis and infection. Reduced by prompt reduction and debridement.
- Non-union and delayed union. Delayed union (>6 months) is seen in approximately 10%. Non-union is rare.
- Malunion. Reduced by appropriate initial care.
- AVN. Occurs in 0–13% of type I, 20–50% of type II and 20–100% of type III fractures. The contribution of non-weight-bearing to the avoidance of late segmental collapse is debated, but a good compromise is to keep the patient in a patellar-tendon bearing cast until revascularization has occurred.
- Post-traumatic arthritis: occurs in the ankle (30%) and sub-talar (50%) joints.

Talar body fractures

These are fractures through the body, and differ from neck fractures because the articular cartilage of the talar dome is involved. The fracture often follows direct compression, resulting from a fall from a height. The plane of fracture can be coronal, horizontal or sagittal.

Features. There are many features in common with neck fractures, including the principles of management – casting of the non-displaced fracture and fixation of the displaced. Approaches through an antero-medial, antero-lateral and medial malleolar osteotomy have all been recommended. There is a high incidence of osteo-necrosis, degenerative change, malunion and non-union following this fracture.

Talar head fractures

These are the result of a compression injury and there may be an associated navicular fracture. Displaced fractures should be reduced, although comminution is occasionally so severe that this is impossible. There is a high incidence of late talo-navicular osteoarthritis.

Talar processes

Fractures of the talar process may involve the lateral or posterior process.

1. Lateral process. This is the second most common fracture of the body of the talus, most often seen in snow-boarders. Most fractures are seen on routine ankle X-rays – the diagnosis should be suspected from clinical examination.

Treatment is in a cast for 6 weeks if the fracture is non-displaced. If displaced, reduction and internal fixation (preferable) or excision (for the comminuted, unfixable fragments) is undertaken.

2. Posterior process. There are two posterior tubercles of the talus, separated by a groove for the tendon of flexor hallucis longus. Injury of the lateral is more common and presents as an ankle sprain. If diagnosed acutely, treatment is in a cast for 4 to 6 weeks. Later treatment is by excision in the symptomatic case. It may be difficult to differentiate a non-united fracture from an os trigonum, but fortunately treatment of both conditions is the same – excision.

Osteochondral fractures

Osteochondral fractures occur in 6.5% of ankle sprains. Classically it was said that lateral lesions were traumatic and medial lesions were 'osteochondritic'. Today most accept that the majority are traumatic. Classification is by Berndt and Harty (1959):

- Stage I: compressed bone.
- Stage II: partially detached fragment.
- Stage III: detached, non-displaced fragment.
- Stage IV: displaced.

For the acutely diagnosed case, stage I and II are treated in a cast for 6 weeks. Stages III and IV are treated by excision or reattachment. Arthroscopic treatment is the preferred method.

Avulsion injuries

Avulsions are relatively common and result from significant ligamentous injuries. Radiographs often reveal a small flake of bone avulsed from the dorsum of the talar neck. The injury is of limited importance and treatment is directed at the soft tissues, with physiotherapy and non-steroidal anti-inflammatory drugs (NSAID).

Further reading

Berndt AL, Harty M. Transchondral fractures of the talus. *Journal of Bone and Joint Surgery*, 1959; **41A**: 988–1020.

Canale ST. Fractures of the neck of the talus. *Orthopaedics*, 1990; **13**:1105–1115.

Canale ST, Kelly FB. Fractures of the neck of the talus: long-term evaluation of 71 cases. *Journal of Bone and Joint Surgery*, 1978; **60A**: 143–156.

De Smet AA, Fisher DR, Burnstein MI *et al.* Value of MR imaging in staging osteochondral lesions of the talus (osteochondritis dissecans): results in 14 patients. *American Journal of Roentgenology*, 1990; **154**: 555–558.

Hawkins LG. Fractures of the neck of the talus. *Journal of Bone and Joint Surgery*, 1970; **52A**: 991–1002.

Related topics of interest

Foot – calcaneal fractures, p. 58; Foot – mid-tarsal fractures, p. 63; Foot – tarsal dislocations, p. 69

FOOT – TARSAL DISLOCATIONS

There are four principal patterns of tarsal dislocation:

- Sub-talar dislocation.
- Total talar dislocation.
- Mid-tarsal injuries.
- Lisfranc injury of the tarso-metatarsal joints.

Sub-talar dislocation

Simultaneous dislocation of the talo-calcaneal and talo-navicular joints has been termed a 'sub-talar' or 'peri-talar' dislocation. The ankle and calcaneo-cuboid joints remain enlocated. The injury is classified according to the direction of displacement of the foot. Medial dislocation, with the talar head prominent dorso-laterally, accounts for 75–85% of cases. Lateral dislocation, with the talar head prominent medially, accounts for almost all the remaining cases, with occasional reports of anterior and posterior dislocation.

1. Mechanism of injury. Inversion of the foot results in medial sub-talar dislocation. Eversion produces a lateral dislocation. In both injuries, the weaker talo-navicular and talo-calcaneal ligaments are disrupted, leaving the stronger calcaneo-navicular ligament intact. Sub-talar dislocations often follow high-energy injuries and are associated with other fractures in 50% of cases. Forty five per cent are open injuries.

2. Radiographic evaluation. The most useful view is an AP of the foot, looking for dislocation of the talo-navicular joint. CT is not helpful acutely, but may define associated fractures.

3. Treatment. Closed reduction under general anaesthesia should be prompt to avoid skin necrosis. Closed reduction fails in 10–20% of cases, as a result of soft tissue or bone interposition. After reduction, the leg is maintained in a below-knee cast for 4 weeks, after which mobilization is commenced to prevent stiffness.

4. Prognosis and complications. Long-term results are variable. Some series report 54% poor results, while others report 88% of patients with no activity restriction at 5 years. The principal complaint is of sub-talar stiffness. When associated with an open wound, there is a high incidence of infection. Osteonecrosis is relatively rare, as are recurrent dislocation and subluxation.

Total talar dislocation

This is a very rare, but devastating injury. Most are open injuries. There is a high incidence of persistent infection (90%), often requiring talectomy and subsequent fusion. Osteonecrosis and arthritis are common sequelae.

Mid-tarsal injury

The mid-tarsal region is a relatively stable area; injuries are rare, but range in severity from a sprain, through subluxation, to the occasional dislocation. The acute diagnosis is difficult, but the consequence of missing the diagnosis is severe for the patient. Diagnosis is based upon careful initial clinical assessment and evaluation of the radiographs.

1. **Classification.** Main and Jowett (1975) identified five patterns of injury, based on the mechanism of injury:

- Medial stress. Inversion of the foot, injuring the mid-tarsal joint. The injury is usually a sprain, but dislocations have been reported.
- Longitudinal stress. A longitudinal force applied through the metatarsal 'splits' the rays and often leads to a longitudinal fracture of the navicular or cuboid.
- Lateral stress. The lateral column of the foot collapses, with the anterior process of the calcaneus, or the cuboid being compressed – the 'nutcracker' fracture.
- Plantar stress. A plantar force is the most common cause of pure dislocation in the mid-foot. The navicular and cuboid are displaced plantarwards.
- Crush injury. High-energy wounds, which are difficult to classify.

2. **Treatment.** The non-displaced injury is treated in a cast for 6 weeks and early diagnosis is important. The displaced injury usually requires reduction and percutaneous wires to hold the reduction.

Tarso-metatarsal joint disruption (Lisfranc's dislocation)

Tarso-metatarsal joint injuries are rare. Intrinsic stability is by bony architecture with the base of the second metatarsal recessed in between the medial and lateral cuneiform bones. There are strong ligamentous connections between the bases of the lateral four metatarsals. Lisfranc's ligament runs between the medial cuneiform and the base of the second metatarsal. There is no ligament attachment between the first and second metatarsals, representing a relatively weak portion in the tarso-metatarsal joint.

1. **Mechanism of injury.** The classic mechanism of injury was twisting, e.g. a mounted rider falling from his horse, trapping and twisting his forefoot, which remains in the stirrup. Today the injury is most commonly sustained through axial loading of the equinus foot (for example tripping on a curb).

2. **Diagnosis.** As with mid-tarsal injuries, a high index of suspicion is required to make the diagnosis. The patient is tender over the mid-foot, with a history of an injury. Twenty per cent are missed at presentation. The problem is not with the frankly dislocated case, but more with the minimally displaced case. The signs of a Lisfranc injury on plain film are (*Figure 1*):

- Fracture of the mid-tarsal bones and the base of the second metatarsal.
- The medial cortex of the intermediate cuneiform and of the second metatarsal should align perfectly, as should the medial cortex of the cuboid and the medial side of the fourth metatarsal.
- A weight-bearing lateral radiograph may show flattening of the arch and subluxation of the joints.

3. **Classification.** Several exist and the simplest is that of Quénu and Küss (1909):

- Homolateral: all five metatarsals displaced in the same direction.
- Isolated: one or two metatarsals dislocate, while the others remain in joint.
- Divergence: displacement of all of the metatarsals in different directions (e.g. the first ray medially and lesser rays laterally).

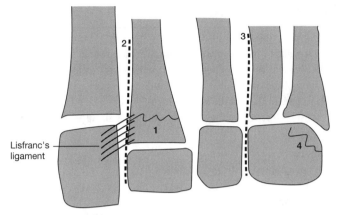

Figure 1. Some of the radiological features in the tarso-metatarsal joint which help to make the diagnosis of a Lisfranc injury. 1. 'Fleck fractures' around the base of the second metatarsal. 2. The second metatarsal medial border should align perfectly with the medial border of the intermediate cuneiform. 3. The fourth metatarsal medial border should align with the medial border of the cuboid. 4. Compression fractures of the cuboid. Oblique views may demonstrate these features more clearly.

4.   *Treatment.* This should be aggressive. The sprain is treated in a non-weight-bearing cast for 6 weeks. Subluxation or dislocation of the joint complex requires anatomical reduction and fixation. Fixation can be with percutaneous wires or more commonly open reduction and internal fixation with small fragment screws. The key to adequate reduction is reduction of the base of the second metatarsal.

5.   *Prognosis.* Anatomical reduction gives rise to good results in 85% of patients. Late arthritis is treated with arthrodesis.

Further reading

DeLee JC, Curtis R. Subtalar dislocation of the foot. *Journal of Bone and Joint Surgery*, 1982; **6A**: 433–437.
Main BJ, Jowett RL. Injuries of the mid-tarsal joint. *Journal of Bone and Joint Surgery*, 1975; **57B**: 89–97.
Merchan ECR. Subtalar dislocations: long-term follow-up of 39 cases. *Injury*, 1992; **23**: 97–100.
Myerson MS. The diagnosis and treatment of injuries to the Lisfranc joint complex. *Orthopedic Clinics of North America*, 1989; **20**: 655–664.
Quénu E, Küss G. Étude sur les luxations du métatarse (luxations métatarso-tarsiens) du diastasis entre le 1. et 2. métatarsien. *Revue de Chirurgie*, 1909; **39**: 281–336.

Related topics of interest

GUNSHOT INJURIES

The prevalence of ballistic injuries in civilian practice has gradually increased, but the majority of surgeons will only have limited experience of treating such trauma. The key to management depends on the state of the soft tissue envelope and the fracture pattern, which are determined by transfer of energy from the missile at the time of injury. The principles of management are broadly similar to open fracture management. A bullet or shrapnel wound may cause:

- A soft tissue wound.
- A vascular injury.
- A transient or permanent neurological deficit.
- A fracture.
- Bacterial contamination.

Ballistics

When a bullet penetrates biological tissue, energy is transferred from the missile to the tissues, which generates a destructive force. The available energy depends upon the mass and velocity ($E = \frac{1}{2}MV^2$). The amount and rate of energy transfer, which cause the soft tissue damage, depends on other factors which include both the type of weapon, the distance from the victim and type of missile. Generally, high velocity weapons (>2000 ft/sec) do more extensive damage. Different types of weapons have a varying muzzle velocity (velocity as the missile leaves the barrel):

- Low velocity (<1000 ft/sec): hand guns.
- Medium velocity (1–2000 ft/sec): magnum handguns and shotguns.
- High velocity (>2000 ft/sec): hunting rifles and military weapons.

Bullets may be of differing mass, shape and composition. Hollow, unjacketed and partially jacketed (dum-dum) bullets cause greater tissue damage.

1. Soft tissue wounds. As a missile passes through tissue, the missile tumbles or spins within its path. This effect and the energy transfer causes temporary cavitation, stretching the surrounding tissues, leading to necrosis and haemorrhage. This effect may draw foreign material (clothing, dirt, etc) into the wound, causing deep contamination. A missile may travel some way into tissue before giving up a maximal amount of energy, so the extent of cavitation varies in the wound track. Missile exit wounds are typically bigger than entry wounds. Military weapons and shotguns fired at close range are generally responsible for the most severe soft tissue injuries.

2. Vascular injuries. Missiles may cause damage to vessels either by effects of cavitation, or direct penetration.

3. Nerve damage. A local blast effect may cause a transient neurapraxia or axonotmesis, as well as a traumatic laceration.

4. Fractures. Missiles cause a fracture with a variable degree of comminution, depending on the rate of energy transfer. The periosteal envelope may be largely intact, or grossly disrupted, again depending on energy transfer.

5. *Bacterial contamination.* Bullets cause contamination, drawing foreign material and fabric into the wound during cavitation, and may carry bacteria.

Wound management

After resuscitation, the limb should be carefully examined, in particular for associated neurovascular compromise. Forensic evidence should be carefully preserved during initial assessment.

1. *Initial treatment.* The wound should be photographed and dressed, preferably after taking a culture swab.

2. *Antibiotic prophylaxis.* Benzylpenicillin (to cover clostridia and β-haemolytic streptococci) and flucloxacillin (to cover staphylococci), or alternatively a cephalosporin, may be used.

3. *Early surgery.* This is required to debride the wound and assess the extent of soft tissue damage. The wound margins should be excised, damaged subcutaneous tissue removed and the muscle inspected. Muscle should be assessed for viability and excised if appropriate. Deep fascia should be incised to accommodate subsequent oedema and soft tissue swelling, to prevent the onset of compartment syndrome. The wound should be irrigated with a generous volume of saline, ideally pulsed lavage. In the presence of a fracture, a minimum of 9 l should be used. The wound is packed with gauze and dressed.

4. *Reinspection.* The wound should be re-inspected 48 hours later under general anaesthesia to confirm tissue viability. At this stage, unless further debridement is required, delayed primary closure can be undertaken. If there is any doubt about tissue viability or swelling, closure should be deferred for two more days. Reconstruction with a skin graft or flap may be required if there is extensive soft tissue loss.

5. *Intra-articular injuries.* These are managed in the same manner, with debridement and irrigation. The synovium and capsule can be closed with drainage, but the overlying skin should initially be left open.

6. *Embolization.* Bullets lodged in the great vessels may embolize, proximally or distally.

Fracture management

The same principles used for the care of open fractures apply. Depending on the site of the fracture and extent of contamination, internal fixation may be appropriate. If in doubt, or the soft tissues are poor, an external fixator should be applied. External fixation is a quick means of fracture stabilization and can always be adjusted at a later date, or exchanged for an IM nail within 3 weeks, if the soft tissues are healthy.

Non-operative management

Less severe gunshot wounds can be managed without major surgery and there are good reports from North America with this approach. All wounds should be cleaned and irrigated. Antibiotic prophylaxis is wise and early, close out-patient follow-up is mandatory. Small pellets are often buried in the tissues and in the absence of significant soft tissue disruption can be left undisturbed, as extensive surgical exploration may be more hazardous.

Further reading

Bowyer GW, Rossiter ND. Management of gunshot wounds of the limbs. *Journal of Bone and Joint Surgery*, 1997; **79B**: 1031–1036.

Related topics of interest

Open fracture management, p. 156; Principles of soft tissue management, p. 223

HAND – CARPAL DISLOCATION

There are three patterns of carpal dislocation – radiocarpal, transverse and axial. Transverse dislocations, which include lunate and perilunate dislocations, are of particular interest, representing one end of the spectrum of carpal instability, predisposing to volar and dorsal intercalated segmental instability (VISI and DISI). Pure radiocarpal (wrist) dislocation is rare, as there is usually an associated dorsal or volar (Barton's) fracture.

Anatomy

Understanding the ligamentous anatomy of the wrist is fundamental to appreciating these complex injuries. The ligaments are divided into intrinsic (within the carpus) and extrinsic (radius to carpal) groups.

1. Intrinsic ligaments. These are short, strong ligaments binding each carpal bone to its neighbour, on both the volar and dorsal aspects of the carpus. The most important are the scapholunate and the triquetrolunate, connecting the bones of the proximal carpal row (scaphoid–lunate–triquetrum). Sectioning the scapholunate ligament allows the lunate to extend with the triquetrum (DISI), whereas sectioning the triquetrolunate allows the lunate to flex with the scaphoid (VISI). The ligaments of the distal row (trapezium–trapezoid–capitate–hamate) seldom fail clinically.

2. Extrinsic ligaments. These are dorsal and volar capsular condensations, acting as accessory stabilizers of the intrinsic ligaments, but are also injured in perilunate dislocation. Less emphasis is placed on their repair.

Radiocarpal dislocation

The commonest purely ligamentous radiocarpal injury is ulnar translation. Purely ligamentous dorsal or volar dislocation is rare. Treatment is open repair of the damaged extrinsic dorsal and volar radiocarpal ligaments, supplemented with K-wire stabilization. Radiocarpal fracture dislocation (Barton's fracture) is usually treated operatively.

Transverse dislocation

The lunate is the 'key' to wrist stability. Perilunate dislocations and fracture dislocations are the extremes of carpal instability. Perilunate dislocation can be caused by rupture of the ligaments attaching the lunate to its neighbouring carpals – a 'lesser arc' injury. Dislocation associated with a fracture of the radial styloid, scaphoid, capitate, or triquetrum is classified as a greater 'arc' injury. Ninety five per cent of greater arc injuries involve the scaphoid. Trans–scaphoid–perilunate dislocation is the commonest pattern.

Clinical presentation

The most common mechanism of injury is a fall on the out-stretched hand, which extends with ulnar deviation and supination. The scapholunate, capitolunate and triquetrolunate joints fail in sequence, leaving the lunate free to dislocate. Dorsal perilunate dislocations often reduce spontaneously.

Up to 25% of these injuries are misdiagnosed acutely, although the diagnosis should be suspected clinically from the degree of swelling. Eight per cent are open; neurovascular and tendinous injury occurs and the median nerve is most commonly affected.

Imaging

1. **The two most important X-rays are the PA and lateral,** with the wrist in neutral. There are two patterns of lunate dislocation. Most commonly the lunate remains aligned with the radius – *perilunate dislocation.* Alternatively, the lunate displaces in a volar or dorsal direction, the carpus aligning with the radius – *lunate dislocation.* The principles of treatment of both injuries are the same and recognition of associated fractures is essential.

2. **An acute dislocation that reduces spontaneously,** or an isolated ligament rupture, is difficult to diagnose. Malalignment between the proximal and distal carpal rows on the PA X-ray raises suspicion, but the lateral X-ray is more useful. The alignment of the radius, lunate, capitate and metacarpals should be confirmed. Arthrography, CT, MRI and wrist arthroscopy are valuable diagnostic tools.

3. **DISI is associated with widening of the scapholunate interval** by >2–3 mm ('Terry Thomas' sign), and a 'cortical ring' sign caused by excessive scaphoid flexion on PA X-ray. On the lateral, the lunate lies volar to the capitate, is extended (>10°) and the scapholunate angle is increased. In VISI the lunate lies dorsal, flexed (>15°) and the scapholunate angle is <30°.

4. **In summary,** a scapholunate angle <30° (VISI) or >80° (DISI) is abnormal and an angle of 60–80° is equivocal.

Treatment

The aim of treatment is to reduce frank dislocation and prevent progression to chronic instability, caused by failure of ligamentous healing. A spectrum of treatment modalities, from plaster to ORIF, is used.

The majority of perilunate dislocations are unstable, irreducible or open. In these cases the reduction can be held with K-wires, or open ligamentous repair undertaken. With dorsal dislocation a palmar approach usually suffices; in other cases combined palmar and dorsal approaches are necessary. The palmar approach allows decompression of the median nerve, repair of the palmar ligaments, and scaphoid fixation. The dorsal approach allows better visualization of the joints and repair of the dorsal ligaments.

Some consider open ligament repair is indicated in all cases, even if normal alignment is achieved after reduction in plaster, because ligamentous healing is unpredictable and the results of closed treatment are also unpredictable.

Prognosis

Closed treatment of perilunate dislocation has been associated with loss of position in 60% of cases, whereas with internal fixation reduction is maintained in 75%. Failure of ligamentous healing can manifest as chronic DISI or VISI deformities. These patients typically have wrist pain, popping, catching and weakness. Even with good early management, 50% of perilunate dislocations develop degenerative change.

Axial

Longitudinal separation of the finger rays follows high-energy trauma. The ulnar or radial rays typically separate from the long finger ray, which usually remains intact. The majority of these injuries are open, necessitating debridement and stabilization. Arterial and nervous (usually ulnar) injury is frequent. The prognosis is determined by the severity of the soft tissue injury and return to work often limited by diminished grip strength.

Further reading

Herzberg G, Comtet JJ, Linschield RL *et al.* Perilunate dislocations and fracture dislocations: a multicenter study. *Journal of Hand Surgery*, 1993; **18A**: 768–779.
Nugent IM, Ivory JP, Ross AC. Carpal instability. In: *Key Topics in Orthopaedic Surgery*. Oxford: BIOS Scientific Publishers, 1995; 78–80.
Ruby LK. Carpal instability. *Journal of Bone and Joint Surgery*, 1995; **77A**: 476–487.

Related topic of interest

HAND – CARPAL FRACTURES (EXCLUDING SCAPHOID)

Carpal fractures are usually the result of a fall on the out-stretched hand. Non-scaphoid fractures are rare, as 79% of carpal fractures involve the scaphoid. Of the remainder, 14% involve the triquetrum and 2% the trapezium. Avascular necrosis (AVN) has been reported with the scaphoid, lunate, capitate and pisiform.

Triquetrum

Triquetrum fractures may occur in association with perilunate dislocation. Other fracture patterns are caused by impingement of the ulnar styloid, or dorsal avulsion in wrist flexion. Treatment in a cast for 4–6 weeks is usually adequate.

Trapezium

There are three main fracture patterns:

- Fractures of the body.
- Marginal fractures of the trapeziometacarpal joint.
- Fractures of the trapezial ridge.

Trapezial dislocation occurs and is most commonly volar. Diagnosis may be difficult and special radiographic views helpful. Carpal tunnel radiographs are necessary to show fractures of the ridge.

Undisplaced fractures are treated in a cast for 4–6 weeks. Displaced body fractures often extend into the joint and require ORIF. Ridge fractures that remain symptomatic are excised. With dislocation, an attempt at closed reduction is made and if this fails, open reduction and K-wire fixation is required. This is covered in more detail in the topic 'Hand – thumb fractures and dislocations', p. 97

Lunate

Acute lunate fractures are a rarer cause of presentation than Kienbock's disease, but the relationship between the two is unclear. The blood supply is from both the dorsal and palmar aspects. Fractures can be of the dorsal horn, volar horn, or body. Fractures of the body are most frequently transverse.

Diagnosis and treatment. Acute diagnosis can be difficult, as the fracture may not be visible on plain X-ray. Bone scintigraphy, tomography, MRI or CT can confirm the diagnosis, if the clinical findings and plain X-rays are suggestive. Failure to diagnose the acute injury may delay presentation until Kienbock's disease becomes established.

An acute fracture should be treated in a cast and followed up with repeat radiographs, or preferably tomograms. The aim is to detect collapse of the lunate into itself, as collapse increases the incidence of non-union and AVN. When collapse occurs, treatment is ORIF of the fracture and reduction of the compressive forces across the joint. Compressive forces can be reduced by the correction of any ulnar minus deformity with ulnar lengthening, or preferably radial shortening. External fixation of the wrist in distraction has been advocated.

Trapezoid

Isolated fracture of the trapezoid is rare. The fracture is usually part of a more complex injury, such as axial dislocation or dislocation of the index finger ray. Plain radiographs may be difficult to interpret. Treatment is with a below-elbow cast for 6 weeks.

Capitate

Fractures of the capitate are rare, but there are two principal points of interest. Firstly, the proximal portion of the capitate is intra-articular and therefore at risk of AVN or non-union. This is treated by bone grafting, arthrodesis or excision. Secondly, capitate fractures are most commonly associated with a perilunate injury and manifest as a combined capitate and scaphoid waist fracture. The proximal capitate fragment rotates through 90° to 180°. This 'scaphocapitate' syndrome is treated with ORIF.

Hamate

Hamate fractures are either of the articular surface, body or hook. The hamate rarely dislocates. Fractures and dislocations are usually the result of high-energy trauma (crush or blast) and associated with axial dislocation of the fifth ray.

Fractures of the hook occur at the base, often as a result of racquet sports or golf. Presentation is with local tenderness and the injury is best visualized on a carpal tunnel radiograph. When diagnosed acutely, treatment in a cast for 6 weeks is appropriate. Left untreated, non-union is common, which may cause chronic pain, ulnar nerve symptoms, or flexor tendon attrition. Treatment is by excision, or ORIF and bone grafting.

Pisiform

The pisiform can be fractured, subluxed or dislocated. Radiological imaging requires a carpal tunnel view, or lateral view of the wrist with the forearm in 30° supination. Symptomatic non-union or post-traumatic arthritis is treated by pisiform excision and reconstruction of the flexor carpi ulnaris.

Related topics of interest

Hand – carpal dislocation, p. 75; Hand – thumb fractures and dislocations, p. 97

HAND – FINGER DISLOCATIONS AND LIGAMENT INJURIES

The joints of the fingers are primarily stabilized by soft tissues, rather than bone. The volar plate and two collateral ligaments form a ligamentous box around the joint. Disruption of two of the three structures is necessary for dislocation.

The proximal interphalangeal joint (PIPJ) is the most commonly injured and functionally the most important joint in the hand. The distal interphalangeal joint (DIPJ) is protected by a shorter lever arm, and the metacarpo-phalangeal joint (MCPJ) by the adjacent tendons and the deep transverse metacarpal ligament connecting the volar plates.

PIPJ injury

Dorsal, volar, rotatory and lateral dislocations of the PIPJ occur.

1. Dorsal dislocation is caused by hyperextension, typically in a sporting accident. The major structure injured is the volar plate, which may be avulsed with a fragment of bone visible on a lateral X-ray. Treatment is mobilization with neighbour strapping for 3 to 6 weeks. Neighbour strapping prevents hyper-extension. Left untreated, the PIPJ can hyperextend and a swan-neck deformity develops. Rarely the volar plate or flexor tendons become interposed in the joint and surgical removal is required.

In cases where >30% of the volar lip of the middle phalanx is avulsed, the joint is potentially unstable. A large single fragment can be surgically reattached. More commonly, the fragment is comminuted and these unstable injuries can be treated non-operatively with an extension block splint. The extension block is discarded at 4 weeks and neighbour strapping is then used to prevent hyperextension. Alternatively, the bony fragments may be excised, and the volar advanced and reattached (volar plate arthroplasty of Eaton). The Eaton procedure can be used for late presentation – after 2 weeks.

2. Volar dislocation is rare. Significantly the injury is often associated with avulsion of the central extensor tendon slip, sometimes with an attached bony flake. The integrity of the central slip must be tested. If it is not intact, the PIPJ is splinted in extension for 4 to 6 weeks, preventing the development of a boutonnière deformity.

3. Rotatory dislocation presents with one condyle of the proximal phalanx buttonholed through a tear in the extensor hood, trapped between the central slip and the lateral band. Open reduction is frequently required.

4. Lateral dislocation is primarily a collateral ligament injury and complete rupture is diagnosed clinically by opening of the joint >20° on stress testing. Treatment is with neighbour strapping for 3 to 6 weeks. The chronic (>6 weeks) case may require surgical reconstruction if symptomatic.

DIPJ injury

DIPJ dislocation is rare and typically dorsal. Treatment consists of reduction and early mobilization. Dorsal avulsion and volar fracture/subluxation occurs with mallet finger (see the topic 'Hand – phalangeal fractures', p. 88).

Irreducible and open dislocations require operative treatment. The FDP, volar plate, bony fragments or capsule can all block reduction.

MCPJ injury

Dorsal, volar and lateral dislocations of the MCPJ occur. Dorsal is the most common.

1. ***Dislocation can be 'simple' or 'complex' (irreducible)*** and differentiating the two is important, to avoid making a simple injury complex. The simple dislocation appears more dramatic, with the finger in 60° or more of hyperextension, compared to a few degrees with the complex. In complex dislocation, the metacarpal head is buttonholed through the capsule, often with puckering of the palmar skin.

The simple dislocation is reduced by flexing the wrist and finger. Distraction of the joint should be avoided as this may allow the volar plate into the joint. Complex dislocation usually requires open reduction. A palmar approach is used with great care to avoid the neurovascular bundle. Both injuries are mobilized with neighbour strapping after reduction.

2. ***Volar dislocation*** is extremely uncommon, reduction can be blocked by the volar plate or dorsal capsule.

3. ***Lateral dislocation*** is treated by immobilization in 30° of flexion for 3 weeks. If a bony fragment is displaced by >3 mm, surgical reattachment should be considered.

The locked MCPJ

The MCPJ can become locked and should be differentiated from trigger finger, which involves the PIPJ. The cause of locking is usually a collateral ligament catching on an osteophyte or prominent metacarpal condyle. Presentation can be acute following trauma.

Treatment is either an attempt at gentle closed reduction, inflation of the MCPJ with local anaesthetic, or surgical excision of the bony block.

Complications of finger joint dislocations

The principal complications are swelling and stiffness. It takes 1 year for the swelling to resolve. Stiffness may be very prolonged.

Persistent stiffness is best avoided by early mobilization (less than 4 weeks). Should stiffness become a problem, treatment is initially with physiotherapy and dynamic splintage. If this fails, particularly in the PIPJ, surgical treatment with collateral ligament and volar plate release is performed. This increases the range of movement (up to 100%) without leading to instability.

Related topics of interest

Hand – phalangeal fractures, p. 88; Hand – thumb fractures and dislocations, p. 97

HAND – METACARPAL FRACTURES

Hand fractures are common, accounting for 30% of all fractures, and most are treated non-operatively, with the emphasis on functional recovery.

Indications for operative treatment are:

- Malrotation.
- Intra-articular fractures.
- Open fractures.
- Associated neurovascular or tendon injury.
- Bone loss.
- Polytrauma.
- Multiple fractures in a single hand.

Classification

Metacarpal fractures are classified according to:

1. **Anatomical location** – head, neck, shaft and base. The neck is the weakest and most frequently fractured site.

2. **Fracture configuration** – transverse, oblique, spiral and intra-articular.

Clinical examination and imaging

Examination includes assessment of the tendon and neurovascular structures. Rotational alignment of the digits is important. With the fingers in extension, the plane of the fingernail reflects alignment. Normally aligned fingers should point towards the scaphoid in full flexion and do not converge on a single point, the scaphoid tubercle, as sometimes depicted. However, a subtle deformity in extension becomes more obvious and disabling in flexion, and the fingers may even cross. Radiographs in two planes are mandatory – usually AP and oblique. A true lateral helps diagnose carpo-metacarpal dislocation.

Treatment

1. **Head fractures** are rare. The most common pattern is the comminuted fracture, which is the most difficult to treat. An attempt should be made to reduce and stabilize the fragments, through a dorsal approach. Tooth lacerations over the MCPJ, sustained while punching, should be formally explored. It is not uncommon for the tooth to penetrate the joint, causing an osteochondral fracture and significant risk of severe infection.

2. **Neck fractures** are usually of the fifth metacarpal and the result of a punching injury ('boxer's fracture'). The distal fragment is typically volarly angulated and up to 70° of angulation is well tolerated, allowing non-operative treatment with one week of splintage for analgesia, followed by mobilization. Residual angulation can leave a dorsal bump and prominence of the metacarpal head in the palm. Malrotation or lateral angulation requires manipulation. Pseudoclawing, with MCPJ extension and PIPJ flexion, may occur and is considered an indication for reduction by some authors.

Closed reduction is usually possible and achieved by flexing the MCPJ and PIPJ to 90° – the *Jahss 90–90 method*. Percutaneous wires are used to hold reduction, with wires passed transversely into the fourth metacarpal or along the metacarpal intramedullary canal. The finger should not be immobilized in the Jahss position, as this risks dorsal skin necrosis and interphalangeal joint stiffness. A fracture of the neck of the other metacarpals is less common and angulation is less well tolerated. Angulation of >15° in the ring or middle fingers requires reduction.

3. **Shaft fractures** are prone to three principal complications:

- Malrotation – any degree of which is unacceptable.
- Shortening – <5 mm is acceptable.
- Angulation (transverse fractures), with a dorsal bump – 30° in the small, 20° in the ring and 5° in the long and index finger is functionally acceptable. Some patients find the dorsal bump cosmetically unacceptable.

If the position of the fracture is acceptable, a light hand cast or a splint with the MCPJs flexed 70° is applied. Where the position is unacceptable, percutaneous wires can be used securing the metacarpal to its neighbour.

There is an increasing trend towards ORIF, although only 10% of metacarpal fractures are irreducible or unsuitable for percutaneous wires. Dorsal plating gives the strongest biomechanical fixation. In some cases interfragmentary compression screws alone can be used, if the fracture is not comminuted. The fragment must be at least three times the size of the screw to avoid splintering and at least two screws should be used. Excellent results have been reported using the AO mini-fragment instrumentation, allowing anatomical reduction and early mobilization.

External fixation is used in fractures with a major soft tissue injury or bone loss. External fixation of the metacarpals leads to more stiffness than when applied to the phalanges.

4. **Basal fractures** are easily overlooked on initial X-ray and often the result of crush injuries. These are treated as shaft fractures. Rotational malalignment must be corrected.

5. **Avulsion fractures** at the base of the index and long fingers by the extensor carpi radialis longus and brevis tendons have been reported. Unless there is a symptomatic bony prominence, treatment is non-operative.

Complications

Complications are usually the result of malunion. Residual angulation requires an opening (bone graft and the risk of non-union) or closing (shortening) osteotomy. Opening osteotomy is usually preferred. Rotational malalignment is best treated by avoidance through careful initial management.

Carpo-metacarpal dislocation

These injuries are caused by high-energy trauma or punching and are usually fracture dislocations, with dorsal displacement in the majority. With dislocation of the small finger carpo-metacarpal joint (CMCJ), the ulnar nerve may be damaged. At presentation, the diagnosis is suspected clinically from the deformity. Oblique radiographs may mask the injury and a true lateral of the hand should be obtained.

The majority of dislocations are treated by closed reduction with percutaneous K-wire stabilization. Maintaining reduction in cast alone is difficult. Open reduction is occasionally required.

Paediatrics

The physes of the finger metacarpals are at the distal end. Fractures of the child's metacarpals are classified into head, neck, shaft and base fractures. Treatment is along similar lines to the adult, except for growth plate injuries. Most fractures can be treated non-operatively, but head splitting Salter–Harris III and IV injuries may require ORIF.

Further reading

Ashkenaze DM, Ruby L. Metacarpal fractures and dislocations. *Orthopedic Clinics of North America*, 1992; **23**: 19–33.

Drenth DJ, Klasen HJ. External fixation for phalangeal and metacarpal fractures. *Journal of Bone and Joint Surgery*, 1998; **80B**: 227–230.

Firoozbakhsh KK, Moneim MS, Howey T *et al.* Comparative fatigue strengths and stabilities of metacarpal internal fixation techniques. *Journal of Hand Surgery*, 1993; **18A**: 1059–1068.

Related topics of interest

Hand – carpal dislocation, p. 75; Hand – thumb fractures and dislocations, p. 97

HAND – NEUROVASCULAR AND SOFT TISSUE INJURIES

Fingertip injuries

Fingertip injuries account for 45% of all hand injuries presenting to the accident department. Various treatment procedures are popular.

1. Non-operative treatment, with healing by secondary intention, gives good results in wounds of <1 cm^2 and the wound contracts up to 90%. Non-operative treatment in larger wounds can lead to hypersensate scars. Exposed bone can be trimmed; however, shortening the distal phalanx by $>50\%$ leads to a hook-shaped nail.

2. Skin grafts can be used as a composite graft to replace the fingertip, particularly in infants. Alternatively the tip can be 'defatted' and used as a full thickness graft. Grafting can lead to instability and surrounding hypersensitivity. The graft is insensate.

3. V–Y advancement can be performed with the remaining pulp, maintaining sensibility. A single palmar 'V' (Atasoy) or two laterally based 'V's can be raised. Moberg developed a flap with two deep incisions dorsal to the neurovascular bundle, advancing the whole pulp down to the level of the flexor sheath.

4. Cross finger or thenar flaps can be used to cover a defect, but are insensate. The cross finger flap has the disadvantage of jeopardizing an adjacent, normal finger and leaves an unsightly dorsal scar. Both these flaps are little used today as the finger must be immobilized with a flexed PIPJ, which can cause long-term stiffness.

Nail bed injuries

Subungual haematomas should be drained using a heated sterile paper clip or mini power drill to penetrate the nail. Some advocate nail removal and surgical nail bed repair if the haematoma involves $>50\%$ of the nail. The nail should always be replaced or the nail bed splinted.

Fifty per cent of nail bed injuries are associated with distal phalangeal fractures. The fractures do not usually require treatment, but the nail bed must be restored by suturing. The nail is temporarily sutured in place as a splint.

Bite wounds

These are serious injuries; firstly the wound is a crush injury, and secondly the oral microbial flora is virulent. Resulting infections can be destructive, with a mixed flora of aerobes and anaerobes.

The incisor bite wound over the MCPJ from punching is particularly dangerous. There is often a laceration of the extensor tendon, which moves when the hand is extended, covering the deeper wound. The MCPJ can be penetrated, sustaining a chondral injury. Only careful exploration will reveal all the components of this injury, and the missed joint penetration can lead to a septic pyarthrosis and joint destruction.

High-pressure injection injuries

The injection of material into the hand under pressure can be devastating. The entry wound may be small, but intense pain may persist for several hours or days. Organic solvents (grease, paint and paint-thinner) are the most dangerous, with amputation rates of 16–48%.

Best results are achieved by massive debridement with wide exposure. Debridement is repeated and delayed primary closure performed only when the wound is clean. Mobilization commences early. With such a regime, 64% of patients regain normal hand function, but 16% still require amputation.

The mangled hand

Management of the mangled hand is important and critical to the patient's ability to self-care and work. Upper limb prostheses do not function as effectively as lower limb prostheses and consequently salvage is attempted in the majority of cases. The management principles are:

- Primary debridement.
- Re-establishment of skeletal stability, arterial inflow and venous outflow. Nerves may be repaired at this stage.
- Skin cover using grafts, local or distant flaps.
- Early mobilization and specialist hand therapy.
- Late surgical reconstruction to improve function may be required, including nerve repair or grafting and tendon grafting or transfer.

Replantation

1. *Thumb, multiple finger, hand and wrist amputation.* Replantation should be attempted, although traumatic amputation is not an indication for surgical replantation in all cases. Children do well after replantation.

2. *Distal phalangeal amputation.* Replantation remains controversial.

3. *Polytrauma.* Replantation in such patients is inappropriate.

4. *Old age, smoking and crush injuries.* These are poor prognostic indicators.

5. *Warm ischaemia time.* This is 12 hours for fingers and 6 hours for the hand – muscle halves the viability time. The ischaemia time is doubled when the part is kept cold (not frozen).

6. *Replantation* is performed in the following order (BEFVANI):

- Bone.
- Extensor tendon.
- Flexor tendon.
- Vein.
- Artery.
- Nerve.
- Integument.

7. *Post-operative mobilization* should commence early. Bony fixation is achieved with K-wires in the digit, or screws and plates proximally. Fingers are not

always replanted to their original site. If the index finger is mangled, it may be preferable to replant an amputated, but intact, ring finger to replace the index.

Revascularization

Revascularization is performed microsurgically. In the presence of vascular or nerve loss, interposition grafts may be needed. Controversy surrounds repair of the single severed digital artery, but cold intolerance may be reduced. Digital nerves should be repaired up to the level of the DIPJ.

Thumb reconstruction

The thumb provides 40% of hand function. Maintenance of a sensate, mobile thumb of normal length and power is important. Good cosmesis and quick rehabilitation are also desirable. Thus replantation of traumatic thumb amputations at all levels should be attempted. If the amputated part is inadequate, a hallux or second toe transfer can be performed, or the index finger can be pollicized.

Surprisingly some studies show that 80% of people return to work after thumb amputation, whether the thumb is replanted, or not. The functional results are most dependent on the re-establishment of 2-point discrimination.

Further reading

Levin LS, Condit DP. Combined injuries – soft tissue management. *Clinical Orthopaedics*, 1996; **327**: 172–181.

Martin C, Gonzalez del Pino J. Controversies in the treatment of fingertip amputations. Conservative versus surgical reconstruction. *Clinical Orthopaedics*, 1998; **353**: 63–73.

Related topics of interest

Hand – finger dislocations and ligament injuries, p. 80; Hand – tendon injuries, p. 93; Principles of soft tissue management, p. 223

HAND – PHALANGEAL FRACTURES

Most phalangeal fractures can be treated non-operatively, like metacarpal fractures, with the emphasis on functional recovery.

The indications for operative treatment are:

- Malrotation.
- Intra-articular fractures.
- Subcapital and peri-articular fractures.
- Open fractures.
- Associated neurovascular or tendon injury.
- Bone loss.
- Polytrauma.
- Multiple hand fractures.

Clinical examination and imaging

Careful examination is mandatory to assess neurovascular and tendinous integrity. Assessment for malrotation and shortening of the finger is important. Malrotation in extension is greatly magnified in flexion. AP and lateral radiographs should be obtained.

Principles of treatment

1.   Displacement and stability determine management. Transverse fractures are more stable than spiral or oblique fractures. Undisplaced, stable fractures are treated non-operatively. Only 15% of displaced fractures are stable after closed reduction, so percutaneous K-wire fixation is frequently required. If open reduction is necessary, stable fixation to allow early mobilization gives the best result.

2.   Treatment of the soft tissues is important and some series identify the severity of soft tissue, rather than bony injury, as the most important factor in determining outcome. The incidence of stiffness increases if the hand is immobilized for more than 4 weeks.

Fractures of the proximal and middle phalanges

Deformity depends on the relation of the fracture to the inserting tendons. Fractures of the proximal phalanx present with flexion of the proximal fragment due to the pull of the interossei. In the middle phalanx, angulation of the fragments is determined by the position of the fracture relative to the central slip of the extensor tendon which inserts proximally and the FDS which inserts along much of the volar aspect.

1.   Shaft fractures. Undisplaced, stable shaft fractures are treated with mobilization of the fingers by 'neighbour strapping'. Closed reduction and immobilization is suitable for fractures that are displaced, but stable on reduction. The MCPJ is immobilized at 70°–90° of flexion, with the interphalangeal joints in extension – the *intrinsic plus* position. The collateral ligaments are at their maximum length and splinting in this position prevents contracture. Burkhalter recommended dynamic splintage – a dorsal extension block splint, allowing finger flexion.

If the fracture is unstable following closed reduction, percutaneous K-wires, an external fixator, or screws and plates should be used. Percutaneous K-wires leave the soft tissue envelope intact by transfixing deep structures, but may not achieve precise fracture reduction. Plates provide the strongest fixation, but are bulky and require more extensive soft tissue dissection. External fixation has a role in the comminuted fracture, or in the presence of gross soft tissue contamination.

2. Subcapital fractures of the proximal phalangeal neck. These should be reduced and fixed with K-wires. More common in children, the phalangeal head is typically 60° or more dorsally angulated. Reduction is usually easy, but lost without fixation.

3. Intra-articular fractures. Undisplaced intra-articular fractures are rare and can be treated non-operatively, but should be closely reviewed with X-rays. Condylar fractures need accurate reduction, by open or closed means, and then stabilization with wires or screws. A pure dorsal approach, splitting the extensor tendon, is favoured. Avulsion fractures around the base of the middle phalanx are associated with injury of the central slip, collateral ligaments or volar plate, and are discussed in the topic 'Hand – finger dislocations and ligament injuries', p. 80.

Comminuted intra-articular fractures are difficult to treat and not readily amenable to ORIF. Recently dynamic external fixators have been used for this injury.

Fractures of the distal phalanx

1. Tuft fractures. The role of surgery is to repair the nail bed and drain a sub-ungual haematoma.

2. Transverse fractures. If displaced, reduction and splinting, or K-wire fixation are required. The distal fragment angulates in a volar direction, from the pull of the flexor digitorum profundus (FDP). If the nail root is avulsed, the bed should be repaired, replacing the nail as a splint. If the nail bed becomes entrapped in the fracture, non-union follows.

3. Mallet finger. This is either a purely tendinous injury, or associated with a distal phalangeal fracture and DIPJ subluxation. Most authors recommend splint-age of the DIPJ in extension (Stack splint) for 6 to 10 weeks. The indications for ORIF include displacement of the bony fragment by >3 mm, avulsion of >30% of the joint surface or volar subluxation. Surgery is technically difficult and does not always improve the outcome, so most mallet fingers, whether of bony or tendinous origin, are treated by splintage. The prognosis after distal phalangeal fractures is disappointing, with 70% of patients reporting stiffness, pain and diminished sensibility at 6 months.

4. Associated tendon injuries. The FDP and extensor tendons can be avulsed from the distal phalanx, with or without a bony fragment. FDP avulsion, 'jersey finger', occurs with a variable-sized fragment of bone (see topic 'Hand – tendon injuries', p. 93).

Complications

1. ***Malrotation*** is corrected by phalangeal or metacarpal osteotomy. Metacarpal osteotomy causes less stiffness and allows correction up to 20°.

2. ***Angulation*** can be corrected by an opening wedge and bone graft, or a closing wedge. Shortening is difficult to correct. Osteotomy, arthrodesis or arthroplasty can correct intra-articular malunion.

3. ***Non-union*** is rare and usually atrophic. When non-union occurs, early treatment at about 4 months is advised, avoiding excessive splinting and consequent stiffness. Radiological union occurs later (4–5 months) than clinical union in the hand.

4. ***Stiffness*** is prevented by avoiding immobilization for >4 weeks. When stiffness occurs it can be caused by capsular or tendinous adhesions, and initially is treated with physiotherapy and splinting. Tenolysis can be undertaken when active movement is less than passive, indicating tendon rather than capsular adhesion.

5. ***Infection*** follows 2% of open fractures.

Further reading

Agee J. Treatment principles for proximal and middle phalangeal fractures. *Orthopedic Clinics of North America*, 1992; **23**: 35–40.

Buchler U, Gupta A, Ruf S. Corrective osteotomy for post-traumatic malunion of the phalanges in the hand. *Journal of Hand Surgery*, 1996; **21**: 33–42.

Hastings H, Ernst JMJ. Dynamic external fixation for fractures of the proximal interphalangeal joint. *Hand Clinics*, 1993; **9**: 659–674.

Related topics of interest

Hand – finger dislocations and ligament injuries, p. 80; Hand – tendon injuries, p. 93

HAND – SCAPHOID FRACTURES

The scaphoid is the most common carpal bone to fracture and the fracture predominantly occurs in young adult men. The mechanism of injury is usually a fall onto the radial aspect of the palm, resulting in extreme dorsiflexion in radial deviation. The presentation of wrist pain and tenderness in the anatomical snuffbox after a fall is synonymous with a scaphoid fracture until proven otherwise.

Investigation

Four standard X-rays which identify 70% of fractures are recommended: neutral PA, lateral, 45° supinated PA, and ulnar deviated PA long axis view. Another 20% may become evident on re-X-ray at 10 to 14 days with fracture osteopaenia. An isotope bone scan undertaken after 48 hours will confirm those not evident on initial X-ray.

Classification

Site and stability, or displacement, may classify acute fractures.

1. Site
- 70% middle third or waist.
- 20% proximal third.
- 10% distal pole or tubercle.

2. Stability
- Stable: undisplaced.
- Unstable: >1 mm step or offset, abnormal angulation.

Management

1. Stable fractures are traditionally placed in a short forearm cast with slight wrist flexion and radial deviation, including the thumb. The significance of positioning is not clear. Union occurs in 95% at 8–10 weeks.

2. Unstable fractures should be reduced by closed or open means and stabilized by K-wire or Herbert screw fixation – a headless compression screw of differential pitch.

Union rate

The time to union, and union rate, depends upon the site and stability of the fracture, and delay in diagnosis or immobilization (*Table 1*). Union rate in the unstable fracture is 65%.

Table 1. Time to union and percentage union at different sites

Site	Time to union (weeks)	Percentage union
Distal	6	98
Waist	9–12	90
Proximal	16–20	70

Complictions

1. *Non-union* is defined as a failure of progression of fracture healing on three separate monthly X-rays; after treatment for 6 months the overall rate is 10%. In about half of these, the fracture was undiagnosed or not treated initially. The natural history of non-union is controversial. It is not clear how many develop symptomatic degenerative osteoarthritis or carpal collapse.

If asymptomatic, the risk of degeneration should be discussed and observed. If symptomatic, consider open Russe cortico-cancellous bone graft +/– restoration of anatomy and fixation; this has a 90% success rate. An assessment of proximal pole vascularity is essential either by pre-operative MRI or intra-operatively. Thirty per cent may be avascular and grafting may not be successful.

2. *AVN*. Five to ten per cent overall. The anatomy of the scaphoid blood supply leaves the proximal pole at risk of AVN. The principal blood supply enters through the dorsal waist and there are intraosseous canals running up and down the scaphoid. A third of people lack canals to the proximal pole, thus a third of proximal pole fractures have no blood supply and risk AVN. Early identification and separation from delayed or non-union is difficult – MRI is helpful.

Procedures for AVN include bone graft and staple or screw fixation, vascularized bone graft, excision of proximal pole, radial styloidectomy for radio-carpal osteoarthritis, proximal carpal row carpectomy and arthrodesis.

Further reading

Proctor M. Non-union of the scaphoid: early and late management. *Injury*, 1994; 5: 5–20.

Related topics of interest

Hand – carpal dislocation, p. 75; Hand – carpal fractures (excluding scaphoid), p. 78

HAND – TENDON INJURIES

Flexor tendons

The majority of flexor tendon injuries follow a laceration. The anatomy is complex. A synovial sheath surrounds the tendons, containing synovial fluid for nutrition and lubrication. A fibro-osseous tunnel encloses the sheath, consisting of five thickened annular (A) bands, and three cruciform (C) pulleys. The A2 and A4 pulleys are the most important in preventing bow stringing and overlie the shaft of the proximal and middle phalanges respectively.

Flexor tendon injuries are classified according to the anatomical zones of injury; from distal to proximal these are (*Figure 1a*):

- Zone I: FDP injuries distal to the FDS insertion
- Zone II: Bunnell's 'no man's land', from the level of the distal palmar crease (A1 pulley) to zone I, containing the FDP and FDS decussation in a tight canal.
- Zone III: the palm.
- Zone IV: the carpal tunnel.
- Zone V: proximal to the deep transverse ligament.

Similar zones are described in the thumb, prefixed by 'T'.

Clinical examination

FDS flexes the PIPJ and when examining FDS function, the other fingers should be held in extension, to eliminate the action of FDP. FDP flexes the DIPJ and is examined with the remainder of the fingers held in extension. Closed avulsion of the FDP ('jersey finger') is easily overlooked.

Techniques of repair

1. Primary repair. Multiple suture techniques are described (Bunnell, modified Kessler, Tsuge, Kirihmayer, etc.) and the principle is to place a core stitch in the

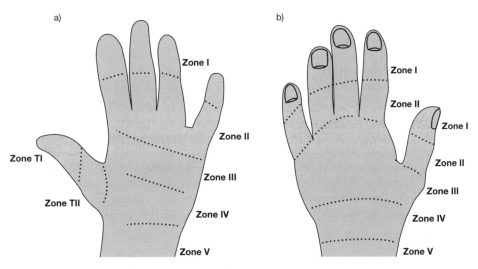

Figure 1. Flexor and extensor tendon injury zones in the hand. (a) Flexor surface. (b) Extensor surface.

palmar aspect of the tendon, preserving the dorsal blood supply. The core stitch is reinforced by a circumferential (Lembert) suture to reduce gapping. Monofilament is favoured and the repair should be secure enough for early mobilization.

2. Delayed repair. Primary or delayed primary repair gives the best results. The only exceptions are with massive hand trauma (when bony stability, vascularity and soft tissue cover take priority) or late presentation.

3. Late reconstruction. When primary repair is not possible, a free graft (palmaris longus, toe extensors) from the palm to distal phalanx is used. If there is extensive damage to the pulley system, staged repair is used. In the first stage, a silastic or silicone rod is implanted under the remnants of the pulley system and left *in situ* for 3 months while passive movement is instituted. The rod is removed and a tendon graft passed through the newly created 'flexor sheath'.

Partial laceration

Partial laceration weakens the tendon, causing rupture or triggering. Repair can cause adhesions, but is recommended for lacerations of 60% of the tendon or more.

Rupture by zone

1. Zone I. FDP avulsion is most common in the ring finger. The tendon usually retracts after rupturing in mid-substance or avulsing a fragment of bone. The bony fragment often lodges in the A4 pulley, or at Camper's chiasma, but can retract into the palm, avulsing the vinculae with the blood supply. Retraction may be visible on plain X-ray, ultrasound scan or MRI. When retracted into the palm, surgery should be performed in the first week, as the tendon contracts and after this grafting is required. In other cases, primary repair may be possible for 3 months. Repair is by suture (if the stump is >1 cm long), pullout suture into bone, or screw if the bony fragment is large enough.

2. Zone II. Repair in this zone is technically demanding. Both the FDP and FDS should be repaired if possible, and the A2 and A4 pulleys preserved.

3. Other zones. The same principles of repair apply.

Principles of mobilization

Early mobilization increases the tensile strength and vascularity of the repair, reduces adhesions and gives superior clinical results. The repair is weakest at 7 to 10 days.

Kleinert described an extension block splint with a rubber band to passively flex the fingers. Recently, attention has turned to active flexion. In the Duran programme, passive flexion is used for the first 4 weeks, protecting the repair with an extension block splint, and active flexion is introduced over the ensuing fortnight. Grip-strengthening exercises and lifting is avoided for 3 to 4 months. Early controlled active mobilization (Belfast regime) gives better results still.

Outcome

At 6 months, recovery of the range of movement is 90% of what can be expected. Tenolysis is seldom considered before 6 months.

Techniques for late reconstruction include DIPJ fusion, tendon transfer and tendon grafting. With modern rehabilitation, good and excellent results have increased from 50% to 95%.

Extensor tendons

Extensor tendon injuries have long been the Cinderella of hand injuries. There is growing realization that this confidence is ill-founded, with only 60% good or excellent results. Loss of flexion is more of a problem than loss of extension.

The extensor system is divided into zones; from distal to proximal these are (*Figure 1b*):

- Zone I: distal to the central slip of the PIPJ.
- Zone II: MCPJ to the central slip.
- Zone III: distal to the extensor retinaculum.
- Zone IV: under the extensor retinaculum.
- Zone V: in the forearm.

Clinical examination

Clinically a mallet deformity is obvious. A closed boutonnière is more difficult to diagnose, especially in the absence of bony avulsion from the middle phalanx. The diagnosis is confirmed by dorsal tenderness and swelling. Boye's test examines the integrity of the central slip – passive flexion of the MCPJ extends the PIPJ, unless the central slip has ruptured.

Repair by zone

1. Zone I. Mallet finger. Closed treatment in a splint. See 'Hand – phalangeal fractures', p. 88.

2. Zone II. Rupture of the central slip leads to development of a boutonnière deformity, with subluxation of the lateral bands. Closed treatment with a spring-loaded dorsal (Capner) splint holds the PIPJ in extension and is worn for 6 weeks, during which the DIPJ is actively and passively flexed. Indications for operative treatment are a large bony avulsion, which should be reduced, or an open injury, often communicating with the joint.

3. Zone III to V. Injuries are repaired with standard suture techniques and simple post-operative splinting. Particular care should be taken with human bite wounds over the MCPJ, which often penetrate the joint. The wound should be extended; the joint exposed, debrided and irrigated. Closure and tendon repair is delayed.

4. Following surgery. The traditional position for immobilization of extensor tendon injuries is with the wrist in 40° of extension and the MCPJs in slight flexion. However, finger flexion is frequently compromised by such a regime and dynamic splinting is favoured for injuries in zones III, IV and V. The splint consists of a volar block to flexion and an outrigger allowing passive finger extension.

Further reading

Baktir A, Turk CY, Kabak S *et al*. Flexor tendon repair in zone II followed by early active mobilisation. *Journal of Hand Surgery*, 1996; **21B**: 624–628.

Ip WY, Chow SP. Results of dynamic splintage following extensor tendon repair. *Journal of Hand Surgery*, 1997; **22B**: 283–287.

Related topics of interest

Hand – neurovascular and soft tissue injuries, p. 85; Hand – phalangeal injuries, p. 88

HAND – THUMB FRACTURES AND DISLOCATIONS

This topic deals with bony and ligamentous injuries of the thumb. The thumb is mobile in three planes and consequently sustains some injuries, which differ from those in the fingers.

Phalangeal fractures

Phalangeal fractures in the thumb are similar to, and treated with the same principles as, phalangeal fractures in the fingers. Avulsion of a fragment of bone from the base of the proximal phalanx occasionally occurs with a gamekeeper's thumb and should be reattached if displaced (see below).

Metacarpo-phalangeal joint dislocation

MCPJ dislocation is usually dorsal and can be simple or complex (irreducible). Simple dislocation is treated with closed reduction and early mobilization. After reduction, a removable spica is applied. It is important to assess integrity of the collateral ligaments after reduction.

Complex dislocations require open reduction. The features of complex dislocation are identical to those seen in the finger – skin dimpling, deformity and sesamoid entrapment. The volar plate and FPL may be entrapped in the joint.

Gamekeeper's (skier's) thumb

Injury of the ulnar collateral ligament (UCL) of the MCPJ, from a sudden abduction injury, was initially described in gamekeepers, but is now more common in skiers. When completely ruptured or detached, the UCL often rolls back on itself and becomes entrapped in the rolled-back position, superficial to the adductor and extensor aponeurosis – the 'Stener' lesion. The Stener lesion occurs in approximately 50% of cases and when present leads to a failure to heal by conservative means.

1. Clinical examination should stress the ligament in both 30° flexion and full extension. Instability of >30° is indicative of complete UCL rupture. Examination under local anaesthetic, stress radiographs, ultrasound, MRI, arthrography and arthroscopy have all been tried to better differentiate the complete and partial tear. Unfortunately none are 100% sensitive and specific. Most practitioners favour clinical examination and possibly stress radiographs.

2. Partial tears are treated non-operatively in a thumb spica for 3 weeks.

3. Complete tears are treated operatively. Occasionally there is a piece of bone large enough to be reattached, but the usual pattern is a direct avulsion from bone. Mid-substance tears are repaired directly. The volar plate and dorsal capsule should be inspected and approximated if torn, avoiding undue tension.

4. Chronic tears are commonly seen and can be reconstructed by repairing the ligament remnants, using a free tendon graft, or a local tendon. The technique of Neviaser is popular, using a capsular flap reinforced by adductor pollicis.

Radial collateral injury

Radial collateral injuries are rare compared to UCL injuries and are usually treated non-operatively. Complete ruptures are sometimes treated operatively, particularly in the presence of volar subluxation on the lateral X-ray.

Metacarpal fractures

There are three regions of the thumb metacarpal – the head, shaft and base. Green and O'Brien classified four types of base fractures:

- Type 1: an avulsion of the volar lip and subluxation of the carpo-metacarpal joint, equivalent to the Bennett's fracture.
- Type 2: a comminuted fracture of the base of the metacarpal, involving the joint surface (Rolando fracture).
- Type 3: extra-articular fractures of the metacarpal base.
- Type 4: epiphyseal injuries.

1. *Head fractures* are rare. If the fragments are large enough, anatomical reduction and internal fixation are required.

2. *Shaft fractures* (types 3 and 4) are most common at the metacarpal base. Determining whether a fracture is extra- or intra-articular can be difficult. As the thumb is so mobile, deformity is functionally well tolerated, although the cosmetic result may be less favourable. Angulation of <30° is treated in a moulded thumb spica. Angulation of >30° can lead to hyperextension of the MCPJ and closed reduction with K-wiring is recommended.

3. *Intra-articular fractures* (types 1 and 2) generally require surgical treatment. A Bennett's fracture is a fracture/subluxation. The volar lip fragment remains attached to the trapezium by the anterior oblique ligament and the metacarpal base is subluxed radially, proximally and dorsally by the abductor pollicis longus. The head of the metacarpal is adducted by adductor pollicis, which further levers the base away from the volar fragment. The aim of treatment is to reduce the joint, but the value of this is debatable. Although the development of radiological arthritis has been shown to correlate with the quality of the reduction, studies demonstrate 92% of patients are asymptomatic at 10 years.

Many treatment methods have been proposed, varying from the application of a well-moulded cast, to open reduction and internal fixation. The usual technique is percutaneous K-wiring. With the thumb **ad**ducted and pressure applied to the metacarpal, reduction is held by two wires passed into the trapezium, trapezoid or second metacarpal. ORIF is rarely required.

A Rolando fracture is more difficult to treat and is fortunately rare. Ideally, treatment is by ORIF. This may be so technically difficult that it is preferable to use limited internal fixation and an external fixator across the joint, or to use the 'bag of bones' technique, with early mobilization.

Carpo-metacarpal dislocation

This is a rare injury and reflects pure avulsion of the anterior oblique ligament. If dislocated, the joint should be reduced and held in a spica. Supplementary K-wires may be required to hold the reduction. Subluxation is often overlooked and the most helpful X-ray is a stress radiograph taken with both thumbs pushing against one another. If the thumb subluxes, immobilization in a spica for 4 weeks is appropriate.

Further reading

Cannon SR, Dowd GSE, Williams DH *et al.* A long-term study following Bennett's fracture. *Journal of Hand Surgery*, 1986; **15B**: 58–61.

Stener B. Displacement of the ruptured ulnar collateral ligament of the metacarpophalangeal joint of the thumb. A clinical and anatomical study. *Journal of Bone and Joint Surgery*, 1962; **44B**: 869–872.

Related topics of interest

Hand – metacarpal fractures, p. 82; Hand – phalangeal fractures, p. 88

HEAD INJURIES

Head injuries generally follow high velocity trauma. An altered level of consciousness is the hallmark, usually evident immediately, which may progress within hours. Occasionally, late complications become evident after a few weeks. Sixty per cent of all road trauma deaths are due to head injury. Immediate action, to prevent anoxia, maintain cerebral perfusion, reduce cerebral compression and prevent infection, are the aims of treatment. Rehabilitation following a major head injury requires prolonged, expensive, intensive, multidisciplinary therapy.

Nature of injury – anatomy, physiology and pathology

1. Skin. A head injury may include a scalp laceration and haemorrhage can be significant, especially in children.

2. Bone. There may be an associated skull fracture, linear or depressed, closed or open. Depressed skull fractures can be associated with epilepsy, more commonly in children, and even without neurological compromise, may need elevation if the depression is greater than the thickness of the skull. Basal skull fractures may not be seen on X-ray and are characterized by CSF leakage from the ear (otorrhoea) or nose (rhinorrhoea), periorbital bruising and intracranial gas. The use of prophylactic antibiotics (penicillin and sulphadimidine) is controversial.

3. Meninges. The dura, arachnoid and pia mater form the meninges.

- Extradural haematomas follow haemorrhage of meningeal vessels, between the skull and dura mater, into the potential extradural space. These occur more frequently in younger patients, after lower velocity trauma. Deterioration can be rapid, and if treated early, is reversible. A declining level of consciousness in a previously alert patient is a neurosurgical emergency.
- Acute subdural haematomas follow violent deceleration and are often associated with intracerebral damage.
- Chronic subdural collections are usually of insidious origin, with minor trauma in the elderly, and may cause late effects at 2 to 6 weeks.

4. Brain. Brain tissue may be damaged by direct trauma, intracerebral haemorrhage, or by the effects of intracranial collections, causing initially local and subsequently generalized compression. A diffuse or focal brain injury follows.

Diffuse brain injuries are either:

- Concussion with a good prognosis.
- Diffuse axonal injury, characterized by prolonged coma and a variable, often poor, outcome.

Focal injuries with localized damage can cause a generalized effect. These include:

- Contusion – single or multiple. Contusion may be at the site of impact (coup injury) or opposite the site (contracoup injury), or a combination.
- Intracranial haemorrhage.
- Acute extradural (1% of all head injuries).

- Subdural – usually acute, occasionally chronic.
- Subarachnoid.
- Intracerebral haemorrhage.
- Impalement and bullet wounds: rare in the UK and often fatal.

5. _Level of consciousness._ This may be altered either by direct injury to the cerebral cortex, or secondary to the effects of rising intracranial pressure, and the resulting diminished cerebral blood flow and tissue oxygenation. The intracranial pressure (ICP) is proportional to the sum of the volume of CSF, blood and brain (Monroe–Kellie hypothesis). Intracranial haemorrhage can be accommodated by reducing the volume of CSF and venous blood, for a collection of up to 50 ml. Larger collections raise the ICP and diminish cerebral perfusion pressure (CPP) (CPP = BP – ICP). An ischaemic brain injury is likely if the ICP falls below 60 mmHg. The arterial blood volume is regulated by arterial pCO_2 and can be decreased by hyperventilation. This is critical to head injury management.

Assessment of injury

Ongoing assessment is vital to determine any deterioration. The Glasgow Coma Scale (GCS) (*Table 1*), based on the best visual, verbal and motor responses, scored out of 15, is a quantitative measure of consciousness. (A score of 3 corresponds to no response and brainstem death.) Full neurological assessment includes briskness and equality of the pupillary response to light, and peripheral neurological status.

The GCS score can be used to categorize patients and is a guideline for management. Patients with a score of 14 have a minor head injury and can often be discharged from an accident department, if they have suitable supervision at home and no skull fracture. Patients with a score of ≤8 have a major head injury, are in coma and require neurosurgical consultation, investigation including CT scan, and treatment. Patients between these two levels, a score of 9 to 13, have a moderate head injury requiring close observation, a CT scan and neurosurgical referral.

Treatment

Treatment of the trauma victim is aimed at resuscitation and treatment of all injuries according to clinical priority, starting with maintenance of the airway, stabilization of the cervical spine, high-flow oxygen, breathing and circulation.

After resuscitation, treatment priorities of a head injury are maintaining cere-

Table 1. The Glasgow Coma Scale

Best visual response (eye opening)	Score	Best verbal response	Score	Best motor response (to painful stimuli)	Score
Spontaneously	4	Orientated	5	Obeys commands	6
To verbal command	3	Confused	4	Localizes	5
To painful stimuli	2	Inappropriate words	3	Withdraws	4
No response	1	Incomprehensible sounds	2	Flexes	3
		No response	1	Extends	2
				No response	1

bral perfusion, controlling ICP, and constant reassessment. A severe head injury requires controlled ventilation, ICP monitoring, nursing care, drug therapy and possibly surgical intervention.

In moderate and severe head injuries, drug therapy may be valuable, including:

- Diuretics. 20% mannitol, 1 g/kg. Loop diuretics such as frusemide, are seldom given.
- Anti-epileptics for a fitting patient: initially diazepam 10 mg and if ineffective, phenytoin 1 g at 50 mg/min, followed by 100 mg 8-hourly.
- Steroids are seldom administered.

Definitive management is undertaken in a neurosurgical centre for the majority of cases. The indications for surgical intervention, in addition to controlled ventilation and hypocapnia, depend upon the pathology. There are seldom indications for the inexperienced to perform blind burr holes.

Depressed skull fractures need careful assessment and possibly elevation. Open depressed fractures require surgical debridement and meticulous dural repair.

Treatment of orthopaedic injuries

Stabilization of orthopaedic injuries is vital, but this does not always equate with the immediate need for prolonged surgery, which may destabilize cerebral perfusion, unless the fracture is open or limb viability dubious. The most suitable window of opportunity for open surgical long bone fixation is often at the time of admission, or following emergency neurosurgery, if the clinical situation and surgical facilities allow. However, stabilization such as external fixation, plaster or possibly traction, can rapidly be applied and an anatomical reduction deferred for a few days, until the clinical situation permits. The consequences of intramedullary reaming at 1 to 6 days following a major head injury may be catastrophic.

Prognosis

The duration of post-traumatic amnesia is a good clinical guide to the severity of a head injury. Recovery following a major head injury is usually exponential, with the greatest recovery in the first 6 months. It may continue for many years.

Fitting, epilepsy and driving (UK DVLA regulations)

An epileptic fit following a head injury may lead to the suspension of a driving licence. In the UK the fit should be reported to the DVLA, who consider each case. The general rules are:

- An immediate fit following a head injury does not lead to suspension of a private driving licence.
- An early fit, within the first 24 hours, leads to suspension of a private driving licence for 6 months.
- Any subsequent fit is considered by the DVLA under the same criteria as epilepsy due to other causes and the licence suspended until a 12 month fit-free period has elapsed.
- Different regulations apply to vocational (HGV and public transport) driving licences, and the licence is usually withdrawn for 10 years.

Further reading

Cummins BH. The management of head injuries (Parts 1 and 2). *Current Orthopaedics*, 1992; **6**: 165–172, 240–244.

Kirkpatrick PJ. On guidelines for the management of the severe head injury. *Journal of Neurology, Neurosurgery and Psychiatry*, 1997; **62**: 109–111.

Related topics of interest

Polytrauma – management and complications, p. 200; Polytrauma – resuscitation and ATLS, p. 209

HIP DISLOCATION

Traumatic dislocation of the hip is a violent injury and usually occurs in young patients following major trauma. The dislocation may be anterior, posterior or central, often with an acetabular rim or femoral head fracture and neurological injury. The dislocation should be reduced as an orthopaedic emergency as the prognosis is proportional to the time interval before reduction.

Fifty per cent of patients have other fractures and 30% have soft tissue injuries of the knee from the dashboard.

This topic discusses hip dislocation, femoral head and acetabular rim fractures; major acetabular fractures are covered in 'Pelvis – acetabular fractures', p. 185.

Classification

Anterior dislocation (10–15%) may be superior or inferior, classified by Epstein as type I or II, respectively, with subtype A for no associated fracture, subtype B for an associated femoral head fracture, and subtype C for an associated acetabular rim fracture.

The Thompson and Epstein classification includes five configurations for posterior dislocation: type I with no associated fracture or very small fragments; type II with a large single posterior rim fracture; type III with a comminuted rim fracture; type IV with an acetabular floor fracture; and type V with a femoral head fracture.

Thompson and Epstein type V fractures (5–10%) have been subdivided by Pipkin into: type I with a caudad head fragment (below the fovea centralis); type II with a cephalad fracture (above or including the fovea centralis); type III with a femoral head and neck fracture; and type IV with an associated acetabular rim fracture.

Central fracture dislocations are usually more complex fractures, involving the anterior or posterior column, and should be considered within the Letournel and Judet classification.

Radiology

The diagnosis can be confirmed from plain AP pelvic radiographs, of sufficient quality to exclude a large rim fragment. Following reduction, radiographs are taken and any rim or head fracture investigated with a CT scan. Only if the injury appears unusual should a CT scan be obtained before closed reduction – another CT scan is likely to be required after reduction. Post-reduction CT helps plan surgery and show intra-articular loose bodies.

Treatment

The injury follows major trauma, so initial treatment is directed at assessment and resuscitation of the patient. Neurological injuries must be assessed and documented. The dislocated hip should be reduced as an emergency and other fractures addressed subsequently.

*1. **Closed reduction*** should be performed within 6 hours of the dislocation. This can sometimes be achieved in the emergency room, with adequate analgesia, but often a full general anaesthetic is required. With a posterior dislocation, greater mechanical advantage for traction can be achieved with the patient on the operating room floor. If the reduction is stable, 2.5 to 5 kg of skin or skeletal traction should be applied.

AP X-rays will confirm the reduction, and when there is doubt about the congruity of the reduction, a CT scan should be obtained.

2. **Immediate open reduction** is required when the dislocation cannot be reduced or the hip is grossly unstable. The joint should be opened, the hip reduced and the rim fracture stabilized.

3. **Retained loose fragments** should be removed by arthrotomy or hip arthroscopy. Fragments can abrade the articular surface and accelerate post-traumatic degenerative change.

4. **Significant rim fractures** require open reduction and internal fixation under appropriate conditions. Where there is less than one third of the posterior rim remaining, the hip may be unstable. Fragments are usually posterior, often comminuted, and should be stabilized with interfragmentary screws and a reconstruction plate. In the presence of extensive comminution, restoration of stability and bone stock for a subsequent reconstructive procedure may necessitate iliac crest bone graft.

5. **Large head fragments** require open reduction and fixation, or removal if not involving the weight-bearing area. This is best performed through an anterior approach to the joint, as cephalad fragments are attached to the ligamentum teres and cannot be adequately visualized or reduced through a posterior approach. The fragment can be fixed with small fragment screws, Herbert screws or absorbable pins.

6. **Mobilization** can start after closed or open reduction as soon as pain allows. In the past, patients with a simple dislocation have been treated with bed rest and traction for 6 weeks prior to mobilization. This is unnecessary and patients should start to move the hip early and be mobilized when their pain permits, usually around 5 to 10 days, with 5 kg partial weight-bearing for 6 weeks, increasing to full weight-bearing over the next 6 weeks.

Where fixation is tenuous, a longer period of traction may be required.

Prognosis

The prognosis is related to the period of dislocation, velocity of the trauma and extent of any associated fracture. A simple dislocation carries a better prognosis than a large rim fracture, and a delay in reducing the hip of greater than 24 hours carries a poor outcome.

Excellent or good results, in terms of pain, return to function and degenerative change, can be expected in 75% of patients with an anterior dislocation and 68% of patients with a type I posterior dislocation. Only 30% of patients have a good result with a type V fracture/dislocation.

Avascular necrosis and post-traumatic osteoarthritis may occur up to 5 years after a dislocation.

Complications

- Avascular necrosis: 10–35% (6–24% following type I).
- Post-traumatic osteoarthritis: 20–30%.
- Heterotopic bone formation: 3%.
- Sciatic nerve palsy: 10–19%.

Further reading

Epstein HC. *Traumatic Dislocation of the Hip*. Baltimore: Williams and Wilkins, 1980.

Related topics of interest

Pelvis – acetabular fractures, p. 185; Pelvis – ring fractures, p. 189

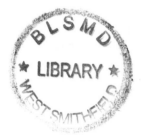

HUMERAL FRACTURES – DISTAL

Fractures of the distal humerus in adults may be extra-articular or intra-articular. Supra-condylar fractures are extra-articular. Intra-articular fractures include transcondylar, inter-condylar, condylar (medial or lateral), epicondylar fractures and isolated fractures of the articular surface. The principles of management are closed treatment wherever possible and ORIF for displaced, unstable or intra-articular fractures. Fractures around the elbow are associated with stiffness and restricted long-term mobility, so early mobilization should be encouraged to optimize outcome.

Fracture patterns

1. Haemarthrosis of the elbow, without a demonstrable fracture, is indicative of a significant soft tissue or bony injury. The haemarthrosis may be aspirated under aseptic conditions, relieving pain and increasing range of movement.

2. Supracondylar fractures are extra-articular and most commonly have an extension (or Malgaigne) deformity, often with a rotational element. Neuro-vascular impairment should be excluded. Undisplaced fractures can be treated conservatively in a long arm cast, with mobilization starting within a couple of weeks, subject to satisfactory radiological appearances. Displaced fractures tend to be unstable, requiring manipulation and percutaneous pin fixation or ORIF, followed by early mobilization. Flexion injuries are rare, less than 4%, but the principles of treatment are similar.

3. Transcondylar fractures are less common and slightly more distal than supra-condylar fractures, but are treated in the same manner. However, the fracture is more unstable than a supracondylar fracture, especially in the rotational plane. The threshold for pin fixation or ORIF is lower, as the potential for non-union is higher.

4. Intercondylar fractures have a 'T' or 'Y' fracture pattern passing between and separating the condyles. These are classified by AO as 13-C1, 13-C2 or 13-C3 and by Riseborough and Radin as: type I, undisplaced; type II, displaced non-rotated; type III, displaced rotated; and type IV, severely comminuted. Undisplaced frac-tures can be treated by mobilization after two weeks in a plaster cast. Displaced fractures require ORIF if the soft tissues permit, through a posterior approach with olecranon osteotomy. Intra-articular open injuries are not a contraindication to ORIF, with appropriate wound management.

Severely comminuted fractures in the elderly are often best treated by traction followed by mobilization, the 'bag of bones approach', to optimize function. Occasionally, an early elbow replacement may be indicated.

5. Isolated condylar fractures follow the Milch classification, with type I frac-tures passing through the capitellum, or medial condyle, leaving the trochlear ridge intact, and type II fractures passing close to the trochlear sulcus, including the trochlear ridge in the fracture fragment. Type II fractures are associated with dislocation of the elbow and collateral ligament rupture. Condylar fractures are uncommon in the adult, with lateral fractures more common than medial.

Undisplaced medial fractures should be immobilized in pronation and lateral fractures in supination for a period before mobilization. Displaced fractures need ORIF; lag screws alone often provide sufficient fixation.

6. *Intra-articular fractures* are rare and follow a fall on the outstretched hand, more commonly involving a shear fracture of the capitellum than trochlea. Capitellar fractures are either type I, with a large osteochondral fragment extending into the trochlea, or type II, with minimal subchondral bone. Undisplaced fractures can be treated by early mobilization. Unstable fragments need ORIF with a lag or Herbert screw. Some comminuted fractures with minimal subchondral bone, or fractures in the elderly, are best treated by excising the fragment and starting early mobilization. The outcome is similar to a radial head fracture.

7. *Epicondylar fractures* may occur in younger adults and are treated conservatively. These can be confused with delayed closure of the ossification centre. The medial epicondyle is the more commonly affected. Occasionally, persistent ulnar nerve symptoms require surgery, or an unsightly lump necessitates late excision of the bone fragment.

Internal fixation of distal humeral fractures

For intercondylar fractures this is achieved by a posterior approach, osteotomizing the olecranon, once the ulnar nerve has been exposed and protected. A chevron osteotomy of the olecranon should be performed through the non-articular segment. The olecranon should first be predrilled for reattachment with a 6.5 mm lag screw and tension band wire. The olecranon is then reflected proximally with the triceps tendon. Pre-operative planning is essential, as surgical reconstruction of the fracture is challenging. The distal intra-articular fragment should be reconstructed and thereafter reattached to the humerus with a double plate technique, adhering to AO principles. DCPs or malleable pelvic reconstruction plates are favoured, in planes at 90° to each other. One third tubular plates are not strong enough. A large defect of the articular surface should be filled with iliac crest bone graft. Finally, the olecranon is reattached. Non-union of the olecranon occasionally complicates the procedure.

Surgery is best performed within 48 hours of the fracture or at 10 days, as the swelling starts to subside. With rigid fixation, mobilization can commence when wound healing is satisfactory. Good or excellent results are reported in 75% of cases – defined by a stable elbow, minimal pain, flexion from 15° to 130° and a return to pre-injury activities.

Condylar fractures should be addressed through a medial or lateral approach.

Complications

1. *Early complications* are vascular compromise and nerve damage. A vascular injury should be treated by immediate reduction of a displaced fracture and further assessment with an arteriogram and vascular surgical opinion if required. A forearm compartment syndrome may occur, progressing to Volkmann's ischaemic contracture if unrecognized.

2. Late complications include non-union, malunion and joint stiffness. Non-union should be addressed in the usual manner. Malunion may lead to an obvious visible deformity or reduced range of movement. An osteotomy is occasionally required if the deformity is great or a progressive ulnar nerve lesion develops. Joint stiffness may improve with time, but an extensive soft tissue release may be required, although the results are poor. Heterotopic bone formation and myositis ossificans can compromise joint movement.

3. Surgery carries the attendant risks of infection and neurovascular damage.

4. Established non-union can be addressed by total elbow replacement, and the mid-term results in these difficult circumstances are good.

5. Osteoarthritis. Mild post-traumatic degenerative change occurs in 50% of intra-articular distal humeral fractures at 6 years. Advanced changes occur in about 10%.

Further reading

Asprinio D, Helfet DL. Fractures of the distal humerus. In: Levine AM, ed. *Orthopaedic Knowledge Update Trauma*. Rosemont: American Academy of Orthopaedic Surgeons, 1998; 35–45.

Helfet DL, Schmeling GJ. Bicondylar intra-articular fractures of the distal humerus in adults. *Clinical Orthopaedics*, 1993; **292**: 26–36.

Jupiter JB. Complex fractures of the distal part of the humerus and associated complications. *Journal of Bone and Joint Surgery*, 1994; **76A**: 1252–1264.

Müller ME, Allgöwer M, Schneider R, Willenegger H. *Manual of Internal Fixation*. Berlin: Springer-Verlag, 1991; 446–452.

Related topics of interest

Elbow dislocation, p. 109; Humeral fractures – shaft, p. 113; Paediatric humeral condylar fractures, p. 169; Paediatric humeral supracondylar fractures, p. 172; Radius and ulna – fractures around the elbow, p. 236

HUMERAL FRACTURES – PROXIMAL

Proximal humeral fractures constitute 5–7% of all fractures and 76% of all humeral fractures in people over 40 years of age. In the elderly this fracture is associated with osteoporosis and there are 70% as many proximal humeral fractures as femoral neck fractures.

Anatomy

The proximal humerus has an anatomical and surgical neck. The anatomical neck encircles the base of the articular surface. The surgical neck is the more distal and closely related to the axillary nerve. The axillary nerve runs through the quadrangular space (border humeral shaft, teres minor, long head of triceps and teres major), supplying the teres minor and deltoid muscles and the 'badge' area of skin over the deltoid. The surgical neck is the most frequently fractured.

The blood supply of the head is primarily from the anterior circumflex humeral artery, although the postero-medial vessels can sustain it.

The proximal humerus was divided into four bony parts by Codman – the head, greater tuberosity, lesser tuberosity and shaft. The rotator cuff inserts to the greater (teres minor, supraspinatus and infraspinatus) and lesser (subscapularis) tuberosities. The direction of pull of these muscles determines the displacement of bony fragments after fracture – postero-superiorly for the greater and antero-medially for the lesser tuberosity. The bicipital groove separates the two tuberosities. The pectoralis major muscle inserts to the humeral shaft distal to the surgical neck and displaces the shaft medially. The humeral head lies under the acromial arch and one of the aims of treatment is to maintain enough space under the arch to prevent subsequent impingement.

Classification

The most common classification is that of Neer, defining the fracture according to the number of the four osseous parts which are displaced. Displacement is defined as separation >1 cm, or angulation >45°. There is a further category for fracture dislocation, where the head is dislocated outside the joint. Splitting or impaction of the articular surface is recognized, quantifying impaction according to the percentage of head involvement.

Clinical and radiological assessment

Clinical evaluation includes neurovascular assessment, as neurological injury is reported in up to 36% of patients and vascular injury in 5%. Radiological evaluation includes AP, scapular lateral and axillary views. The axillary view defines displacement of the lesser tuberosity and injury to the humeral head. This is obtained by abducting the arm, positioning the X-ray tube in the axilla and the plate superiorly.

Treatment

1. Non-operative management. This is suitable for the 80–85% of proximal humeral fractures which are impacted and non-displaced. A sling is used until pain allows pendular (Codman) exercises after 7 to 14 days, followed by more vigorous mobilization and physiotherapy.

2. *Operative management.* The aim of surgery is to re-establish proximal humeral anatomy, with an intact rotator cuff which does not impinge. Care must be taken not to devascularize fragments, or leave hardware that interferes with shoulder motion.

- Two-part fractures of the surgical neck can usually be treated conservatively, although occasionally removal of an interposed bicipital tendon is required. Greater tuberosity fragments displaced by >1 cm require ORIF and rotator-cuff repair.
- Three-part fractures have a better outcome if the bony anatomy can be restored. Plate and screw fixation is associated with AVN rates of 30%, which has led to a move away from plate fixation to less invasive techniques. Closed reduction and percutaneous pinning is technically demanding, but useful in selected patients. ORIF using wires and tension bands is gaining popularity. This technique reduces impingement and disturbance to blood supply.
- Four-part fractures have a poor result with non-operative management, which led Neer to introduce the hemiarthroplasty in the 1950s. This gives a pain-free shoulder, with active forward flexion to 90° or more. The technique is technically demanding – the rotator cuff should be reattached and the natural humeral head retroversion of 35° maintained. Recent publications indicate the rate of AVN following these fractures is not as high as previously thought and so reconstruction with wires and tension-band fixation has become more popular. The results of early hemiarthroplasty are better than those of delayed primary arthroplasty, or late arthroplasty to revise failed internal fixation.

3. *Fracture/dislocation.* Fracture of the greater tuberosity often reduces after closed reduction of the shoulder, but failure of the fragment to reduce requires ORIF and cuff repair. Care should be taken not to convert a non-displaced fracture dislocation into a displaced injury during manipulation. Two- or three-part fracture dislocations can be treated by ORIF. Four-part injuries generally have a poor prognosis due to AVN and are treated by hemiarthroplasty.

4. *Impaction or splitting of >45% of the articular surface.* This is an indication for prosthetic replacement.

Complications

- **Neurological:** up to 36% of patients have neurological impairment. The axillary nerve is the most commonly injured, but injury to the suprascapular, musculocutaneous and radial nerves have been reported. Ninety per cent recover spontaneously within 4 months.
- **Vascular:** axillary artery damage occurs in up to 5%, and in 27% of these the distal pulses remain palpable.
- **AVN** is related to the severity of the injury and occurs in 5–15% of three-part fractures and 10–34% of four-part fractures. Recent studies show that these figures maybe an overestimate.
- **Malunion** can lead to impingement of the greater tuberosity and limitation of range of movement.
- **Shoulder stiffness** follows a poor rehabilitation programme, myositis ossificans, malunion and AVN.

Paediatrics

Fractures in children of <5 years are most commonly Salter–Harris type I, and >13 years Salter–Harris type II. Between 5 and 12 years, the physis is seldom involved. The most remarkable factor in these injuries is their ability to remodel, and hence surgical intervention is rarely required.

Further reading

Hawkins RJ, Bell RH, Gurr K. The three part fracture of the proximal humerus: operative treatment. *Journal of Bone and Joint Surgery*, 1986; **68A**: 1410–1414.

Hawkins RJ, Switlyk P. Acute prosthetic replacement for severe fractures of the proximal humerus. *Clinical Orthopaedics*, 1993; **289**: 156–160.

Jaberg H, Warner JJ, Jakob RP. Percutaneous stabilisation of unstable fractures of the humerus. *Journal of Bone and Joint Surgery*, 1992; **74A**: 508–515.

Neer CS. Displaced proximal humeral fractures: I. Classification and evaluation. *Journal of Bone and Joint Surgery*, 1970; **52A**: 1077–1089.

Nugent IM, Ivory JP, Ross AC. Rotator cuff injuries. In: *Key Topics in Orthopaedic Surgery*. Oxford: BIOS Scientific Publishers, 1995; 260–262.

Nugent IM, Ivory JP, Ross AC. Shoulder instability. In: *Key Topics in Orthopaedic Surgery*. Oxford: BIOS Scientific Publishers, 1995; 278–280.

Related topic of interest

Humeral fractures – shaft, p. 113

HUMERAL FRACTURES – SHAFT

The humeral shaft extends proximally from the upper border of pectoralis major insertion to the supracondylar ridge distally. Shaft fractures constitute 3% of all fractures and most are treated conservatively. The principal issues are avoidance of non-union, radial nerve palsy, and the role of IM nailing.

Clinical examination and imaging

1. Diagnosis. This rarely presents a challenge, except in the unconscious. The neurovascular status of the limb should be documented before any manipulation. Radiological evaluation consists of full-length AP and lateral radiographs, including the shoulder and elbow.

2. Proximal fragment displacement. This depends upon the fracture location relative to muscular insertions. In the more proximal fracture, the rotator cuff abducts and rotates the proximal fragment, while in slightly more distal fractures, pectoralis major serves to adduct. In more distal fractures the deltoid abducts the proximal fragment.

Classification

The humerus is divided into thirds for descriptive purposes and the fracture described according to configuration (transverse/spiral/oblique etc.). The AO numeric code for the humeral shaft is '12'.

Management

1. Non-operative treatment. This is associated with good or excellent results in 95% of patients. Acceptable displacement includes <3 cm shortening, <20° of antero-posterior angulation and <30° varus – valgus angulation. Mean time to union is 6 weeks, with 95% of fractures united at 10 weeks and 90% of patients having normal function at 10 weeks. The most favoured methods of splinting are:

- Hanging cast over the upper arm and forearm. The length of the sling or collar 'n' cuff controls varus/valgus alignment. The position of a loop on the forearm controls AP alignment. A heavy cast can distract the fracture, predisposing to non-union, particularly in transverse fractures.
- U slab. This is bulky and predisposes to axillary irritation, but is useful acutely.
- Functional cast brace. Described by Sarmiento, a cast brace consisting of pre-fabricated anterior and posterior shells secured with a Velcro strap can be applied after 1–2 weeks in a U-slab, when the swelling has decreased. Early mobilization of the elbow and shoulder is encouraged. The brace is progressively tightened as swelling decreases and discontinued after a minimum of 8 weeks.

2. Operative treatment. The indications are: open fractures, floating elbow, bilateral humeral fractures, polytrauma, vascular injury, intra-articular extension, inability to maintain reduction and delayed or non-union. The methods of internal fixation are:

- A compression plate and screws using a broad 4.5 mm plate. Two surgical approaches are popular. Either an antero-lateral approach extended proximally to the shoulder and distally to the elbow, or a posterior approach, allowing exposure of the elbow through an olecranon osteotomy – the radial nerve must be identified. Proximal extension is limited by the axillary nerve and circumflex humeral vessels. Complication rates average 10%, the most serious being non-union (2%) and radial nerve palsy. A low threshold for acute bone grafting is advised.
- External fixation with a conventional or ring fixator may be applied. Conventional fixators are associated with pin-tract problems, soft tissue transfixion and non-union. The use of ring fixators is not widespread.
- IM nailing is increasingly favoured. Traditional non-locked and flexible nails (Enders, Rush, Kuntscher) were used with variable results. Biomechanically superior locked nails are now available, but their role in the management of humeral shaft fractures has not been fully determined. Debate concerns the direction of insertion: antegrade is complicated by rotator-cuff impingement and axillary nerve damage, while retrograde is complicated by fracture extension into the distal humerus and loss of elbow extension. IM nailing is most suitable for fractures >2 cm distal to the surgical neck and >3 cm proximal to the olecranon fossa.

Complications

1. **Radial nerve injury.** Such injury occurs in 2–20% of cases and, while classically associated with the 'Holstein–Lewis' fracture (spiral fracture of the distal third), is more common following middle third fractures. Neurapraxia or neurotemesis is the most common and 90% resolve without treatment. The recommendation is to wait 3 to 4 months for spontaneous resolution. In the absence of recovery at this stage, the nerve is explored – EMG or nerve conduction studies can help determine the presence or absence of recovery.

Acute exploration is indicated in open injuries – 64% of open injuries involve nerve damage or nerve interposition.

With post-manipulation palsy, many surgeons advise exploration despite the fact that the majority recover spontaneously.

2. **Vascular injury.** This can follow direct trauma or compartment syndrome, most commonly in proximal and middle third fractures, and requires urgent treatment. The role of arteriography is controversial. In many cases the clinical picture is sufficiently clear to make the delay in treatment caused by angiography difficult to justify. The ischaemia time should be kept below 6 hours.

3. **Non-union.** Defined as >4 months without healing. The incidence is 0–15%. It is most common in the proximal and distal thirds. Predisposing factors are systemic (age, diabetes, nutritional status, etc.) and local (transverse fracture, distraction, soft tissue interposition, inadequate immobilization). Treatment is operative with a plate and bone graft (union rate 89–96%) or reamed, locked IM nail (union rate 87%). The complication rate is lower with nailing (12% versus 21%). Closed insertion of the IM nail is advocated if technically possible.

Pathological fractures

A non-reamed, locked IM nail gives the best biomechanical fixation. For proximal and distal fractures a plate can be used, possibly with methylmethacrylate augmentation.

Paediatrics

There is little difference between the paediatric and adult fracture, with the emphasis being on non-operative management. Radial nerve palsy occurs in children and guidelines for management are similar to those in adults.

Further reading

Ingman AM, Waters DA. Locked intramedullary nailing of humeral shaft fractures. Implant design, surgical technique and clinical results. *Journal of Bone and Joint Surgery*, 1994; **76B**: 23–29.

Rosen H. The treatment of non-unions and pseudarthroses of the humeral shaft. *Orthopedic Clinics of North America*, 1990; **21**: 725–742.

Sarmiento A, Horowitch A, Aboulafia A *et al*. Functional bracing for comminuted extra-articular fractures of the distal-third of the humerus. *Journal of Bone and Joint Surgery*, 1990; **72B**: 283–287.

Related topics of interest

Humeral fractures – distal, p. 107; Humeral fractures – proximal, p. 110

IMAGING IN TRAUMA

Clinical assessment should be undertaken before imaging. For major trauma, initial imaging is undertaken simultaneously with resuscitation; and AP chest, AP pelvis and lateral cervical spine X-rays are mandatory.

Good quality, correct exposure plain radiographs should include the joint above and the joint below an injury. However, this rule is broken with many obvious intra-articular or peri-articular fractures, such as the distal radius, elbow, hip, tibial plateau, ankle, etc. This is acceptable, provided there are no other adverse clinical findings.

In addition to plain X-rays at presentation, further imaging may be required to determine management and plan operative procedures.

Additional imaging modalities include:

- Special plain radiographs – obliques, tomograms, stress views.
- Fluoroscopy.
- Computerized tomography.
- Magnetic resonance imaging.
- Ultrasound.
- Arthrography.
- Isotope scintigraphy.
- Arteriography.

Special plain radiograph views

*1. **Additional plain views*** are often of benefit, to demonstrate the characteristics and extent of an injury, and to plan the surgical approach to management. Examples include X-rays such as axial views of the glenohumeral joint, a tunnel view of the wrist for hamate fractures, a tunnel view of the knee for condylar fractures and loose bodies, 15° oblique views of the tibial plateau, 60° pelvic inlet and outlet views for pelvic fractures and 45° Judet views for acetabular fractures.

*2. **Tomograms*** may be used to demonstrate the extent of a fracture, or degree and direction of articular displacement, by imaging a thin horizontal slice of bone which is in focus, with the rest of the bony structure blurred out of focus. A large dose of irradiation is required and many centres now favour the use of spiral CT imaging for this purpose. The technique remains of value in demonstrating odontoid peg fractures, in the lateral plane.

*3. **Stress views*** are helpful in the diagnosis of soft tissue ligamentous injuries, most notably for collateral ligament injuries in the thumb, knee and ankle.

Fluoroscopy

Fluoroscopy is the examination of a bone or joint, under X-ray video images. This technique is useful to demonstrate the presence or absence of a fracture, such as a proximal femoral or proximal humeral fracture, as the structure can be manipulated and the extent of displacement or degree of instability established.

Computerized tomography

1. Computerized axial tomography generates transverse images of a structure, which is especially valuable for imaging the axial skeleton and intra-articular fractures of the shoulder, hip, knee and calcaneum.

2. Modern spiral imaging with sophisticated computer software means exposure to irradiation is kept relatively low and 3D images can be constructed from planar images. Some software allows integration with machine tools or lasers to produce a resin model of the bone structure, which again helps plan surgical reconstruction.

Magnetic resonance imaging

MRI is of limited benefit in acute trauma care. However, MRI generates excellent images of the axial skeleton and spinal cord, which is relevant in spinal trauma, especially the cervical spine, and some brachial plexus injuries. MRI is valuable in some acute soft tissue injuries to the knee or shoulder. In the acute setting, there may be evidence of bone bruising or oedema following peri-articular injuries. Diagnostic information may be obtained with stress fractures and occult fractures.

MRI is a valuable prognostic indicator to demonstrate recovery or avascular necrosis following peri-articular injuries, such as femoral head fractures, and is more reliable than isotope scintigraphy. Non-ferrous fixation devices are required to prevent signal voids during imaging.

MRI is more frequently applied to the diagnosis of chronic shoulder, spinal and knee conditions.

Ultrasound

Ultrasound should not be underestimated as a diagnostic tool in acute trauma care. Soft tissue injuries are excellently demonstrated, such as muscle tears, partial quadriceps or Achilles tendon ruptures, and ulnar collateral ligament ruptures in the thumb. An acute effusion or haemarthrosis can be demonstrated and aspirated, most usefully around the hip joint. Ultrasound can also be used to subsequently assess the healing process following a muscular or tendinous injury.

Arthrography

Arthrography is a valuable aid in paediatric trauma, as cartilaginous structures may not be visible on plain X-rays, and is an especially useful adjunct in demonstrating the extent of elbow fractures.

Isotope scintigraphy

Isotope scintigraphy contributes to the early management of trauma, most commonly following possible scaphoid fractures. [99]Technetium-labelled methylene diphosphonate is administered and uptake imaged at various phases with a gamma camera. It is a useful adjunct in acute assessment of the paediatric or adult hip following a possible injury, with equivocal radiological findings and for the diagnosis of stress fractures. Sensitivity is good, but specificity is poor. Localization can be improved by co-registration with plain X-rays on computer software to localize a lesion.

Arteriography

Displaced fractures in the vicinity of a vessel relatively tethered to bone, where the distal circulation is in jeopardy, may require imaging of the vascular structures. Typical injuries include displaced fractures of the distal or proximal humerus and fractures or fracture-dislocations around the knee.

Further reading

Burnett SJD, Stoker DJ. Practical limitations of magnetic resonance imaging in orthopaedics. *Current Orthopaedics,*1995; **9**: 253–259.

INFECTION AND TRAUMA

This chapter deals with viral and bacterial infection in the trauma patient, and discusses the implications of HIV and viral hepatitis for the surgical team.

Bacterial infection

Wound contamination is defined by the presence of bacteria, not clinical indicators of infection. The bacterial count is important, with >100 000 micro-organisms per gram necessary to cause infection (β-haemolytic streptococci can cause infection at lower levels). The number of bacteria required to cause infection can be reduced if there is local (e.g. necrotic tissue, foreign bodies), or systemic immuno-compromise. For example a silk stitch in a wound reduces the number of staphylococci required to cause infection by 10 000 times.

The mean infection rate after an open fracture is 16%. (Gustilo–Anderson grade I: 7%; grade II: 11%; grade IIIA: 18%; grade IIIB/C: 56%.)

When a fracture is internally fixed, a closed injury is converted to an open one. All possible measures should be taken to avoid infection – careful soft tissue handling, no touch technique, etc. Studies both recommend and discourage prophylactic antibiotic use, but the evidence probably favours prophylaxis. The first dose of antibiotics is the most critical and should be given 10 min before tourniquet inflation.

Reduction of wound infection

The factors that help to reduce wound infection after an open injury are:

1. Debridement to remove bacteria, dead tissue, etc. Wound debridement should be undertaken early, as bacterial counts increase rapidly from 100 per gram at 2 hours, to over the 100 000 threshold at 5 hours.

2. Copious irrigation – preferably with large volumes of pulsed lavage saline (>9 l). The addition of antibiotics to the irrigation is controversial.

3. Systemic antibiotics are an adjunct to debridement, as dead tissue is not perfused.

Tetanus

1. Clostridium tetani is an anaerobic gram-positive rod, widespread in the environment and particularly in human or animal faeces. Deep anaerobic wounds containing necrotic tissue are the ideal environment for multiplication.

2. The disease is caused by the exotoxin *tetanospasmin*. There are two forms of the disease, local and systemic. Local disease is rare and causes muscle spasms. Systemic disease causes muscle spasm, trismus and dysphagia, progressing to generalized convulsions. The mean incubation period is 1 week and the mortality from systemic disease 20–60%.

3. Treatment is with penicillin, streptomycin and immunoglobulin. Surgically, the wound should be debrided; otherwise, treatment is supportive, particularly of the airway.

4. Prophylaxis consists of:

- Adequate wound debridement.
- Tetanus toxoid (0.5 ml i.m.) for patients who have not had a booster in the last 5 years.
- Tetanus immunoglobulin (250 units i.m. at a different site to the toxoid) for patients who have not been immunized in the last 10 years. This should be considered in all patients with tetanus-prone or farmyard injuries.
- Consider adding penicillin or oxytetracycline.

Gas gangrene

Clostridium perfringens and *Clostridium septicum* (anaerobic gram-positive rods) are the most important pathogens in man. These organisms produce several exotoxins, including lecithinase, causing cell wall destruction and tissue death, with the production of carbon dioxide and hydrogen sulphide.

Gas in the tissues is not diagnostic of gas gangrene, as gas is also seen in necrotizing fasciitis, anaerobic cellulitis and infected vascular gangrene, or from an open wound. The diagnosis is principally clinical. There is a history of a deep wound, usually of the buttock or thigh, less than 3 days previously. Local pain and swelling are severe, with a serosanguineous discharge. The patient is apprehensive and fearful of dying. Initially there is no pyrexia, but the patient is tachycardic. The production of gas is rarely abundant, but the systemic toxaemia leads to haemolysis, renal and hepatic failure.

Modern treatment, with mortality <10% includes:

- Repeated surgical debridement and fasciotomy.
- Antibiotics (penicillin).
- Supportive measures.
- Hyperbaric oxygen.

There is no immunization against the microbe or toxins. Prophylaxis consists of adequate initial wound debridement and prophylactic antibiotics.

Viral infection

Human immunodeficiency virus (HIV)

HIV is a retrovirus, synthesizing DNA from its own RNA, and causes lysis of the CD4 (T helper) lymphocyte. CD4 counts are an indicator of disease activity. In urban areas 10% of trauma patients may be HIV positive.

The seroconversion rate by inoculation is 0.4% per incident. The risk of seroconversion after parenteral exposure is 0.1% and 0.6% after mucous membrane exposure. An infective dose may be carried by 0.3 ml of blood. Trauma surgery has one of the highest incidences of blood contact during operative cases (48%) and the cumulative lifetime risk for a surgeon has been estimated at 1–4%. Surgeons should protect themselves by taking 'universal precautions', including wearing double or impervious gloves, boots, impervious gowns or aprons and space suits. Sharp instruments should not be passed from hand to hand and suturing with hand needles should be avoided.

In operating on HIV positive patients for trauma (not patients with full-blown AIDS), the infection rate is 16%, as opposed to 5% in controls. In open fractures the infection rate is 55%, so open treatment must be performed with great discretion.

Hepatitis

Five types of hepatitis virus account for 95% of cases. Types A and E are parenterally transmitted.

Hepatitis B is transmitted much more readily than HIV. Exposure results in infection in 10–30% following a needle-stick injury, with 1% dying acutely of fulminant hepatitis and 15–25% dying prematurely from cirrhosis or hepatocellular carcinoma. Five to ten per cent become chronic carriers. Recombinant vaccine is safe and has 95% seroconversion rates.

Hepatitis C is the principal cause of non-A, non-B hepatitis. Spread is blood-borne with the highest levels in haemophiliacs and drug abusers. The sero-conversion rate after exposure is <10%, although 60% of those infected develop chronic liver disease and many of these progress to chronic hepatitis or cirrhosis after several years. Hepatitis C may also be a cause of hepatocellular carcinoma. No vaccine is available against hepatitis C.

In hepatitis D, the delta agent coats itself with hepatitis B surface antigen, and thus only occurs in the presence of hepatitis B. Hepatitis D often results in severe acute hepatitis or rapidly progressive chronic liver disease.

Further reading

Behrens FF. Fractures with soft tissue injuries. In: Browner BD, Jupiter JB, Levine AM, Trafton PG, eds. *Skeletal Trauma*. Philadelphia: WB Saunders, 1998; 391–419.

Nugent IM, Ivory JP, Ross AC. Osteomyelitis. In: *Key Topics in Orthopaedic Surgery*. Oxford: BIOS Scientific Publishers, 1995; 208–210.

Thomas HC. Clinical features of viral hepatitis. In: Weatherall DJ, Ledingham JGG, Warrell DA, eds. *The Oxford Textbook of Medicine*. Oxford: Oxford University Press, 1996; 2061–2069.

Related topics of interest

Infection control and viral prophylaxis, p. 122; Open fracture management, p. 156

INFECTION CONTROL AND VIRAL PROPHYLAXIS

Infection control is summarized by the phrase 'prevention is better than cure'. Patient and healthcare workers in trauma surgery are exposed to high risks of bacterial and viral infection.

Infection control

Prevention of bacterial infection is by reducing the inoculum and assisting the host's natural defences, *before*, *during* and *after* surgery.

Reducing the inoculum

*1. **Ward hygiene and management.*** Reducing the bacterial inoculum starts with procedures such as separating pre-operative patients from infected cases and reducing the opportunity for blood or airborne contamination. Screening for concurrent sepsis, practised in elective surgery, is not always possible.

- Soiled skin is cleaned and casts removed prior to entering the operating theatre.
- Reducing skin-scale loads is useful, but antiseptic baths do not reduce sepsis rates and risk colonization with resistant bacteria.
- Shaving is undertaken immediately prior to surgery. Earlier shaving increases skin colonization with *Staphlococcus aureus* due to multiple small abrasions.

*2. **Theatre design is aimed at reducing contamination.*** Theatre blocks are located away from thoroughfares and wards, with designated clean and dirty areas. Pressurized ventilation systems reduce airborne infection.

*3. **Ventilation systems.*** There are several types, with variable methods of airflow delivery and filter pore size. Ultra-clean air filters (pore size 0.5 μm), laminar flow and 200 air changes/hour reduce infection rates by 50%. Efficiency is measured by air changes/hour and particles/m^3, or colony forming units/m^3.

- The *plenum system* is most commonly used. Filtered air is injected through theatre ceiling vents at a higher pressure than surrounding rooms, providing 30 changes/hour, exiting through balanced flap valves in the walls. Turbulent airflow is contaminated by convection currents and recirculation.
- *Laminar or linear flow* is low velocity, low turbulence air movement. Filtered air passes into the theatre over a large ceiling or wall diffuser, creating a continuous bank of air with unidirectional movement. This bank of air passes the operating site once, removing airborne particles, with minimal recirculation. Vertical delivery is more effective than horizontal, reducing particles by 98% and 90%, respectively. Hanging side 'curtains' improve efficiency by reducing entrainment of particles at the periphery. Three to four hundred changes/hour and particle counts of 10–20/m^3 are optimal.
- *Ex-flow, or exponential ceiling flow* is the most effective system. Air enters over a large area in the manner of linear flow, with high pressure in the centre, reducing peripherally. Particle counts are typically 2–8/m^3.

- *UVC light units* are more effective than linear flow units, but a major health risk to personnel.

4. *Theatre personnel* are the principal source of bacteria; the number of personnel in theatre should be minimized and they should be adequately clothed. Skin scales are 12 μm in size, carry an average of four bacteria/scale and easily transgress standard cotton theatre garments with a pore size >80 μm. Humans disperse 3000–60000 bacteria per person per minute, increasing with activity and higher in men! Tightly weaved material and newer fabrics have a smaller pore size. Exhaust suits reduce infection rates by >25%.

5. *Meticulous hand washing* with alcoholic chlorhexidine solutions reduce bacterial counts most effectively – 97% with a single wash, 99% with subsequent washes.

- Nailbrushes should only be used on nails, as skin abrasion brings bacteria to the surface.
- Rings are associated with increased glove perforations.
- Double-gloving is recommended in trauma surgery.

6. *Skin preparation* with alcoholic chlorhexidine or povidone iodine solutions removes 98% of bacteria.

- Adhesive drapes secure drapes in place and prevent scales moving to the wound site, but have not been shown to reduce infection.
- Newer, tightly woven drapes are more effective at reducing contamination than cotton drapes.

7. *Surgical technique*, with careful non-traumatic tissue handling, meticulous haemostasis and adequate drainage reduce haematoma formation – an ideal bacterial culture medium.

8. *Pulsed saline lavage* reduces wound bacterial counts by 80%, more with aqueous chlorhexidine. Debridement of contaminated wounds is fundamental to open wound management.

9. *Dressings* should only be changed when there is concern or heavy soiling. Sutures and drains are removed at the earliest opportunity.

10. *Poor general health, malnutrition and immunocompromise* increase infection rates and measures to minimize these should be undertaken. Major surgery is avoided at the peak metabolic response to trauma, i.e. 2–5 days.

Enhancing the defence

1. *Antibiotic prophylaxis* for 16 hours is effective in trauma and elective surgery, and should be broad-spectrum, covering organisms likely to be encountered. In prolonged surgery, (more than 2 hours), the antibiotic half-life should be considered and additional doses given.

2. *Antibiotics* are given 10 min before tourniquet inflation.

Viral prophylaxis

Viruses presenting a risk to healthcare personnel are HIV and Hepatitis B and C.

HIV

The retrovirus HIV synthesizes DNA within CD4 lymphocytes. CD4-lymphocyte death occurs, leading to impaired immunological function and infection susceptibility. The risk of infection after hollow needle-stick injury exposure is 1:200. The lifetime risk to a surgeon depends on the prevalence of HIV and the size of the inoculum – the minimum inoculum is estimated at 0.1 ml, and the risk may be 1–4%. Worldwide, 35 health staff, including 4 surgeons, have become infected with HIV through blood contact. No vaccine exists and prophylaxis depends on prevention of exposure.

Hepatitis B

Hepatitis B is transmitted more easily than HIV and the minimum inoculum required is 0.004 ml. The risk of infection after hollow needle-stick exposure is 1:3. Vaccination is a requirement for all UK surgeons. Failure to develop antibodies occurs in 10%. Antibody levels are checked and boosters required every 5 years.

Hepatitis C

Hepatitis C is responsible for most post-tranfusional hepatitis. Those with any hepatitis C antibody are infectious. Transfusion donors are screened. There is no vaccine as yet.

Prevention of exposure

The mainstay of prophylaxis is prevention of exposure. Universal precautions are mandatory during surgery on infected, or high-risk, patients. These should include most trauma cases, as there is a large exposure to blood and seldom a reliable history. Precautions include:

- Impervious gowns.
- Face visors.
- Double gloves.
- Kevlar gloves.
- Filtered space suits.
- Non-touch sharps handling.

Further reading

Burnstein RL, Rosenberg AD, Stehling L. Blood transfusions/HIV/hepatitis. In: Kasser J. *Orthopaedic Knowledge Update 5.* Rosemont, IL: American Academy of Orthopaedic Surgeons, 1996; 47–52.

Irvine GB. Prevention of infection in orthopaedic surgery. In: Barrett D, ed. *Essential Basic Sciences for Orthopaedics.* Oxford: Butterworth-Heineman, 1994; 148–156.

Related topics of interest

Infection and trauma, p. 119; Principles of soft tissue management, p. 223

INTRAMEDULLARY IMPLANTS – REAMED AND UNREAMED

The use of IM implants has revolutionized long bone fracture care. However, the merits of reamed compared to unreamed implants are controversial and good indications for plate fixation remain. An IM implant, with a central location in the bone, has a biomechanical advantage over an eccentrically located plate. Load sharing is improved and the bending moment reduced.

Principles of IM implants

The fracture is reduced by traction, either on an orthopaedic operating table, or with a distractor. Through an entry site remote to the fracture, the canal is entered and the nail inserted. If reaming is desired, a guide wire is passed and the canal expanded by serial reaming. Depending on the flexibility of the nail, the canal should be reamed to a diameter 0.5 to 1.5 mm greater than the intended implant. If the fracture configuration is unstable, the nail should be locked proximally and distally. If closed reduction cannot be achieved, the fracture site must be opened.

Implant designs

The strength or stiffness of a nail depends upon:

- Diameter.
- Length.
- Shape.
- Cross-sectional characteristics.
- Material.

Nails may be solid or cannulated, and cannulated nails may be rigid or slotted. Most nails are cylindrical, but some have a cloverleaf shape on cross section, which increases stiffness. The construction of the nail affects its stiffness too. Unreamed nails are generally of a smaller diameter, but solid, to give adequate stiffness with a reduced diameter. For a given material, the stiffness of the nail is proportional to the fourth power of the radius ($radius^4$). Fixation is enhanced by maximizing the length of close contact between the implant and endosteal bone – the need for endosteal contact, and hence the diameter of the implant, is reduced by interlocking screws.

The effects of IM instrumentation

1. Closed IM nailing causes minimal disturbance of the soft tissue at the fracture site. Reaming throws out bone graft into the fracture site, which may assist fracture union. However, reaming disturbs the endosteal blood supply and generates heat, causing local necrosis. Studies suggest better blood supply to a fracture site, for a greater period of time, after nail compared to plate fixation.

2. Instrumenting the canal, with a broach, reamer, or unreamed nail increases the intramedullary pressure to >1000 mmHg, which also causes necrosis. Instrumentation of the canal releases medullary products, especially marrow fat, into the circulation, which can have serious respiratory consequences. The release is greater after reaming. A distal venting hole in the bone has limited benefit. The effects of embolic phenomenon are greater if nailing is delayed beyond 48 hours after the fracture and greater during instrumentation of pathological fractures. This is demonstrated with transoesophageal echocardiography.

3. **The harmful effects of reaming** have stimulated interest in unreamed implants. An unreamed implant possibly does less damage to the endosteal blood supply, but the implants usually have less torsional and bending rigidity. Provided the nail is not too flexible, this may help fracture healing and revascularization is more rapid.

4. **Unreamed femoral and tibial nails** are valuable in polytrauma and for open fractures, but fixation with these implants should not be considered as reliable as reamed implants.

5. **Infection rates** with reamed and unreamed implants are similar, but the infection rates may be higher with stainless steel implants.

Dynamization

There was a vogue for removing locking screws at 6 weeks in the past, after stability had been achieved by early bone healing. Dynamization allows greater consolidation of the fracture site. This is no longer regarded as necessary. Ninety eight per cent of femoral fractures heal without dynamization. Consideration should be given to removing locking screws at 6 to 8 weeks after unreamed tibial nailing, if there are no signs of healing and if there is any fracture distraction.

Alternatives to IM nailing

Protagonists of plate fixation claim that plating is a quick surgical procedure, the endosteal blood supply is not damaged and blood loss is minimal if a tourniquet is used. A 'minimally invasive plating technique' or 'bridge plating', through a limited surgical exposure with subcutaneous tunnelling may be a good compromise.

Future advances

Traditionally, nailing has been carried out using an antegrade approach for all bones except the humerus and the approach for the humerus is controversial. Supracondylar femoral nails have been introduced and longer femoral nails for retrograde insertion are available. Small IM devices, allowing static locking, are being developed for narrow long bones, such as the radius and ulna.

Plating

This remains the treatment of choice for:

1. **Humerus.** In polytrauma, intra-articular extension and some radial nerve lesions.

2. **Femur.** In pre-adolescent children, fractures with associated vascular injury, ipsilateral pelvic or acetabular fractures, and some polytrauma cases.

Further reading

Chandler RW. Biologic consequences of intramedullary surgery. In: Rockwood CA, Green DP, Bucholz RW, Heckman JD, eds. *Fractures in Adults*. 4th Edn. Philadelphia: Lippincott-Raven, 1996; 203–217.

Christie J, Robinson CM, Pell ACH *et al*. Transcardiac echocardiography during invasive intramedullary procedures. *Journal of Bone and Joint Surgery*, 1995; 77B: 450–455.

Kottmeier SA. Femoral shaft fractures. In: Dee R, Hurst LC, Gruber MA, Kottmeier SA, eds. *Principles of Orthopaedic Practice*, 2nd Edn. New York: McGraw-Hill, 1997; 483–494.

Pell ACH, Christie J, Keating JF *et al*. The detection of fat embolism by transoesophageal echocardiography during reamed intramedullary nailing. *Journal of Bone and Joint Surgery*, 1993; 75B: 921–925.

Related topic of interest

Biomechanics of fracture implants and implant removal, p. 19; Intramedullary nailing techniques, p. 128

INTRAMEDULLARY NAILING TECHNIQUES

The vast majority of the intra-operative complications and problems associated with intra-medullary nailing can be avoided by diligent pre-operative planning.

Pre-operative planning

Care should be taken in ensuring that the fracture configuration is such that IM fixation is appropriate. Most IM implants can be locked proximally and distally with screws to control rotation and prevent shortening. It is imperative to ensure that there is adequate distance between the proximal and distal extension of the fractures, to allow stable cross screw fixation.

Intra-articular extension may preclude the use of nailing techniques, although prior lag screw fixation of such fractures may be appropriate.

Equipment

Ensure the correct equipment and nails are available. Templates are available to measure the canal width and tables are available to estimate, with a reasonable degree of certainty, the length of nail required. In the femur and tibia, this correlates with the patient's height.

Timing of surgery

Patients with multiple injuries may develop adult respiratory distress syndrome (ARDS), fat emboli or bleeding disorders. Open fractures should be stabilized within 6 to 8 hours, after adequate debridement and irrigation of the soft tissues and fracture site.

Operative technique

1. Positioning. Careful positioning on a traction table is important, in order to reduce the fracture, allow appropriate surgical access and facilitate the entry portal.

2. Traction. In the lower limb, a skeletal traction pin in the distal femur or proximal tibia for femoral fractures, and calcaneum for tibial fractures, is useful to assist fracture reduction in traction. If there is any knee joint damage, a distal femoral pin should be used for femoral fractures, but this can interfere with nail and locking screw placement. A greater traction force can be applied with skeletal traction and rotation is easier to control. With some fractures, and greater experience, traction in a boot may be suitable for femoral shaft fractures.

3. Fracture reduction. Accurate closed fracture reduction with traction, under image intensification, eases the operation. Malreduction can be overcome intra-operatively with the use of a curved ball-tipped guide wire, but often an assistant is required to manually reduce the fracture to allow passage of the guide wire into the other segment.

The aim of most IM nailing techniques is to perform closed reduction and metalware insertion, without the need to expose the fracture. Opening the fracture causes a great deal of soft tissue damage around the fracture site, with resultant damage to the vascularity of the bone, which may delay healing. Care and time should therefore be taken to set the limb up on traction and achieve reduction prior to passage of the guide wire, obviating the need to open the fracture secondarily.

4. Entry portal. Care must be taken in developing this portal. The entry portal affects nail placement, fracture reduction and overall alignment. Malpositioning can result in fractures of adjacent bone, or damage to the soft tissues at the entry portal.

5. Reaming. When using a reamed nail, care should be taken not to over-ream so as to weaken the cortex. Over-reaming not only removes excessive quantities of bone, but may also result in thermal necrosis, increased operation time and blood loss, and additional comminution of the fracture fragments. However, the medulla must be over-reamed adequately for the safe passage of the nail – generally 0.5 mm for slotted nails and 1–1.5 mm for rigid nails.

Complications

1. Fat emboli. Identification of patients at risk (polytrauma, ARDS, pulmonary injuries, hypovolaemia) will alert one to this serious complication. Excessive reaming in these cases should be avoided, as this has been associated with increased fat and platelet aggregates as shown on transoesophageal echocardiography. Unreamed nails still cause fat emboli.

2. Implant size and length. The biomechanical characteristics of modern nails is such that smaller, stronger nails can be used with safety. Interlocking of these nails is recommended as there is a 98% union rate in the static mode, whereas shortening or mal-rotation can occur when leaving the nail unlocked.

Smaller diameter nails can be associated with a higher incidence of screw breakage, if the patient is allowed to weight-bear prematurely. Progressive weight-bearing should begin when callus is visible.

3. Infection. This is low in closed fractures (1–2%), but obviously greater in those with open fractures or those with significant soft tissue injuries.

Normal sterility and care with soft tissue handling reduces the infection rate. Treatment in the early stages can be with simple i.v. antibiotic therapy, but an exchange nailing procedure may be required for those with delayed union and infection.

4. Non-union and delayed union. The incidence of non-union in femoral fractures is relatively low (2%). Dynamization of the fracture fragments is rarely needed. Bone grafting of large defects may be required.

5. Malunion. The incidence of significant malunion in femoral fractures is rare, although approximately 2% of patients will have >20° malunion. This can be avoided by accurate reduction at the time of fracture fixation.

Angular malunion is more common in the proximal and distal segments of the bone, where it is difficult to obtain accurate reduction.

6. Neurovascular injuries. Traction injuries, as a result of adduction of the limb around a fixed perineal post in femoral fractures, can result in sciatic or pudendal nerve palsies.

Two-thirds recover completely, but in one third of cases there is a residual deficit. Care should be taken in positioning of the patient to avoid excessive traction, especially in femoral fractures.

7. *Implant failure.* The frequency of nail breakage is now reducing with the advent of stiffer implants. Fractures are more common through screw holes.

Related topics of interest

Femoral fractures – shaft, p. 49; Humeral fractures – shaft, p. 113; Intramedullary implants – reamed and unreamed, p. 125; Tibial shaft fractures, p. 291

KNEE – ACUTE COLLATERAL LIGAMENT INSTABILITY

These injuries are conveniently classified into either medial or lateral collateral ligament complex injuries. There may be associated cruciate or meniscal damage.

The medial collateral ligament (MCL) originates from the medial epicondyle of the femur and is inserted approximately 4 cm distal to the medial joint line on the proximal tibia. The MCL has classically been described as consisting of three layers: the first, and most superficial, is the crural fascia; the second, the superficial medial collateral (the primary static stabilizer to valgus stress); and the third, the menisco-tibial and menisco-femoral portions of the deep medial collateral ligament.

The superficial medial collateral (second layer) consists of vertical and oblique portions. The vertical fibres remain taut throughout the range of motion, while the oblique portions become lax with flexion. These oblique fibres are considered to be a separate entity and have been called the posterior oblique ligament.

The lateral collateral ligament (LCL) originates on the lateral epicondyle of the femur and is inserted into the head of the fibula. Injuries to the lateral side of the knee joint are considered as an injury to the complex rather than a single injury to the LCL (which is relatively rare). Again, the complex can be considered to consist of three layers: the first layer includes the ilio-tibial tract and superficial portion of the biceps femoris; the second layer includes the extracapsular lateral collateral ligament itself; and the third layer includes the joint capsule and arcuate ligament, as well as the popliteal tendon.

Medial collateral complex injuries

The MCL acts to resist external torque and valgus moment. Testing of the MCL should be undertaken in 20° to 30° of flexion. When tested in extension, the anterior and posterior cruciate ligaments (ACL and PCL) contribute to stability.

Isolated disruption of the MCL usually occurs as a result of a direct blow to the lateral aspect of the knee, in a slightly flexed position. As a result there is a valgus stress to the knee joint. Patients may describe a 'popping' or 'pulling' sensation on the medial side of the joint. Only 10% of MCL ruptures are the result of non-contact injuries. When the deforming force includes a rotational component, associated injuries to the cruciate ligaments may occur.

Classification

Typically, sprains of the ligament are graded according to the American Medical Association recommendations. A grade I tear is a result of damage to a minimum number of fibres with localized tenderness, but no discernible instability or laxity on testing. Grade II tears result in more ligamentous fibres being damaged with resultant localized swelling and possible mild laxity, but no significant clinical instability. Grade III tears involve disruption of a greater number of fibres with definite clinical laxity. These sprains can be further divided according to the amount of laxity as noted on clinical stress testing and assessed by opening of the joint line:

- Grade I: <5 mm.
- Grade II: 5–10 mm.
- Grade III: >10 mm.

Treatment

The majority of collateral ligament injuries can be treated non-operatively. Minor sprains, without significant instability, are treated with simple rest, ice, and compression bandages in the acute stages. Early physiotherapy may reduce the swelling, strengthen the quadriceps and hamstrings, and allow patients to return to activities more quickly.

More significant sprains (still with no significant instability) can be treated in a brace to allow the pain to settle and movement to commence.

Patients with significant instability should be mobilized in a hinge brace blocked at 30° flexion, which is removed at 3 to 6 weeks. Several studies have confirmed that healing of the MCL is improved with physical activity and early mobilization. Mobilization leads to higher load:failure ratios than in MCL injuries treated by immobilization.

Operative treatment of isolated MCL injuries is rarely necessary, although when associated with other significant injuries, it can be considered. Avulsions from the origin or insertion can be repaired with bone anchoring devices, and midsubstance tears can be sutured directly.

Treatment of the chronic, isolated MCL rupture is difficult. Simple reapproximations tend to elongate and stretch, especially when associated with antero-posterior instability. Augmentation with semitendinosis has been advocated, as has a bone–patellar tendon graft.

Lateral collateral complex injuries

The LCL is the primary ligament restraining lateral opening of the joint, and the ilio-tibial tract, popliteus tendon, arcuate ligament and capsule provide additional stability. This lateral capsular ligamentous complex has been shown to contribute to rotational stability of the knee.

Significant injuries to the lateral complex can result in marked instability. Isolated injuries of the LCL are relatively rare (20%) and can be treated non-operatively. Those in association with other ligamentous injuries should be stabilized early and primary re-attachment or re-suture is advocated.

Chronic LCL instability is often difficult to correct. Transfer of a portion of the biceps femoris muscle with tenodesis to the lateral epicondyle can restore some stability.

Combined tears of collateral and cruciate ligaments

Combined MCL and ACL injury is reasonably common. This is associated with a tear of the lateral meniscus in 50–60% and of the medial meniscus in 15–20%. Generally, the acute reconstruction of both ligaments is associated with an unacceptably high prevalence of stiffness, so repair is avoided. The vast majority of patients can be treated with cast immobilization for 4 to 6 weeks to allow the MCL to heal, followed by physiotherapy and rehabilitation. Subsequent rotatory instability can be addressed with ACL reconstruction, not less than 6 weeks after the original injury.

When the MCL injury is associated with a PCL injury, there has often been significant subluxation or dislocation. It may be possible to re-attach or reconstruct the PCL initially, but it is imperative to stabilize the collateral ligament and the posterior oblique ligament to ensure stability of the joint.

LCL complex injuries in association with PCL injuries can result in significant disability. The PCL should be repaired or reconstructed and the lateral complex repaired.

Complications

Although MCL injuries are relatively common in isolation, more significant injuries may well have resulted in damage to other structures within the knee. Ten per cent have associated meniscal damage and there should be a high index of suspicion for associated cruciate ligament injuries.

Operative repair of either collateral ligament can result in significant knee stiffness, and early physiotherapy is essential.

Further reading

Grood ES, Noyes FR, Butler DL, Suntay WJ. Ligamentous and capsular restraints preventing straight medial and lateral laxity in intact human cadaver knees. *Journal of Bone and Joint Surgery*, 1981; **63A**: 1257–1269.

Hughston JC, Andrews JR, Cross MJ, Moschi A. Classification of knee ligament instabilities. Part I: the medial compartment and cruciate ligaments. Part II: The lateral compartment. *Journal of Bone and Joint Surgery*, 1976; **58A**: 159–179.

Scuderi GR, Scott WN, Insall JN. Injuries of the knee. In: Rockwood CA, Green DP, Bucholz RW, Heckman JD, eds. *Fractures in Adults*, 4th Edn. Philadelphia: Lippincott-Raven, 1996; 2067–2074.

Shelbourne KD, Patel DV. Management of combined injuries of the anterior cruciate and MCLs. *Journal of Bone and Joint Surgery*, 1995; **77A**: 800–806.

Vailas AC, Tipton CM, Matthes RD, Gart M. Physical activity and its influence on the repair process of MCLs. *Connective Tissue Research*, 1981; **9**: 25–31.

Related topics of interest

Knee – cruciate ligament instability, p. 134; Knee – meniscal injuries, p. 144

KNEE – CRUCIATE LIGAMENT INSTABILITY

The anterior cruciate ligament (ACL) is one of the most commonly damaged ligaments of the knee and accounts for up to 50% of documented ligamentous knee injuries. The posterior cruciate ligament (PCL) is rarely injured and represents only 9–20% of injuries.

Anterior cruciate ligament

Clinical history

Injury to the ACL is fairly typical and patients often describe a non-contact, deceleration, twisting injury or occasionally a hyperextension injury. In over half of the cases patients will hear a 'pop' or feel something tear within the knee. There is an inability to continue playing sport or continue with their activity, followed by rapid swelling within the first 4–6 hours. Despite this typical history, the diagnosis is made in less than 10% of cases by the primary attending physician.

It is well-documented that up to 80% of patients attending the accident and emergency room with an acute haemarthrosis have sustained an injury to their ACL. Of these cases, 60% will have associated pathology within the knee at the time of initial presentation. This is either chondral damage, typically to the lateral femoral condyle, or a meniscal tear. The incidence of a meniscal tear increases with time and up to 80% of patients will have a meniscal tear within the first 3 years following the original injury. In contrast to the normal pattern of meniscal tears within the knee, the lateral meniscus is injured more frequently than the medial.

Clinical findings

The initial physical examination may be difficult because of swelling, pain and hamstring spasm, all of which can interfere with mechanical stability testing. Ligamentous examination involves the determination of anterior tibial translation in relation to the femur, and is best performed by the Lachman test. The anterior draw, pivot shift, flexion/rotation draw, Slocum and jerk tests have all been described.

It is rare that the ACL is injured in isolation and care should be taken in examining the medial, lateral, postero-lateral and postero-medial structures.

Instrument testing, using measuring devices (e.g. KT2000), can grade the degree of anterior translation and can be used to compare the side to side difference. The accuracy of these devices, however, has been questioned.

Plain radiographs can indicate a Segond fracture (a small capsular fracture of the margin of the lateral plateau) or an avulsion of the ACL attachment. The routine use of MRI is probably unnecessary. The reported accuracy for the diagnosis of a cruciate ligament tear is approximately 90–95%. The advantage of MRI, however, is in detecting other associated ligamentous, meniscal or chondral damage.

Management

1. Initial treatment is based on the reduction of pain and swelling, and the early restoration of normal joint movement. Thereafter, there is debate as to the need and timing of reconstruction surgery. Noyes has suggested a rule of thirds. One third of patients will be able to compensate and pursue normal recreational sports and will not require surgery. A further third will be able to compensate, but would have to reduce their sporting activities with the possible avoidance of jumping, pivoting or cutting exercises. The final third of patients do poorly and develop instability with not only sporting activities, but with the simple activities of daily living. In this group of patients early surgery will be required.

Daniel has suggested that early reconstruction reduces the risk of secondary degenerative change and the incidence of further meniscal damage. There is, however, at this stage, no evidence to suggest that an early reconstruction will allow the patient to return to unrestricted sporting activities without further problems, such as developing osteoarthritic change or a further meniscal tear.

2. *Conservative treatment* involves the re-education of the quadriceps and hamstring muscles. Emphasis should be placed on the hamstrings as they can restrict the amount of anterior tibial translation on the femur.

3. *Operative treatment* has traditionally used either an intra-articular reconstruction, an extra-articular reconstruction, or a combination of both. Isolated extra-articular reconstruction may be useful in the skeletally immature, when there is concern about damage to the growing physis. In isolation, extra-articular reconstruction is prone to failure within 3 to 5 years.

Primary intra-articular repair often fails unless there is clear evidence of bony avulsion from either the femoral or tibial attachments, where this can be re-apposed. In the majority of cases a reconstructive technique is required and a bone–patellar–tendon–bone or hamstring graft is the most frequently used method of reconstruction. These grafts may be used in conjunction with an extra-articular tenodesis (MacIntosh type) to augment stability.

Results

The results of conservative treatment depend upon patients' expectations and a desire to return to sporting activities. Low demand patients, who do not desire a return to sporting activities, do well without operative repair.

The results of operative reconstruction obviously vary, but the majority of studies suggest that 80–90% of patients can return to their pre-injury sporting activities. Long-term osteoarthritic degeneration is largely dependent on the state of the menisci, and when these can be resutured in preference to a partial or total meniscectomy, the risk of long-term degenerative change is lessened.

Patellar fractures, patellar tendinitis, patellar tendon ruptures and donor site pain have all been reported following bone–patellar–tendon–bone graft harvest.

Posterior cruciate ligament

Clinical history

The PCL is often injured in motor vehicle accidents as a result of a direct injury against the dashboard, when the knee is flexed to 90°. Falls on the flexed knee with the foot in plantar flexion, or forced hyperextension on the knee, can similarly result in PCL injuries. In isolation, even with total disruptions, there is often little long-term instability. When associated with postero-lateral or postero-medial injuries, stability of the knee is dramatically reduced.

Dashboard injuries are associated with injuries to the patellar tendon, patella and patello-femoral articulation. In those ruptures sustained as a result of a fall or twisting injury, 80% of patients may sustain a posterior third medial meniscal injury and the majority have anterior cruciate or medial collateral ligament tears.

The diagnosis is often relatively easily made on the history, but the posterior sag or posterior draw test, with the knee between 70 and 90° of flexion, is indicative of a tear of the PCL. The degree of posterior sag is graded according to the displacement of the tibia posteriorly on the femoral condyle. The reverse pivot shift test (with the tibia held in external rotation) helps identify postero-lateral corner injuries. Care should be taken in assessing damage to the postero-medial structures on valgus stress tests. Radiographic evaluation, with or without a posterior stress test, may show the degree of posterior subluxation. MRI not only demonstrates the cruciate injury, but again also helps to delineate other injuries within the knee.

Management

Non-operative treatment of isolated PCL tears is often successful. The initial aim is to reduce swelling and pain, and restore normal joint kinematics. Early active and isometric quadriceps exercises are used. Rarely is surgical treatment of the isolated PCL rupture necessary. In cases with associated ligamentous injury and gross instability or dislocation, reconstruction of the cruciate could be considered. In those cases with bony avulsion from the femoral or tibial attachment this can be fixed directly. In chronic cases, an autograft of patellar tendon, hamstring or an allograft can be used.

Results

The results of PCL reconstruction have been reported as poor, whereas conservative treatment of the isolated tear is generally adequate.

Further reading

Dandy DJ, Hobby JL. Anterior cruciate ligament reconstruction. *Journal of Bone and Joint Surgery*, 1998; **80B**: 189–190.

Dandy DJ, Pusey RJ. Long-term results of unrepaired tears of the PCL. *Journal of Bone and Joint Surgery*, 1982; **64**: 92–94.

Daniel DM, Fithian DC. Indications for ACL surgery. *Arthroscopy*, 1994; **94**; 434–441.

Noyes FR, Barber-Westin SD. A comparison of results in acute and chronic ACL ruptures of arthroscopically assisted autogenous patellar tendon reconstruction. *American Journal of Sports Medicine*, 1997; **25**: 460–471.

Noyes FR, Mooar PA, Matthews DS, Butler DL. The symptomatic anterior cruciate-deficient knee. Part I: the long-term functional disability in athletically active individuals. *Journal of Bone and Joint Surgery*, 1983; **65A**: 154–163.

Related topics of interest

Knee – acute collateral ligament instability, p. 131; Knee – haemarthrosis, p. 142

KNEE – DISLOCATION

Traumatic dislocation of the knee is relatively rare, but is a severe and potentially limb-threatening injury. High-energy trauma, usually an RTA, is the most common cause. Dislocation may occur following lesser injuries, such as a fall or sporting accident.

Classification

Several classifications are described relating to energy, position or ligament involvement. The simplest and most frequently used is that describing position, based on the displacement of the tibia with respect to the femur:

- Anterior: 35%.
- Posterior: 25%.
- Lateral: 10%.
- Medial: 5%.
- Rotatory: 5%.
- Occult: 20% (spontaneous reduction).

A classification based on the involved anatomical structures (torn ligaments) is complicated, but more relevant for surgical planning, prognosis and outcome comparison.

Mechanism and anatomical involvement

1. Anterior dislocation is principally a hyperextension injury, following a direct force to the anterior thigh with the foot fixed (for example on the floor). Hyperextension of >30° results in sequential disruption of the posterior capsule, PCL and ACL. Damage to the popliteal artery occurs with hyperextension beyond 50°.

2. Posterior dislocation may result from a dashboard-type injury, where the force is directed posteriorly on the flexed knee. The PCL is first disrupted, followed by the ACL and eventually the artery.

3. Lateral dislocation results from valgus stress, often with the tibia fixed and the thigh adducted. The MCL, postero-medial capsule and meniscal attachments are first disrupted, followed by the ACL and PCL.

4. Medial dislocation results from a varus force to the thigh, but may involve a rotational component. Lateral side structures are ruptured first.

5. Rotatory dislocation is usually associated with a twisting injury, on a fixed foot. The ACL, PCL and MCL or LCL may be disrupted, with rotation occurring on the intact collateral.

6. Open injury to the knee occurs in 30% of cases.

Assessment

This includes stability, vascularity and nerve function.

1. Stability. Gross deformity is the most striking feature on presentation, leaving little doubt of the diagnosis. However, the diagnosis of a true knee dislocation may initially be missed, as spontaneous reduction and re-alignment of the limb at the scene of the accident occurs in 20%.

Clues to the severity of the injury may be found on examination in extension. Significant varus or valgus instability in extension, indicates tears of the cruciate ligaments, as well as the corresponding collateral ligament. Exaggerated hyper-extension (recurvatum) implies combined cruciate and capsular instability.

2. Vascularity. This must be carefully assessed. Colour, temperature, capillary return, pedal pulses and non-invasive vascular studies, such as doppler ultrasound, must be undertaken in all cases. The presence of peripheral pedal pulses does not exclude a vascular injury.

3. Neurological function. This must be carefully assessed. The incidence of nerve injury is 25%.

Investigations

1. Plain X-rays should be undertaken following immediate reduction of the gross deformity. Bony avulsions of ligaments or capsule are often seen.

2. Early MRI is useful to assess complex ligament disruption and plan surgery.

3. Arteriography is required for vascular compromise. Some authors feel that an arteriogram is mandatory in all cases after reduction of a knee dislocation. The importance of recognizing a vascular injury cannot be underestimated.

Management

Priorities are reduction, revascularization and ligament stabilization.

1. Closed reduction and examination under anaesthetic is undertaken as soon as possible. Open reduction is required for open or irreducible cases. Most irreducible cases are due to the medial femoral condyle button-holing through the medial capsule.

2. Non-operative management. Stabilization and treatment of these injuries is controversial. Closed treatment requires 4 to 6 weeks immobilization. Less than 4 weeks results in chronic instability, but more than 6 weeks leaves a stiff joint. Closed treatment may be appropriate for dislocation associated with arterial injury or polytrauma, using a cast or preferably an external fixator. Subsequent stiffness is helped by manipulation and arthroscopy.

3. Surgical management aims to stabilize the knee and allow earlier mobili-zation. No studies have compared open with closed management. Timing of surgery depends on the condition of the patient and the limb. The first priority is to reduce the joint and re-establish limb perfusion. Controversy surrounds acute versus delayed ligament reconstruction. Meniscal re-attachment, and capsular and collateral ligament repairs should be undertaken acutely, as primary repair is often easier than secondary repair. Direct suture fixation of intraligamentous tears, in combination with ligament fixation to bone (using appropriate devices), is preferable. Subsequent immobilization in a cast brace with early passive motion is recommended. Delayed cruciate ligament reconstruction can be considered in patients with rotatory instability thereafter. Severe arthrofibrosis is associated with acute collateral and cruciate ligament reconstruction.

Associated injuries

1. ***Vascular injury*** to the popliteal artery occurs in 40% of dislocations. Early recognition is essential as popliteal artery occlusion for >8 hours is associated with a subsequent amputation rate of 85%. After closed reduction of a dislocation, the distal pulses return in only 10%. Intimal tears of the popliteal vessels may precipitate thrombus and subsequent arterial occlusion. The collateral circulation is often inadequate to maintain long-term viability in the presence of popliteal artery disruption.

Surgical exploration and revascularization should not be delayed. The reduced knee is bridged with an external fixator to facilitate vascular repair, and a four-compartment fasciotomy performed.

2. ***Neurological injury*** affecting the common peroneal nerve is seen in 25% and is often an axonotmesis. Primary exploration of the nerve and grafting has not been shown to be effective. Secondary exploration after 3 months has similarly produced poor results.

Complications

1. ***Early.*** Vascular, neurological, skin breakdown and infection.

2. ***Late.*** Stiffness, instability, degenerative change and foot drop.

Proximal tibio-fibular joint dislocation

This rare injury may occur in isolation or in association with major trauma. Classically known as 'horseback rider's knee', the injury more often follows parachute jumping. The mechanism is axial force on a knee flexed beyond 80°. Hyperlax individuals (Ehlers–Danlos) are more susceptible. The four types include: subluxation, postero-medial, antero-lateral and superior dislocation.

Closed reduction is usually successful and most are stable, allowing early mobilization. Complications include a peroneal nerve palsy which is usually transient.

Further reading

Kennedy JC. Complete dislocation of the knee joint. *Journal of Bone and Joint Surgery*, 1963; **45A**; 889–904.

Schenck RC, Hunter RE, Ostrum RF *et al.* Knee dislocations. *American Academy of Orthopaedic Surgeons Instructional Lectures*, 1999; **48**: 515–522.

Wascher DC, Dvirnak PC, DeCoster TA. Knee dislocation: initial assessment and implications for treatment. *Journal of Orthopaedic Trauma*, 1997; **11**: 525–529.

Related topics of interest

KNEE – EXTENSOR MECHANISM DISRUPTION

The extensor mechanism of the knee comprises the quadriceps tendon, the patella, the medial and lateral retinacular fibres, the patellar tendon and the tibial tubercle. Injuries can occur at any age, but quadriceps tendon avulsion or rupture is more common in mature adults and patellar tendon injuries are more common in younger adults. Disruption of the extensor mechanism is six times more frequent in males than females.

Direct injuries to the anterior aspect of the knee can result in damage to the tendinous attachment to bone, the patella or the tibial tubercle. Similarly, open injuries disrupt not only bone, but soft tissue attachments too.

Investigation

Where the clinical diagnosis is in doubt, plain X-rays may show a high riding patella, or an avulsion fracture. Soft tissue injuries can be delineated further with ultrasound or MRI. Ultrasound is useful to assess subsequent healing.

Avulsion injuries and rupture

Avulsion injuries can occur at the attachment of the:

- Quadriceps tendon to the superior pole of the patella.
- Patellar tendon to the inferior pole of the patella.
- Patellar tendon to the tibial tubercle.

1. Quadriceps tendon avulsion is three times as common as patellar tendon avulsion. These injuries result from forced contraction of the extensor mechanism, with the foot planted on the floor. Injuries to the quadriceps tendon are more common in elderly patients, sometimes with chronic illnesses, and 85% occur in patients over 40.

Quadriceps tendon avulsion occurs close to the superior pole of the patella, but the tendon may occasionally rupture more proximally. This may represent an attrition-type rupture, in the relatively avascular zone of the quadriceps tendon. In partial thickness ruptures, where the medial and lateral quadriceps muscles and retinacular fibres are intact, patients may be able to perform a limited straight leg raise, although a gap will be palpable on direct examination.

2. Patellar tendon avulsion typically occurs in patients under the age of 40 and is not associated with significant chronic illness or tendinitis. This is a rare injury. The most common location is from the inferior pole of the patella, and in skeletally immature patients this may be associated with the avulsion of a sleeve which may include a significant proportion of the chondral surface of the patella. A mid-substance rupture of the patellar tendon seldom occurs, except following penetrating trauma.

3. Treatment depends on the degree of disruption and the ability/inability to perform a straight leg raise, or achieve active knee extension.

When undisplaced, an avulsion can be treated in an extension cast or brace for 4 to 6 weeks before mobilization. When displaced, the avulsed fragments should be re-attached anatomically and held with screws, wires or strong bone sutures. The joint should be immobilized, depending on the quality and method of the fixation, to allow healing prior to starting rehabilitation.

Rupture of the quadriceps or patellar tendon should be repaired when the patient is unable to perform a resisted straight leg raise or actively extend the knee. Direct repair, using non-absorbable materials is preferable. Augmentation of patellar tendon repair with a wire around the patella and through the tibial tuberosity facilitates early mobilization, while protecting the repair. In those patients presenting late with quadriceps tendon ruptures, the operative repair is often complicated by the contraction of the quadriceps muscle proximally. If it is impossible to re-approximate the torn portions of the quadriceps tendon, a reinforcement of the repair with a Scuderi flap can be considered. V–Y advancement flaps, with attachment of the lengthened tendon to the patella via bone drill holes, has also been advocated.

Care should be taken when attempting to re-attach the tibial tubercle in the skeletally immature, as there is a risk of further damage to the growing physis.

Fractures

1. Tibial tuberosity. Tibial tuberosity fractures can follow a direct injury, but again are more common as a result of an avulsion. These have been classified by Ogden, according to the size and displacement of the fragment.

2. Patellar fractures. Patellar fractures are classified according to the degree of displacement and extent of comminution. A sleeve fracture may occur in children, with a sizeable portion of articular cartilage.

3. Treatment. Undisplaced fractures that have not disrupted the continuity of the extensor mechanism, and therefore allow some active knee extension and a straight leg raise, can be treated in an extension cast or brace. Active quadriceps rehabilitation is instituted at an early stage. When stable with minimum disruption, a cast may not be necessary provided patients are carefully supervised.

Sleeve fractures in children require reduction and fixation. Displaced fractures in adults require open reduction and internal fixation (see 'Knee – patellar fractures', p. 146).

Further reading

Houghton GR, Ackroyd CE. Sleeve fractures of the patella in children. *Journal of Bone and Joint Surgery*, 1979; **61**B: 165–168.

Ogden JA. *Skeletal Injury in the Child*, 2nd Edn. Philadelphia: WB Saunders, 1990.

Ogden JA, Tross RB, Murphy MJ. Fractures of the tibial tuberosity in adolescents. *Journal of Bone and Joint Surgery*, 1980; **62**A: 205–215.

Scuderi C. Ruptures of the quadriceps tendon. *American Journal of Surgery*, 1958; **95**: 626–635.

Siwek CW, Rao JP. Ruptures of the extensor mechanism of the knee joint. *Journal of Bone and Joint Surgery*, 1981; **63**A: 932–937.

Related topics of interest

Knee – acute collateral ligament instability, p. 131; Knee – cruciate ligament instability, p. 134; Knee – haemarthrosis, p. 142; Knee – meniscal injuries, p. 144; Knee – patellar fractures, p. 146

KNEE – HAEMARTHROSIS

Haemarthrosis of the knee is extremely common. Approximately 400 per 300 000 population attend Accident and Emergency Departments annually with such a complaint.

Classification

1. ***Primary (spontaneous) haemarthrosis*** occurs without trauma. Disorders of coagulation, such as haemophilia or anticoagulant therapy, may result in spontaneous haemarthrosis. Unless controlled with prophylactic treatment, or early medical intervention, this can result in extensive damage to the joint and secondary osteoarthritic changes.

Vascular tumours or malformations within the knee, although rare, can occur and bleed spontaneously following mild trauma. Arteriography is often required to confirm the diagnosis, followed by appropriate surgery.

2. ***Secondary haemarthrosis*** is a result of trauma:

- Eighty per cent follow damage to the ACL.
- Ten per cent follow dislocation of the patella.
- The remaining 10% include peripheral third meniscal separations, capsular tears, and osteochondral or osteophyte fractures.

Mechanism

In young patients, a sporting injury is common (70%), especially from netball, soccer or skiing. In the elderly, a fall is more common.

In the majority of cases there is a characteristic history of non-contact injury, twisting on the semi-flexed knee. Damage to the cruciate ligament can occasionally occur following hyperextension, or direct contact. The patient often describes hearing something 'go', being unable to continue playing and swelling within the first 4 to 6 hours. The rapid onset of swelling distinguishes haemarthrosis from an effusion, which is more often associated with a torn meniscus and characteristically does not develop for at least 6 hours following injury, or until the next day.

Investigations

Plain X-ray may reveal fractures or the fluid level of a lipohaemarthrosis. MRI may be increasingly available, but is unlikely to alter the management when compared with experienced clinical examination. Indications for MRI include: children, elite athletes, multiple ligament disruption and inconclusive examination.

Management of primary haemarthrosis

Adequate medical prophylaxis in those patients with a bleeding disorder, or rapid treatment of this disorder after an acute haemarthrosis, will lessen the chance of ongoing damage within the joint. Aspiration of the joint can be considered, although this risks further bleeding.

Management of secondary haemarthrosis

1. ***Initial management.*** The objectives are to alleviate initial symptoms, make a diagnosis and plan definitive treatment. Initial management consists of aspiration and re-examination.

2. *Aspiration* relieves tension, and hence pain, in the capsular lining. This reduces quadriceps and hamstring spasm, allowing better clinical examination. The aspirate is inspected for fat globules, which indicate exposure of cancellous bone and a fracture.

3. *Examination* attempts to make a definitive diagnosis and three groups emerge:
- A clear diagnosis.
- No diagnosis despite adequate examination.
- No diagnosis, but inadequate examination.

Where there is a clear diagnosis, specific treatment is commenced. When the diagnosis is unclear, despite adequate examination, an expectant policy is adopted, with mobilization, physiotherapy and subsequent re-evaluation. In those patients where examination has been inadequate, further investigation may be required to confirm the diagnosis, with EUA, arthroscopy or MRI.

4. *Arthroscopic assessment and irrigation* are difficult acutely, but allow a more accurate diagnosis. In cases with a peripheral third meniscal separation, direct meniscal suture can be performed.

5. *Definite indications for acute arthroscopy* include:
- Locked knee.
- Osteochondral fracture.
- Severe grinding on Lachman test.

6. *Relative indications for acute arthroscopy* include:
- Fat in the aspirate: concern over possible osteochondral fracture.
- Elite athletes: to confirm a diagnosis and optimize recovery.

Further reading

Allum R. The management of acute traumatic haemarthrosis of the knee. *British Journal of Hospital Medicine*, 1997; **58**; 138–141.

Lu KH, Hsiao YM, Lin ZI. Arthroscopy of acute knee haemarthrosis in road traffic accident victims. *Injury*, 1996; **27**; 341–343.

Maffulli N, Binfield PM, King JB *et al*. Acute haemarthrosis of the knee in adults. A prospective study of 106 cases. *Journal of Bone and Joint Surgery*, 1993; **75**: 945–949.

Related topics of interest

KNEE – MENISCAL INJURIES

The meniscus, once considered a vestigial structure, is now known to contribute not only to the load sharing, but also to the stability of the knee. When the knee is loaded in full extension, 70% of the compressive load through the lateral compartment is transmitted through the lateral meniscus and up to 50% of the medial load through the medial meniscus. The meniscus also provides secondary stability in resisting anterior tibial translation and this is especially important in the cruciate-deficient knee. Fairbank (1948) documented the degeneration of the knee following total menisectomy. Degeneration is more frequent with damage of the lateral meniscus.

Meniscal tears are caused by axial loading with rotational force. Damage to the meniscus can occur in isolation or in combination with ligamentous or chondral surface damage. In general, traumatic tears of the menisci occur in younger individuals and degenerative tears in patients over 35 years old. Degenerative tears are frequently associated with significant chondral damage.

Diagnosis

1. **Symptoms** are usually as a result of mechanical irritation within the knee, including 'locking', 'clicking', 'grinding' or 'giving-way'. Pain, although a frequent feature, is not always consistent. An effusion is common on the day following the original injury, but may settle completely.

2. **Physical signs** include the meniscal provocation tests of McMurray, Apley and Steinman. Joint line tenderness is frequently noted, but no single test is pathognomonic of a meniscal tear.

3. **MRI** is a useful diagnostic aid for selected patients, when the clinical signs are equivocal.

Classification

For ease of classification the meniscus is divided into anterior, middle and posterior thirds. The tear pattern is generally classified in accordance with the location in the meniscus and the type of tear. Further classifications relate to the vascularity of the meniscus. The peripheral or outer third of the meniscus is vascularized, whereas the middle two-thirds are not. Tears in the outer third may heal primarily or may be amenable to secondary suture.

Tears are further classified according to whether the tear pattern is vertical, longitudinal, radial or oblique. Vertical tears in the mid-substance of the meniscus usually extend to produce the classic bucket-handle tear, which can be well localized to the posterior third, the posterior/middle third or throughout the whole of the meniscus. Radial tears are more commonly found in the lateral meniscus, as are oblique or parrot break tears. Degenerative tears in association with a horizontal cleavage component can result in meniscal cyst formation. These are more commonly noted on the lateral side, although have been reported from the medial meniscus.

Treatment

1. **Symptomatic meniscal tears** warrant arthroscopic treatment, preserving as much meniscal tissue as possible. Tears in the periphery of the meniscus where

there is a reasonable vascular supply, are often amenable to re-suture. Tears in the avascular inner two-thirds are usually excised arthroscopically, leaving a stable rim of peripheral meniscal tissue. Care should be taken to avoid excessive removal of meniscal tissue, especially on the lateral side, in the region of the popliteal hiatus.

2. ***Meniscal repair*** can be performed with sutures or meniscal arrows, using an inside-out, all inside or outside-in technique. The aim of the procedure is to anchor the meniscal tear to the menisco-synovial junction. Meniscal arrows and other such fixation devices have recently been developed to facilitate an 'all inside' technique. Pullout strengths of these devices are inferior to suture techniques.

Results

Partial menisectomy is preferable to total menisectomy, but only 50–60% of people are satisfied with the outcome. Although often satisfied initially, the long-term results of menisectomy can be poor, with osteoarthritic degeneration within the knee. Approximately 44% of patients have pain after excessive or physical work at 8 to 10 years following partial menisectomy.

Further reading

Dixon AK. Magnetic resonance imaging of meniscal tears of the knee. *Journal of Bone and Joint Surgery*, 1996; **78B**: 174–176.

Fairbank TJ. Knee joint changes after menisectomy. *Journal of Bone and Joint Surgery*, 1948; **30B**: 664–670.

Faunø P, Nielsen AB. Arthroscopic partial menisectomy: a long term follow up. *Arthroscopy*, 1992; **8**: 345–349.

Mackenzie R, Palmer CR, Lomas DJ, Dixon AK. Magnetic resonance imaging of the knee: diagnostic performance statistics. *Clinical Radiology*, 1996; **51**; 251–257.

Schumacher SC, Markolof KL. The role of the meniscus in anterior–posterior stability of the loaded anterior cruciate deficient knee. *Journal of Bone and Joint Surgery*, 1986; **68A:** 71-79.

Seedhom BB, Dowson D, Wright V. Functions of the menisci. *Journal of Bone and Joint Surgery*, 1974; **56B:** 381–382.

Shrive NG, O'Connor JJ, Goodfellow JW. Load bearing in the knee joint. *Clinical Orthopaedics*, 1978; **131:** 279-287.

Walker PS, Erkman MJ. The role of the menisci in force transmission across the knee. *Clinical Orthopaedics*, 1975; **109:** 184–92.

Related topics of interest

Knee – acute collateral ligament instability, p. 131; Knee – cruciate ligament instability, p. 134; Knee – haemarthrosis, p. 142

KNEE – PATELLAR FRACTURES

Fractures of the patella account for 1% of all skeletal injuries and occur mostly within the 20–50 year age group. The incidence in males is twice that in females. Patellar fractures are usually the result of direct injuries and can be in isolation or in combination with ipsilateral femoral or tibial fractures. An indirect injury, as a result of tripping or stumbling, can result in avulsion fractures of the proximal or distal poles in adults. In the skeletally immature patient, indirect trauma is associated with a sleeve or chondral surface fracture.

Classification

Patellar fractures can be classified into:

- Transverse: 50–80%.
- Stellate (comminuted): 30%.
- Longitudinal (vertical): 12%.
- Proximal/distal pole (marginal).
- Osteochondral.

Displacement is defined as an articular step exceeding 2 mm, or separation exceeding 3 mm.

Methods of treatment

The history and physical findings are often very typical and there may be extensive contusion of the overlying skin. The treatment depends on the age of the patient and whether the extensor mechanism is intact, as there may be extensive tearing of the medial and lateral retinacular expansions. If the patient can perform a straight leg raise or has active knee extension, the extensor mechanism is intact. Extensor insufficiency with radiographic evidence of fracture displacement is the prime indication for surgical intervention.

1. Non-operative treatment is adequate for non-displaced fractures with a preserved extensor mechanism. If a tense haemarthrosis is present, aspiration is recommended, prior to immobilization in a cylinder or removable brace. Quadriceps exercises are recommended after a period of rest. The brace can be removed after 4 to 6 weeks.

2. Open reduction and internal fixation has been described with a cerclage wire, tension band wire and two Kirschner wires, or lag screw fixation. The surgical approach is through a mid-line incision. In those cases with extensive comminution, removal of the small fragments may be necessary. Immobilization is advisable until wound healing has begun, but early mobilization should be encouraged within a few days.

3. Partial patellectomy with repair of the extensor mechanism is preferable to internal fixation, when it is impossible to obtain a smooth articular surface. Resection of the inferior pole is only indicated in those with severe comminution, as this predisposes the patient to patella baja. Reconstruction of the normal anatomy is the goal in the majority of cases.

4. *Total patellectomy* is indicated in severely comminuted fractures, where there is no possibility of reconstruction.

Prognosis

Undisplaced fractures have a good or excellent outcome in over 90% of cases, with minimal pain and flexion beyond 120°. Displaced transverse and comminuted fractures treated by surgical fixation have excellent results in 40%, good in 45% and fair in 10%. Results are poor in 5%.

The long-term results after partial patellectomy range from 50 to 80% good or excellent. Weakness of the quadriceps mechanism ranges from a 15% to 50% reduction in isokinetic power, compared to the opposite side. The results of total patellectomy are very poor and 40% have an acceptable result. Weakness and instability are major problems, which do not fully recover. The patella should be excised only in exceptional circumstances. Even a single large fragment retained in isolation gives better results than total patellectomy.

Prolonged immobilization after fracture fixation may be detrimental to the long-term function of the knee, and early joint movement is to be encouraged.

In cases followed for several years, patellar arthritic changes ensue in >50% of displaced fractures. Non-union following internal fixation is uncommon (<3%). AVN is rare due to the good blood supply. Irritation from metalware is common and this often needs to be removed.

Further reading

Boström A. Fractures of the patella: a study of 422 patellar fractures. *Acta Orthopaedica Scandinavica*, 1972; **143**(S): 1–80.

Braun W, Weidemann M, Ruter A *et al.* Indications and results of non-operative treatment of patellar fractures. *Clinical Orthopaedics*, 1993; **289**: 197–201.

Carpenter JE, Kasman R, Matthews LS. Fractures of the patella. *Journal of Bone and Joint Surgery*, 1993; **75A**: 1550–1561.

Carpenter JE, Kasman R, Matthews LS *et al.* Biomechanical evaluation of current patella fracture fixation techniques. *Journal of Orthopaedic Trauma*, 1997; **11**: 351–356.

Koval KJ, Kim YH. Patella fractures. Evaluation and treatment. *American Journal of Knee Surgery*, 1997; **10**: 101–108.

Nummi J. Operative treatment of patellar fractures. *Acta Orthopaedica Scandinavica*, 1971; **42**: 437–438.

Related topics of interest

Knee – extensor mechanism disruption, p. 140; Principles of external fixation, p. 214

MYOSITIS OSSIFICANS

Myositis ossificans (MO) is a process of extraskeletal ossification in muscle and soft tissues, which most commonly follows elbow fractures, elbow dislocations and injuries with large haematomas, especially soft tissue injuries of the thigh. Haematoma formation is followed by an invasion of fibroblasts, which undergo metaplasia to osteoblasts and chondroblasts. The term really refers to the formation of bone in striated muscle, but is synonymous with heterotopic bone formation around a capsule or joint following trauma. The reactive bone formed is in effect a 'pseudoneoplastic' condition.

There are three distinct types of MO:

- Myositis ossificans progressiva.
- Traumatic localized MO.
- Non-traumatic localized MO.

Seventy five per cent of the localized types follow trauma, which should be differentiated from osteogenic sarcoma (OS) variants. The following are useful distinguishing features from OS (although it may be difficult to make this distinction, necessitating further investigation):

- MO occurs over the diaphysis (OS over the metaphysis).
- The pain and mass of MO decreases with time (unlike OS).
- On X-ray, the cortex is intact with MO (unlike OS).
- On biopsy, MO has a zonal pattern, with differentiated mature tissue peripherally.

Head injuries, burns and massive trauma are associated with MO. Prolonged immobilization and aggressive passive movement are thought to contribute to MO, while early active movement and indomethacin for 4 weeks are protective.

1. **Myositis ossificans progressiva** is a rare, non-traumatic condition, autosomal dominant with a high mutation rate, related to fibrodysplasia. Early in life, multifocal swellings appear, affecting the head, neck or trunk, followed by ossification of connective tissue in the muscles of the trunk and limbs. The thumbs and toes may be short, due to a short first ray, and are occasionally absent. The condition restricts movement and is usually fatal, due to respiratory compromise.

2. **Traumatic localized MO** is the formation of heterotopic bone in the striated muscle covering a fracture, restricting the movement of nearby joints. The cause is unknown, but may be related to joint movement which is too early and too vigorous.

The most common site is around the elbow, some 3 or 4 weeks after a fracture or dislocation, when movement spontaneously becomes restricted and painful, with X-rays showing calcification anteriorly. Treatment is rest, usually in a plaster cast for a few weeks, before commencing mobilization again. The mass of calcification gradually reduces and movement increases. Late excision may be beneficial.

MO may follow a soft tissue injury, without a fracture, most commonly in the thigh. The process starts soon after injury and is characterized by an enlarged, painful, warm thigh. Radiographic changes are seen within a couple of weeks. A hard mass of calcified tissue eventually forms, which may require excision.

Another common site is around the hip, after a dislocation or acetabular fracture. The incidence after a dislocation of the hip is 2%, but is increased by open surgery. Following an acetabular fracture the incidence is 5%, increasing to 35% after open surgery. The incidence can be reduced by a single fraction of radiotherapy, or preferably indomethacin for 4 weeks after surgery.

Proximal humeral fracture-dislocations are associated with MO, especially when chronically neglected.

3. *Non-traumatic localized MO* occurs spontaneously, without a documented history of trauma. The features are similar to traumatic localized MO, most commonly affecting the thigh of the young athlete.

Histology

A mature lesion of MO has zonal characteristics. Peripherally there is calcified woven bone, with trabeculae radiating towards the centre, where there are areas of immature trabecular bone, with proliferative osteoblasts and osteoclast-like giant cells. Early lesions have scattered fibroblasts and giant cells, in disorganized trabeculae and granulation tissue, which can mimic OS.

Further reading

Miettinen M, Weiss SW. Soft-tissue tumours. In: Damjanov I, Linder J, eds. *Anderson's Pathology*. St Louis: Mosby-Year Book Inc., 1990; 2512–2513.

Torg JS, Thompson TL. Complications of athletic injuries in young adults. In: Epps CH, ed. *Complications in Orthopaedic Surgery*. Philadelphia: Lippincott-Raven, 1994; 880–884.

Related topics of interest

Bone healing, p. 31; Bone structure, p. 34; Elbow dislocation, p. 43

NON-UNION – INFECTED

An infected fracture non-union is a disastrous complication. Management is difficult, prolonged and not always successful. It is important to determine whether the infection is still active, to identify the organism, and to determine whether the non-union is atrophic or hypertrophic and whether there is any sequestrated dead bone. When these factors have been determined, definitive management can be planned. Thirty per cent of non-unions are infected and 70% follow open fractures. The most common site is the tibia (~ 60% of cases). *Staphylococcus aureus* is isolated in 75% of cases.

Aetiology

The specific cause is not always apparent, but is related to injury severity and initial management factors, including:

- High grade open fractures.
- Inadequate debridement.
- Early inadequate internal fixation, especially with rigid plates and screws.
- Wound breakdown.

Assessment

1. History. A thorough and meticulous review of the history of the original injury and all management events, procedures, radiographs, microbiological cultures and antibiotic therapy, is vital to define the aetiology and infecting organisms. Relevant medical history and smoking habits should be reviewed.

2. Examination. An assessment of the local features is undertaken to consider the site of the injury, soft tissue viability, vascularity, sinus tracts, scars and pin sites, neurological function and viability of adjacent joints. Systemic assessment includes consideration of age, medical condition, nutritional status and other limb function.

3. Investigation. Full blood count, erythrocyte sedimentation rate (ESR), C-reactive protein (CRP), albumin and blood cultures are taken as indicators of the severity of infection. Wound swabs and samples are cultured, but often show contaminants only. Plain X-rays, tomograms, CT, MRI, technetium, gallium and indium labelled white cell scintigrams all have a place in the initial investigation. At surgery, methylene blue sinograms assist in identifying the precise location and extent of the infected tissue and dead bone.

Treatment

Treatment options are limb reconstruction or amputation. Amputation and a prosthesis may be the best option in the elderly or those not prepared to tolerate lengthy surgical reconstruction and rehabilitation. The outcome with a prosthesis is surprisingly good.

Reconstruction principles are:

- Debridement of dead tissue.
- Eradication of infection.
- Establishment of a healthy vascular bed with soft tissue cover.
- Bony reconstruction, stability and union.

Surgery may be staged. Quiescent cases without active signs of infection for 3 months may be managed as for a sterile non-union with a single-stage procedure. Active infection requires several stages to eliminate infection prior to achieving stability and union. Techniques vary considerably and depend on many factors including site, soft tissue deficit and bone loss, but in broad terms surgery can be considered in three stages.

Stage 1: Debridement, stabilization and eradication of infection. Radical debridement of all dead tissue, removal of metalwork and initial skeletal stabilization, usually with external fixation, is the first requirement. Dead bone can be difficult to identify, but extensive excision is preferential. Generous samples of tissue must be sent for prolonged enhanced culture before administration of antibiotics. A period of antibiotic administration is undertaken, usually i.v. over 2–6 weeks, augmented by local delivery, through cement beads or gel. Continuous irrigation (Lautenbach) may be utilized for extensive medullary sepsis of the femur. Repeated debridement may be necessary.

Stage 2: Soft tissue and bone reconstruction. Once adequate debridement has been achieved, soft tissue cover and elimination of potential dead space is required. Cancellous bone grafting, wound closure and irrigation may be undertaken. Inadequate soft tissue cover may be addressed by:

- **Papineau open technique** with open wet dressings on the clean cancellous grafted bed. When granulation tissue fills the defect a split skin graft can be applied.
- **Local or free flaps** may be used to reconstruct the soft tissues. Muscle flaps bring in an additional blood supply.

Small bone defects, <6 cm, may be managed by petalling and cancellous bone grafting. Stabilization may be achieved with internal or external fixation depending on the site. Large bone defects are better managed by vascularized graft (fibular) or bone transport with ring frames such as the Ilizarov. Bone transport involves radical bone excision, acute shortening and then a distant corticotomy, followed by distraction osteogenesis. This is attractive but complex, and should only be attempted in experienced hands.

Stage 3: Rehabilitation. Fixators may need to be in place for 6–9 months, with several surgical procedures during this period. Cast support is often required for up to 2 years. A multidisciplinary team approach to patient care and family support is essential in order to cope with the prolonged treatment and complications. Physical therapy is important to limit contractures and joint stiffness.

Complications

Complications are common in this complex management and include:

- Recurrent infection of bone, wound, pin sites, etc.
- Malunion or non-union.
- Soft tissue contracture.
- Neurovascular damage.
- Reflex sympathetic dystrophy.

Further reading

Rosen H. Non-union and malunion. In: Browner BD, Jupiter JB, Levine AM, Trafton PG, eds. *Skeletal Trauma*. Philadelphia; WB Saunders, 1998; 619–660.

Saleh M. Non-union surgery. Parts 1 and 2. *International Journal of Orthopaedic Trauma*, 1992; **2**: 4–24.

Related topics of interest

Bone defects, transport and late reconstruction, p. 25; Non-union and delayed union, p. 153; Principles of external fixation, p. 214

NON-UNION AND DELAYED UNION

Delayed union represents a slower healing period for a given fracture than expected and can be confirmed both clinically and radiologically. The rate of fracture healing is dependent on patient and fracture variables, including the severity of the initial injury, soft tissue damage, location, displacement, comminution, local blood supply, corticosteroids, diabetes, nutritional status, systemic disease and age. Pathological, open and segmental fractures have slower healing rates. Primary ORIF disturbs the soft tissues and prolongs the healing time, as *direct* bone healing occurs after rigid fixation and is slower than *indirect* bone healing with closed treatment.

Delayed union may progress to a state of non-union with failure of healing. Non-union is either hypertrophic (hypervascular) with abundant callus formation, or atrophic (hypovascular) with local bone resorption. In some cases, non-union stabilizes into a fibrous union, alternatively cartilaginous tissue and fluid may occupy the interval between fracture ends creating a pseudarthrosis (false joint).

In addition to the causes of delayed union, other causes of non-union include: infection, inadequate immobilization, failure of a fixation device, soft tissue interposition and aseptic necrosis of peri-articular fractures. There is an association between smoking and non-union. Treatment is by rigid stabilization of the fracture and bone grafting. Loading, micromotion and electrical stimulation are also used to promote healing.

Diagnosis

Delayed union is diagnosed clinically and radiologically. Clinical union occurs when sufficient internal and external callus formation stabilizes a fracture which becomes pain free. Radiological union is generally slower and demonstrated on X-ray by trabeculae crossing the fracture site. Where the diagnosis is in doubt, tomograms or a CT scan may be diagnostic. Measuring fracture stiffness is a more scientific method of assessing fracture healing, but is not currently available for clinical application.

The accepted times for delayed and non-union of common fractures in adults are given in *Table 1*:

Table 1. Times for delayed and non-union (weeks)

Bone	Delayed union	Non-union
Scaphoid	8	16
Clavicle	8	16–26
Ulna	8	16
Humeral shaft	8	16
Tibial shaft	16	36
Femoral shaft	20	44

Management of delayed union

The principle of treatment is to load the fracture and observe progress.

1. Where a locked IM nail has been used, the locking screws should be removed at 12 to 16 weeks if there are scant signs of union. Fifty per cent will progress to union. Metaphyseal and comminuted fractures are at risk of displacing.

2. Delayed union of the tibia may respond to fibular osteotomy and loading. In some series union rates of 75% are reported after fibular osteotomy or partial fibulectomy.

3. Delayed union of the humerus or tibia following conservative treatment may be addressed early by IM nailing.

Management of non-union

Treatment of non-union depends upon the modality of primary treatment and the aetiology of the non-union. In broad terms, the fracture should be exposed, rigidly stabilized and bone grafted with morsellized iliac crest cancellous graft. Interposed soft tissue should be removed. Stripping of periosteum alone may stimulate callus formation and fracture healing.

Infection must be eradicated and treatment may therefore be a staged procedure. Extensive bone loss or infection, sometimes combined with deformity, can be addressed with an Ilizarov fixator or similar ring fixation device to achieve distraction osteogenesis, bone transport and compression. Alternatively a vascularized graft (e.g. fibula) can be used. Allograft bone can also be used. BMP, and electromagnetic stimulation may have more widespread clinical applications in the future to promote union.

1. Non-union after conservative treatment is managed by open reduction, rigid fixation with a DCP or IM nail and bone grafting.

2. Non-union following IM fixation is addressed by exchange nailing, reaming up the intramedullary canal and inserting a larger diameter IM nail. Reaming has an ill-defined osteogenic effect and reamings act as bone graft, so exposing and grafting the fracture site is not always required. However, grafting is advisable and essential with extensive bone loss. Infected non-union can also be addressed by reaming, exchange nailing and antibiotic therapy.

3. Non-union following plate fixation requires revision of the fixation with a new plate or conversion to an IM nail, and grafting.

4. Non-union following external fixation is more challenging. The fixator should be removed and the fracture may heal with loading in a cast. If a fixator is removed, an interval of at least 2 weeks must be allowed for pin site healing before open or IM fixation, as infection may be introduced. Infection rates of 40 to 60% are reported for IM nailing after external fixation. The final option is revision to a more stable frame (e.g. ring fixator).

5. Non-union of peri-articular fractures, especially the proximal humerus and femur, should be addressed by replacement arthroplasty. Some elbow fractures can be treated in this manner with good results.

6. Electrical stimulation by direct current, inductive coupling or capacitive coupling, may accelerate bone healing.

7. Chronically infected non-union requires carefully planned management. Debridement of the infection, removal of any sequestrum and healthy soft tissue cover are prerequisites to union. Some long bone fractures respond to reaming, exchange IM nailing and antibiotic treatment. More resistant cases of infection need a staged procedure with external fixation to stabilize the fracture and followed later by bone grafting.

8. Amputation and a well-fitted orthosis should be considered for some cases of infected non-union and may be more appropriate than prolonged attempts at reconstruction. Amputation has a predictable outcome with rapid recovery and return to society, without extensive hospital treatment, pain and suffering.

9. The tibia is the most common site for non-union and warrants special consideration. The literature suggests a 90% union rate with exchange IM nailing without bone grafting for non-union, with the exception of grade IIIB and IIIC open fractures which require open bone grafting. Exchange nailing should be carried out at 16 to 20 weeks, but is complicated by infection in 10% of cases. Fractures with >30% circumferential bone loss, grade IIIB and IIIC fractures should be grafted at 6 to 8 weeks as part of the primary treatment programme. Reaming and exchange IM nailing of grade IIIB and IIIC fractures may reactivate quiescent infection. For grafting, the fracture is exposed through a postero-lateral approach.

Further reading

Court-Brown C, Keating JF, Christie J, McQueen MM. Exchange intramedullary nailing. Its use in aseptic tibial non-union. *Journal of Bone and Joint Surgery*, 1995; **77B**: 407–411.
Templeman D, Thomas M, Varecka T, Kyle R. Exchange reamed intramedullary nailing for delayed union and non-union of the tibia. *Clinical Orthopaedics*, 1995; **315**: 169–175.

Related topics of interest

Bone healing, p. 31; Infection and trauma, p. 119; Non-union – infected, p. 150

OPEN FRACTURE MANAGEMENT

Open fractures occur in isolation or in combination with polytrauma and are often high energy injuries with associated soft tissue damage. The open fracture is an orthopaedic emergency and immediate treatment is imperative, often in collaboration with plastic surgeons.

Classification

The Gustilo and Anderson classification divides open fractures into:

- Type I, puncture wound <1 cm with minimal soft tissue damage.
- Type II, wound >1 cm with moderate tissue damage.
- Type III, extensive tissue devitalization.

Gustilo, Mendosa and Williams expanded the original classification into: type IIIA, large wound, typically >10 cm, and extensive muscle damage but adequate skin cover; type IIIB, extensive periosteal stripping, with skin damage requiring a reconstructive procedure to close the defect; type IIIC, associated vascular injury requiring repair.

The mechanism of injury, degree of contamination and soft tissue damage are the key to the classification, not the length of visible skin wound. By definition, high energy, segmental or contaminated fractures are type IIIA, wounds requiring a skin graft or flap are type IIIB and high velocity missile wounds are type IIIB or IIIC – small entry wounds camouflage extensive soft tissue damage.

The AO classification distinguishes skin, muscle–tendon and neurovascular damage in separate categories. Skin wounds are: IO1, from inside-out; IO2, <5 cm skin breakage from outside; IO3, >5 cm skin breakage; IO4, considerable skin damage, contusion and loss; IO5, degloving. Muscle-tendon and neurovascular damage are graded from MT1 to MT5 and NV1 to NV5, respectively.

Management

Initial open fracture management includes assessment and resuscitation, soft tissue debridement, and fracture stabilization, which should all be achieved within six hours of the injury. Once the fracture is stabilized, wound care is easier and definitive skin cover can be achieved within a few days.

1. Assessment and resuscitation starts in the emergency department, with appropriate treatment of other injuries. The skin wound is documented, photographed, swabbed for microbiological culture and covered with an aqueous povidone–iodine or saline soaked gauze, which is not removed until definitive treatment in the operating theatre.

Intravenous antibiotics, historically flucloxacillin and benzylpenicillin (although there is a trend in favour of third generation cephalosporins), are started in the emergency department. Contaminated wounds require cover for Gram negative organisms. Tetanus prophylaxis must be considered.

2. Treatment of the soft tissues follows resuscitation, and the patient should be transferred to theatre for debridement and irrigation of the wound. Under general anaesthesia, foreign debris is removed, the skin margins excised and devitalized soft tissues debrided. The wound and fracture should be generously irrigated – minimum 6 l of warm saline. Aqueous chlorhexidine (0.05%) solution is more effective. A pressurized lavage system is preferable to remove debris, but there is some concern this may drive debris into the tissues.

To achieve adequate exposure of devitalized tissue, the wound may need extending with a longitudinal incision. This portion of a wound may be closed primarily, provided there is no skin tension.

3. *Stabilization of the fracture* depends upon the nature of the bone injury. Long bone fractures should be stabilized with an external fixator or IM nail. The choice remains controversial, with good results reported for external fixation and IM nailing up to type IIIB fractures. Unreamed nailing is advocated to reduce damage to the endosteal blood supply, although this subject is similarly controversial. External fixator pins must be carefully placed to avoid jeopardizing subsequent skin cover procedures. The use of plate fixation is contra-indicated, with the possible exception of forearm fractures where muscle cover is adequate. Intra-articular fractures should be reconstructed with the minimum of metalware. Type IIIC fractures, which do not require amputation, should be stabilized with an external fixator.

Some long bone fractures can be treated in plaster, but wound management is awkward.

4. *Skin cover.* There are no exceptions to the rule that skin wounds over an open fracture are not closed primarily. A joint capsule should be closed where possible, leaving the skin wound open. Viable soft tissues are placed without tension to cover the bone and the wound packed with a gauze and bandaged. The wound should be re-inspected within 48 hours, in consultation with the plastic surgeons, under full general anaesthesia in an appropriate operating theatre environment. Small wounds may be left to granulate. Larger wounds may be amenable to secondary closure, if the wound is healthy and the margins are not tight.

Large soft tissue defects require a reconstructive procedure. This may be a split skin graft or complex flap procedure – fasciocutaneous, myofascial, or microvascular free flap. The goal of treatment is to achieve definitive wound closure within 5 days of the injury.

5. *Duration of antibiotic therapy.* For type I, II and IIIA fractures, there is no benefit in giving antibiotics for more than 48 hours. A three-dose regimen may be adequate. More severe fractures require a longer course of treatment, which continues until skin cover is achieved.

Complications

As high energy injuries, open fractures are associated with a higher incidence of delayed and non-union. The incidence of infection is 1.5–2.5% for type II injuries and as high as 19–28% for type IIIB fractures. The overall incidence of non-union is 9%.

Pitfalls

Compartment syndrome necessitating fasciotomy may occur, despite the open injury. Inadequate debridement may lead to delayed wound healing and infection.

Debridement must be thorough and non-viable tissue excised at subsequent wound inspections.

Early wound closure, while desirable, should be delayed if the tissues are swollen or tight. Skin has elastic recoil and a superior cosmetic result can be achieved by securing the skin edges across an open wound with elastic bands stapled to the skin margins.

Neurovascular complications are associated with high-energy trauma. If the distal circulation is dubious, an arteriogram and vascular opinion are required. Nerve injuries should generally be repaired as a secondary procedure at 6 to 12 weeks from injury, although some may be treated earlier if appropriate.

Further reading

The Early Management of Open Tibial Fractures. British Orthopaedic Association and British Association of Plastic Surgeons. London, 1997.

Related topics of interest

Amputation and replantation, p. 158; Intramedullary implants – reamed and unreamed, p. 125; Non-union and delayed union, p.153; Principles of external fixation, p. 214

PAEDIATRIC FEMORAL FRACTURES

Femoral fractures represent 5% of all fractures in children, are generally mid-shaft, and treated by traction or stabilization in a hip spica. However, some femoral fractures are more challenging to manage and warrant special consideration. Under the age of 2 years, 70% are associated with non-accidental injury (NAI). Fractures of the femur are classified by site.

Femoral neck

Proximal femoral fractures are uncommon. Neck fractures follow severe high-energy trauma in 10–15 year olds. In young children NAI should be considered.

1. **Classification**
- Type I – transepiphyseal.
- Type II – transcervical.
- Type III – basicervical.
- Type IV – intertrochanteric.

2. **Undisplaced fractures** can be managed in a hip spica.

3. **Displaced fractures** first require reduction by traction, closed manipulation or open reduction. Stabilization with cannulated screws is advised for children over the age of 6 years. An acute transepiphyseal fracture is similar to a slipped upper femoral epiphysis (SUFE), but a careful history must be obtained to determine whether displacement is acute.

4. **Complications** principally affect type II fractures, with AVN occurring in 40–50%, usually within the first year. The treatment and age-related outcome is similar to Perthe's disease, but the AVN is more extensive. Non-union occurs in 10%. Type IV usually heal well. Growth arrest occurs in 20%, resulting in leg length discrepancy proportional to the age at injury.

Diaphysis

Diaphyseal fractures affect all ages, reflecting skeletal maturity.

- 0 – 5 years: weak cortex:cancellous strength ratio (50%).
- 5 – 10 years (30%).
- >10 years: high energy trauma (20%).

1. **Classification** is by site, displacement and open or closed type. The AO or Winquist and Hansen classification used in adults applies.

2. **Initial management** includes fluid resuscitation, fracture immobilization and treatment of associated injuries. Early immobilization is achieved by skin traction and a Thomas' splint.

3. **Non-operative management** is usually acceptable. In some situations operative fixation is advantageous, but convenience and expense must be balanced against complications.

Patients up to the age of 2 years are managed by Bryant's or 'gallows' traction. Immediate or early 1½ hip spica application with hip and knee flexion may be used.

At <6 months a simple splint or Pavlik harness is suitable for stable fractures. Union is quick and remodelling extensive.

Patients between the ages of 2 and 10 years are treated on balanced traction with a Thomas splint. A hip spica allows early discharge and may be used immediately if shortening is <2 cm, or applied at 3–4 weeks. Most fractures are healed by 6–8 weeks. Some children benefit from gait re-training.

Patients aged from 10 to 15 years are treated in balanced traction. Conversion to a single leg hip spica may be chosen at 4 weeks. Union is achieved at 10–12 weeks.

Patients over >15 years old are managed as adults with an IM nail.

4. Special consideration is needed for subtrochanteric and supracondylar fractures, as muscle forces cause rotation. This is overcome by hip and knee flexion in traction.

5. Indications for operative management are:
- Open fractures.
- Failed closed reduction.
- Loss of reduction.
- Segmental fractures.
- Polytrauma and ipsilateral fractures.
- Neurovascular injury.

6. Operative techniques are similar to adults including:
- Retrograde insertion of flexible nails, avoiding growth plates, is a popular technique and most suitable for 10–15 year olds.
- Rigid IM nails may damage the epiphyseal plate and vascular supply of the femoral head during insertion, and are most suitable for adolescents nearing maturity. Advantages include early mobilization, reduced X-ray exposure and reduced cost, when compared to non-operative management.
- ORIF with a plate is reserved for subtrochanteric fractures and polytrauma victims as an alternative to flexible nails, or following failure of non-operative management.
- External fixation is a relatively safe and reasonable option, most suited to >5 year olds with open fractures and polytrauma.

7. Complications. Length discrepancy with shortening or overgrowth is common, but seldom noticed unless >1.5 cm. Shortening or overlap may be present initially or develop during non-operative management. Fracture healing stimulates growth, resulting in an average overgrowth of 1.5 cm before puberty and less after puberty. Thus anatomical reduction in the young leads to overgrowth, and optimal reduction includes shortening to compensate for the overgrowth.

Malunion and angular deformity depend on age, distance from the physis and plane of deformity. Varus/valgus deformity should be <10°. In the AP plane, 45° remodels in infants, but in adolescents only 10° is acceptable.

Distal femoral epiphyseal fractures

Distal femoral fractures, previously described as 'wagon wheel' fractures as a leg caught between the spokes was the traditional mechanism of injury, are high-energy RTA or sports injuries.

1. Classification. Fractures are described by direction, degree of displacement and Salter–Harris type. S–H II are most common.

2. Management. Undisplaced fractures are managed in a cast for 6 weeks. Displaced fractures require anatomical closed or open reduction. Fixation is advised for displaced S–H II and mandatory for displaced S–H III and IV fractures. Fixation is by K-wires or intra-epiphyseal screws.

3. Complications. These include injury to the popliteal vessels or peroneal nerve. Redisplacement and growth arrest, leading to length discrepancy and angular deformity may occur. Growth disturbance occurs in 30% of displaced fractures, which is significant as the distal femur contributes 70% of femoral growth at an average of 1 cm/year.

Further reading

Kasser J. Femoral shaft fractures. In: Rockwood CA, Wilkins K, Beaty J, eds. *Fractures in Children*, 4th Edn. Philadelphia: Lippincott-Raven, 1996; 1195–1230.

Macnicol MF. Fracture of the femur in children. *Journal of Bone and Joint Surgery*, 1997; **79B**: 891–892.

Stannard JP, Christensen KP, Wilkins KE. Femur fracture in infants: a new therapeutic approach. *Journal of Pediatric Orthopedics*, 1995; **15**: 461–466.

Wilkins KE. Operative management of children's fractures: is it a sign of impetuousness or do the children really benefit? *Journal of Pediatric Orthopedics*, 1998; **18**: 1–3.

Related topics of interest

PAEDIATRIC FOREARM FRACTURES

Fractures of the upper limb account for 70% of children's fractures and the majority involve the distal radius.

The distal radial and ulnar ossification centres appear at 2 and 5 years, respectively, fusing at 18 years. The radial head ossifies at 5 years. Eighty per cent of forearm growth occurs distally.

Site of fracture
- Physis: 15%.
- Metaphysis: 65%.
- Shaft: 20%.

Distal radius and ulna
Distal fractures occur in all age groups, but commonly in boys of 10 to 13 years, after a 'fall on the outstretched hand' during recreational activities.

1. Radial physeal fractures are classified according to Salter and Harris. Most are managed by closed reduction and plaster for 4 to 6 weeks. Fifty per cent translation and 25° angulation may be accepted, if 1 year or more of growth remains. Open reduction is indicated with compartment syndrome, median nerve compression, ipsilateral elbow fractures and failure to obtain acceptable closed reduction. K-wire fixation usually suffices. Growth arrest occurs in 5% of cases.

2. Isolated ulnar physeal fractures are rare. Transepiphyseal fractures are associated with Galeazzi fractures and growth arrest in 50% of cases.

3. Metaphyseal radial fractures occur around puberty. Ninety nine per cent are dorsally angulated. Classification is according to the direction of displacement (dorsal or volar), associated ulnar fractures, and fracture characteristics (buckle, greenstick, complete).

- Buckle fractures are 'compression failure' of one cortex, with a cortical 'crumple' on X-ray. The fractures are stable, requiring 3 to 4 weeks in a cast.
- Greenstick fractures are 'tension failure' in one cortex, hinging on the opposite periosteum. Dorsal angulation of 10° is accepted. Volar displacement is less stable and should be observed closely. Displaced fractures require reduction, 6 weeks in a cast and close follow-up for re-angulation.
- Complete, displaced fractures require reduction and 6 weeks in a cast. Acceptable reduction includes 80% medial–lateral contact, and 50% dorsal–volar contact. Angulation depends on age: if <9 years, 15° in either plane is acceptable; if >9 years, 10° on lateral and <10° on AP is acceptable. A well-moulded below-elbow cast with a 'cast index' of <0.7 (AP diameter/medial–lateral diameter) reduces the incidence of subsequent displacement. Review after 1 week and 2 weeks should be undertaken.
- Some favour percutaneous K-wire fixation of displaced fractures, especially if the ulna is intact.
- Open or percutaneous stabilization is required for open fractures, bifocal fractures, irreducible fractures and where >50% radial translation occurs with an intact ulna.

Shaft (diaphysis) of radius and ulna

Shaft fractures occur in children aged 6–8 years. One bone may be fractured in isolation. There may be a fracture, plastic deformation, or dislocation of the other. Fractures are classified by site (proximal, middle and distal thirds) and by displacement.

1. **Angulation** is the most common deformity, seen clinically and on X-ray.

2. **Rotation** is harder to assess, so the radial bow, cortical width, interosseous gap and orientation of bony landmarks are used. For the radius, when the biceps tuberosity points medially, the radial styloid points laterally. For the ulna, when the coronoid points anteriorly, the ulna styloid is posterior.

3. **Management** depends on displacement. Minimally displaced fractures are managed in an above-elbow cast for 6 weeks, with an X-ray at 1 week. The limits of acceptable displacement are controversial, reducing with age: if <10 years, 15° angulation and if >10 years, 10° angulation. A malrotation of 30° may be compensated for at any age. Complete displacement, or 'bayonet', is acceptable in younger patients, but a well moulded above-elbow cast in neutral or supination is essential, as re-angulation occurs in 7–10%.

4. **Plastic deformation** occurs because of wider haversian canals in the younger bone. Reduction is undertaken with slow steady pressure.

5. **Open fixation** is required for compartment syndrome, associated neurovascular injury, inadequate closed reduction, open fractures, displaced fractures in adolescents and some cases of re-displacement. Open stabilization is by plate, K-wire, or flexible IM nail.

6. **Monteggia fractures** of the ulna with radial head dislocation were classified by Bado (1967) (*Table 1*). Management by closed reduction in a cast with >90° elbow flexion is usually adequate. Open surgery is required for failure of reduction. Complications include a missed diagnosis with a chronically dislocated head, which should be reduced in the young and may need ulnar lengthening. Older patients require excision of the radial head if symptomatic. Posterior interosseous nerve injury occurs in 10%. Exploration and division of the arcade of Fröhse is advised if there is no recovery at 3 months.

Table 1. Bado classification of Monteggia fractures

Type	Frequency (%)	Direction of head dislocation	Apex of fracture
I	70	Anterior	Anterior
II	5	Posterior	Posterior
III	24	Lateral	Lateral
IV	<1	Anterior	Posterior (radius and ulna shaft fracture)

7. **Galeazzi fractures** follow similar treatment principles to adults. Ulnar head dislocation may be dorsal or volar. After reduction, immobilization is in supination for dorsal dislocation and pronation for volar dislocation. Occasionally, ORIF of the radius is required.

Radial neck fractures

Radial neck fractures are uncommon (5% of elbow fractures) and classified as:

- Type I: <30° displacement.
- Type II: 30–60° displacement.
- Type III: >60° displacement.

Type I are the most common, following a fall on the outstretched hand with a valgus force. Type II and III are associated with olecranon fractures or medial epicondyle avulsions. Arthrography is a useful means of outlining the cartilaginous head. Thirty degrees of neck angulation, but only 2 mm of translation, are acceptable and managed non-operatively in a cast for 2 weeks before mobilization. With 30°–60° angulation, closed reduction may be successful. With >60° angulation, reduction with a percutaneous pin or open reduction, stabilizing the head with a wire into the proximal ulna is required.

Proximal ulna

1. Metaphyseal fractures are uncommon and >50% are associated with other elbow fractures. Classification: A, flexion; B, extension; and C, shear. Minimally displaced fractures are casted for 2–3 weeks. Displaced flexion types may require tension band fixation with fine wire or absorbable sutures.

2. Coronoid fractures are classified as: I, tip; II, <50%; III, >50% and may be associated with a dislocation. Most are managed non-operatively.

Further reading

Bado JL. The Monteggia lesion. *Clinical Orthopaedics*, 1967; **50**: 71–86.

Chambers H, Fernando De La Garza J, O'Brien E *et al*. Fractures of the radius and ulna. In: Rockwood CA, Wilkins K, Beaty J, eds. *Fractures in Children*, 4th Edn. Philadelphia: Lippincott-Raven, 1996; 449–652.

Cullen MC, Roy DR, Giza E *et al*. Complications of intramedullary fixation of paediatric forearm fractures. *Journal of Pediatric Orthopedics*, 1998; **18**: 14–21.

Related topic of interest

Paediatric fracture principles, p. 165.

PAEDIATRIC FRACTURE PRINCIPLES

Paediatric bones differ from their adult counterparts in three main ways: the presence of a growth plate, different biomechanical properties and the ability to remodel during growth.

Bone growth

There are two major mechanisms of growth:

1. Intramembranous ossification. The cranial bones, facial bones and part of the clavicle are formed by intramembranous ossification. Cells of mesenchymal origin develop sites of primary ossification in the absence of a cartilaginous precursor. Intramembranous ossification is responsible for the increase in the diameter of long bones during growth.

2. Endochondral ossification. A cartilaginous precursor is replaced by osseous tissue, commencing in the ossification centres. The primary ossification centre of all the long bones is present by the twelfth week *in utero* and secondary ossification centres appear after birth. The exception is the secondary ossification centre of the distal femur, which is present at birth.

The secondary ossification centres lie within the epiphysis. The epiphysis is separated from the metaphysis by the 'physis' or 'growth plate'. The physis is divided into zones based on function. The zones, in order, from epiphysis to metaphysis are:

- Reserve.
- Proliferative.
- Hypertrophic.

Classically, physeal injuries were considered to occur through the zone of provisional calcification, which is a subzone of the hypertrophic zone. In reality, the injuries can occur in any zone.

Paediatric fracture patterns

Paediatric bone is more porous and more elastic, with a thicker periosteum, than adult bone. Thus paediatric bone is less likely to fracture across both cortices and the fracture is less likely to be comminuted. As the child approaches adolescence, the fracture patterns become similar to the adult. The following fracture patterns are not seen in adult bone.

1. Greenstick. An incomplete fracture. The cortex and periosteum remain intact on the compression side.

2. Torus. A buckle fracture secondary to compression. Torus fractures are most common in the porous bone of the metaphysis.

3. Plastic bowing. The bone bends under a compressive load. When the elastic limit of the bone is exceeded the deformity becomes irreversible.

Physeal injuries

1. The physis fails in torsion. The physis is normally stabilized by *mammillary projections* and *lappets*. The *mammillary projections* are interdigitating bumps between the metaphysis and epiphysis. The *lappets* are extensions of the physis up and around the metaphysis. Physeal injuries make up approximately 15% of all childhood fractures and are most commonly seen in the phalanges (37%), distal radius (18%), distal tibia (11%) and distal fibula (7%).

2. Salter and Harris (1963) have classified five types of injury (*Figure 1*). Rang (1969) added a sixth type and Ogden (1981) added types seven, eight and nine.

- Type I (8%). Complete separation of the epiphysis and metaphysis through the physis. This is seen in younger children.
- Type II (73%). A physeal fracture, extending into the metaphysis. A triangular fragment of metaphysis is created – on X-ray this is known as the 'Thurston–Holland' sign.
- Type III (6.5%). A split of the epiphysis, extending into the joint.
- Type IV (12%). A vertical split through the epiphysis, physis and metaphysis.
- Type V (<1%). Compression of the physis. This is often not recognized acutely as the X-ray is normal. The patient presents late with growth arrest.
- Type VI (<0.5%). Injury of the perichondral rim (zone of Ranvier) around the physis.
- Types VII, VIII and IX are discussed in Ogden's paper (see Further reading).

Treatment of physeal injuries

Type I. Closed reduction and immobilization is usually satisfactory. Approximately 3% develop a growth arrest.

Type II. Closed reduction, but a K-wire is occasionally required. Reduction is sometimes blocked by interposed periosteum, particularly in the distal tibia. The wire is best placed through the Thurston–Holland fragment; however, it is permissible to pass a thin, non-threaded wire across the physis. Manipulation after 5–7 days is

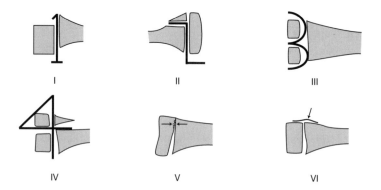

Figure 1. The Salter and Harris classification of physeal fractures. Types I to IV can easily be remembered, although it should be noted that type II is viewed as a mirror image. Type IV is the 'Rang' fracture, with injury of the perichondral rim.

controversial – some consider this will further damage the physis, and prefer to perform a late osteotomy.

Type III. Requires anatomical reduction usually with ORIF. Some authors do not even accept 2 mm of displacement. Fixation is with transverse wires or screws, fixing epiphysis to epiphysis. Growth arrest is common, but frequently unimportant as the fracture occurs around the time of skeletal maturity.

Type IV. As with type 3, this is an intra-articular fracture and often needs ORIF.

Type V and VI. These are diagnosed late.

Complications of paediatric fracture

1. Overgrowth. Particularly in the femur, fracture of the diaphysis may lead to overgrowth of the bone, secondary to disruption of the periosteum, which acts as a restraint to growth.

2. Shortening. Either due to malunion or complete physeal arrest.

3. Malunion. Potential for remodelling is greatest in the younger child, with an injury close to the physis and angulation in the same plane as the major plane of motion of the joint. Rotational deformity does not correct spontaneously.

4. Angular deformity. From partial physeal arrest.

Physeal arrest

Physeal arrest is most commonly secondary to trauma (70%); other causes include infection, irradiation, tumour and developmental abnormalities. Growth arrests occur in the 2 years following injury. The 'transverse lines of Park' or 'Harris lines' are useful markers of growth arrest. A line converging on the physis suggests growth arrest.

1. Complete growth arrest causes shortening and is treated with a shoe-raise or leg lengthening. Alternatively epiphysiodesis or shortening of the opposite side may be performed.

2. Partial growth arrest causes angular deformity or shortening. Ogden and Bright divided partial growth arrest into three patterns:

- Central bridges – shortening with less angular deformity.
- Peripheral bridges – involving the zone of Ranvier, producing angular deformity.
- Linear bridges – more common after Salter–Harris type IV injuries, producing angular deformity and shortening.

In a teenager approaching maturity, surgical treatment may not be required. A leg length discrepancy of 2.5 cm is well tolerated. Menelaus has shown that ultimate discrepancy can be predicted by assuming that the distal femur grows by ⅜ of an inch, and the proximal tibia by ¼ of an inch per year, and that boys stop growing at 16 and girls at 14.

The classic operation for partial arrest is resection of the bone bridge (Langenskiöld), giving the best results when <50% of the physis is involved and there is >2 years growth remaining. Central or linear bridges respond better than peripheral bridges.

Most cases requiring surgical treatment are in the distal femur (35%), distal tibia (30%) and proximal tibia (16%). The bone bridge is localized by X-ray, tomography and CT. Treatment is resection and interposition grafting. Fat has been interposed, but solid, load sharing grafts, such as silastic, elastomer or poly-methylmethacrylate are better.

Further reading

Ogden JA. Injury to the growth mechanism of the immature skeleton. *Skeletal Radiology*, 1981; **6**: 237–253.

Ogden JA. Skeletal growth mechanism injury patterns. *Journal of Pediatric Orthopedics*, 1982; **2**: 371–377.

Peterson HA, Madhok R, Benson JT *et al.* Physeal fractures: epidemiology in Olmsted County, Minnesota, 1979–1988. *Journal of Pediatric Orthopedics*, 1994; **14**: 423–430.

Rang M. *The Growth Plate and Its Disorders.* Baltimore: Williams and Wilkins, 1969.

Salter RB and Harris WR. Injuries involving the epiphyseal plate. *Journal of Bone and Joint Surgery*, 1963; **45A**: 587–622.

Related topics of interest

Paediatric femoral fractures, p. 159; Paediatric forearm fractures, p. 162; Paediatric non-accidental injury, p. 175; Paediatric spine trauma, p. 177; Paediatric tibial fractures, p. 180

PAEDIATRIC HUMERAL CONDYLAR FRACTURES

Twenty five per cent of fractures around the elbow in the child are condylar fractures and 70% of these involve the lateral condyle. The remainder involve the medial condyle or epicondyle. T or Y intercondylar fractures are rare.

As much of the paediatric skeleton is cartilage, radiological interpretation may be very difficult and the extent of the fracture, degree of displacement or rotation easily mistaken. Extreme caution should be exercised, and where the diagnosis is uncertain, an arthrogram or stress X-rays obtained, or the elbow screened under the image intensifier. X-rays of the opposite elbow provide a useful comparison. A missed diagnosis or inappropriate treatment can have severe long-term consequences.

Classification

The *Milch classification* refers to medial and lateral condylar fractures of the humerus, with type I passing through the capitellum or medial condyle, fracturing off the condyle, leaving the trochlear ridge intact. Type II fractures pass close to the trochlear sulcus and include the trochlear ridge, allowing the elbow joint to sublux. Milch type I are Salter–Harris type IV fractures and type II behave as Salter–Harris type II fractures, although some authors classify them as Salter–Harris type IV.

Fracture patterns and treatment

1. Lateral condylar fractures typically occur in the 6-year-old child (*Figure 1*). Milch type I are uncommon and Milch type II more common. The fractures are further divided into non- or minimally displaced (<2 mm), moderately displaced

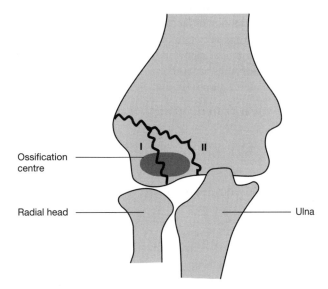

Figure 1. The Milch classification of lateral condylar fractures of the humerus. Note that type I is a Salter–Harris type IV injury, and that type II is a Salter–Harris type II injury.

(>2 mm) and completely displaced. Some displaced fractures are grossly rotated, with the fragment hinging on the collateral ligament complex.

Type I injuries show some metaphyseal bone on X-ray and are usually stable. Undisplaced fractures can be supported in plaster for 3 weeks before starting mobilization. Ten per cent of minimally displaced fractures displace in plaster and check X-rays should be obtained at 5–7 days.

Displaced Milch type I and II fractures require open reduction and fixation, either with smooth K-wires or small fragment screws. Where there is doubt about the degree of displacement or stability, there should be a low threshold for surgical exploration and fixation. The fracture is exposed through a postero-lateral approach, reduced with minimal disturbance of the soft tissues (especially posteriorly) and stabilized. If possible, fixation should be through the metaphyseal bone spike. To prevent rotation, two pins are required and where the metaphyseal spike is small, the pins can pass through the epiphysis, without causing significant growth disturbance in the majority of cases. One transverse and one oblique K-wire provides the greatest rotational stability. Screw fixation through the metaphyseal fragment is more stable, and very good results are reported, without growth disturbance. Overall, 90% of patients have excellent or good results.

Stabilization should be augmented with plaster immobilization. The K-wires are removed at 4 weeks if union is adequate and the elbow mobilized. Delayed or non-union may occur.

2. *Medial condylar fractures* are less common than lateral condylar fractures. The principle of treatment is the same, with a low threshold for stabilization of displaced fractures.

3. *Medial epicondylar fractures* represent 10% of all elbow injuries in the child. The fracture is rare before the age of 10 and usually an avulsion injury which can be treated conservatively. More severe injuries may be associated with elbow dislocation and instability of the lateral collateral ligament complex. The fragment can occasionally become trapped in the joint. On rare occasions with a displacement greater than 1 cm, or elbow instability, screw or K-wire fixation may be required. However, the results of conservative treatment are good. Stiffness can be a problem and early mobilization is recommended.

4. *Intercondylar fractures* are rare (1%) and when displaced, require internal fixation.

Complications

1. *Non-union*, defined as >12 weeks, should be treated by bone graft and revision fixation.

2. *Cubitus valgus* is caused by non-union of a lateral condylar fracture, or occasional growth arrest of the epiphysis. This can be corrected with an opening lateral osteotomy, or a closing medial osteotomy, supplemented with bone graft and fixation. The deformity is greater following Milch type II injuries, and lateral displacement with an opening wedge osteotomy of the distal humerus will be required to prevent an unacceptable cosmetic deformity.

3. _Tardy ulnar nerve palsy_ is a late consequence of cubitus valgus deformity, developing over a period of 2 to 3 decades.

Further reading

Macnicol MF. Indications for internal fixation. In: Benson MKD, Fixen A, Macnicol MF, eds. _Children's Orthopaedics and Fractures._ Edinburgh: Churchill-Livingstone, 1994; 707–720.

Thomas IH. Fractures in children. In: Gregg PJ, Stevens J, Worlock PH, eds. _Fractures and Dislocations – Principles of Management._ Oxford: Blackwell Science, 1996; 237–248.

Related topics of interest

Humeral fractures – distal, p. 107; Paediatric humeral supracondylar fractures, p. 172

PAEDIATRIC HUMERAL SUPRACONDYLAR FRACTURES

Supracondylar fractures account for 65% of fractures around the elbow in the child. With much of the paediatric skeleton being cartilage, radiological interpretation may be difficult and the extent of the fracture, degree of displacement, or rotation, easily overlooked. Caution should be exercised and where the diagnosis is uncertain, an arthrogram can be helpful. X-rays of the opposite elbow provide a useful comparison. Inappropriate treatment, or a missed diagnosis, can cause severe long-term complications. Neurovascular injuries are common and should be carefully assessed.

Supracondylar fractures are more common in boys, in the left arm and around 5 to 8 years of age. Baumann's angle (the angle between the long axis of the humerus and the physeal line of the lateral condyle, with a true AP X-ray), ranges from 64° to 82°, mean 75°.

Fracture patterns and associated injuries

1. *Displacement into extension,* with the distal fragment posterior, is the most common pattern and classified as type I, undisplaced; type II, displaced with the posterior cortical hinge intact; type III, completely displaced. Type III injuries more commonly have postero-medial displacement, but displacement may be postero-lateral. The approach to fixation is different.

2. *Displacement into flexion* occurs in 2 to 6% of cases and requires more aggressive treatment.

3. *Floating elbow* occurs in 5% of cases, with a forearm fracture in addition to the supracondylar fracture. Fixation is usually required.

4. *Neurovascular injuries* occur in a substantial number of patients and include:

- Neurological injury in 3 to 15% of cases. The radial nerve is most frequently involved – 55% radial, 30% median, 15% ulnar. There may be subtle impairment of the anterior interosseus nerve, with weakness of FDP to the index finger and FPL, and normal sensibility. Almost all neurological injuries recover within 2 to 3 months.
- Vascular injury is much higher than the 0.5% reported historically. Figures up to 38% have been reported, including simple compression, spasm, an intimal tear, or rarely complete rupture of the brachial artery. Where there is clinical suspicion of a vascular injury which does not respond to reducing the fracture, further investigation is by Doppler measurement, comparing the wave form with the opposite limb, or arteriography if time permits. Urgent surgical exploration should be undertaken in consultation with a vascular surgeon if the clinical signs are obvious, or if there is any delay with investigation. A digital pulse oxymeter can be misleading and unreliable, as there is usually sufficient collateral circulation to maintain skin perfusion distally. However, there may not be sufficient perfusion of forearm muscle.
- Compartment syndrome occurs in <1%, necessitating fasciotomy for decompression.

Management

1. _Undisplaced fractures_ should be immobilized in a plaster slab, with the elbow flexed 100° and the forearm neutral. Undisplaced fractures can displace and a check X-ray at 1 week is necessary. The plaster can be discarded at 3 weeks and the elbow mobilized.

2. _Displaced fractures_ require urgent treatment and are always easier to reduce and stabilize before swelling obscures the landmarks. Type III injuries are unstable, as are some type II injuries and internal fixation may be required. The literature on this subject is extensive and controversial. Treatment options include:

- Closed reduction and plaster immobilization, with the elbow flexed 110° provided a good pulse is maintained, is suitable for many type II and some type III injuries. The fracture is reduced by traction along the pronated forearm with the elbow extended. The elbow is hyperextended, exaggerating the deformity, then flexed as the distal fragment is manipulated by direct posterior pressure. On a true lateral X-ray, a crescent sign is caused by medial or lateral tilt with the distal humerus overlying the ulna.

- Closed reduction and percutaneous K-wire fixation is favoured where the fracture is unstable. Some units advocate K-wiring of all type III fractures. Crossed K-wires placed from the medial and lateral sides provide the greatest stability and rotational control. However, there is a risk of iatrogenic ulnar nerve damage, and the incidence can be reduced with a small skin incision and dissection down to bone, or by identifying the ulnar nerve with a nerve stimulator and placing the wire anterior to this. The medial wire should be placed first with the postero-medially displaced fracture, and the lateral wire first with postero-lateral displacement. The medial wire should start posteriorly and be directed anteriorly, while the lateral wire should start anteriorly and be directed posteriorly. This procedure is best performed after closed reduction, with the elbow over the image intensifier and the arm abducted. Two parallel wires can be placed from the lateral side, but fixation is less secure. Wires are removed at 3–4 weeks and the elbow mobilized.

- Open reduction and K-wire fixation is occasionally required if the fracture cannot be reduced. Skin puckering at presentation suggests penetration of the brachialis by the humerus, and is a useful indicator that open reduction may be necessary. Postero-lateral displacement should be exposed through an antero-medial approach, visualizing the median nerve and brachial artery. Postero-medial displacement should be exposed through an antero-lateral approach visualizing the radial nerve. A posterior approach violates virgin tissue and should be avoided, as access to anterior neurovascular structures which may be damaged, is compromised.

- Traction. Very swollen limbs, and cases where the radial pulse is jeopardized on flexion, can be treated on traction while swelling subsides, followed by definitive plaster or K-wire fixation. Overhead skeletal traction with a screw in the proximal ulna, or a transolecranon K-wire, gives more control and better results than Dunlop skin traction.

3. _Flexion injuries_ generally require K-wire fixation when displaced, as plaster immobilization in extension is cumbersome and unreliable. There is a higher incidence of cubitus valgus.

Late complications

Good results are reported in over 90% of patients.

1. Cubitus varus occurs when reduction has been inadequate, often because reduction has been lost as the swelling resolves and X-rays in plaster are difficult to interpret, leading to a gunstock deformity which is largely cosmetic. The functional effect is minimal. A closing lateral wedge osteotomy, with rotational correction is occasionally required.

2. Cubitus valgus is less common, with greater functional impairment.

3. Volkmann's ischaemic contracture is seen in <1% of cases.

4. Myositis ossificans is a rare complication, but occasionally follows open reduction.

Further reading

Macnicol MF. Indications for internal fixation. In: Benson MKD, Fixen A, Macnicol MF, eds. *Children's Orthopaedics and Fractures*. Edinburgh: Churchill-Livingstone, 1994; 707–720.
Thomas IH. Fractures in children. In: Gregg PJ, Stevens J, Worlock PH, eds. *Fractures and Dislocations – Principles of Management*. Oxford: Blackwell Science; 237–248.

Related topics of interest

Compartment syndrome, p. 41; Humeral fractures – distal, p. 107; Paediatric humeral condylar fractures, p. 169

PAEDIATRIC NON-ACCIDENTAL INJURY

Non-accidental injury (NAI) is better considered as 'unexplained injury', since this is the usual presentation and proof of NAI may not be confirmed until some time after the acute event.

Incidence

- Proven NAI – 4:10 000 children.
- 'At risk' – 34:10 000 children.

The overall incidence has probably remained unchanged, but NAI receives more publicity from today's media. Eighty per cent occurs below the age of 2 years. In infants of <18 months, one in eight fractures is related to NAI, so vigilance by medical staff is essential. Unrecognized injury is associated with a 20% risk of further injury, including permanent neurological damage and death in 5%.

Presentation and risk factors

1. History. Delayed presentation, inappropriate 'changing' history, social deprivation, unemployment, alcohol, marital instability and premature birth are recognized risk factors, but none of these may be present.

2. Examination. Certain skin and soft tissue lesions are as characteristic as fractures, including trunk bite marks, cigarette burns and bruises of differing ages. Fingerprint bruises on the upper arm or face are more obvious. A generally unhappy face may be a clue. 'Shaken' babies may have subconjunctival haemorrhages or a torn frenulum.

Radiology

A skeletal survey is the best investigation and superior to bone scintigraphy.

1. Less than 2 years of age. Rib, metaphyseal 'chip' and spiral long bone fractures with periosteal reaction, particularly the femur, raise suspicion, as should neurological injury.

- Rib fractures are at the posterior rib angle or costochondral junction and often multiple. Fifty per cent of NAI cases have rib fractures.
- Metaphyseal 'chip' or corner fractures are almost pathognomonic and caused by shearing injuries, which force cartilage into the zone of provisional calcification. Metaphyseal 'chip' fractures appear as a radio-lucency at the physeal–metaphyseal junction and are usually found at the elbow or the knee. There is *no* periosteal reaction and as transient features, 'chip fractures' may appear and disappear over 3 weeks. Repeat X-rays are recommended after 3 weeks in suspicious cases.
- Femoral fractures rarely occur by 'falling from a height' of 1 m in infants.
- Neurological injury, including sub-dural haemorrhages and grey–white matter shearing, may result from shaking.

2. Between 2 and 5 years. Complex skull fractures, spiral humeral fractures and fractures of more than one bone of differing ages are found in this age group. Skull fractures are non-linear, parietal and often depressed.

3. *Older than 5 years.* Injuries tend to mirror direct trauma to the chest and head.

Differential diagnoses

- Haematological disorders such as haemophilia or leukaemia.
- Osteogenesis imperfecta (OI)
- Prematurity and copper deficiency

The chance new presentation of OI (type IV) without a clear positive family history, blue sclera or evidence of progressive deformity is extremely rare, estimated at 1 in 3 000 000 or 1 case every 200 years for the average hospital. Premature infants may have porotic bones or even copper deficiency (TPN fed), but these cases are obvious on further enquiry.

Orthopaedic management

The role of the orthopaedic surgeon is:

- To recognize unusual injury and instigate hospital procedures under the Children's Act (1989), implemented in October 1991, whereby the safety and well-being of the child is paramount.
- Management of the specific injury.

Further reading

Nugent IM, Ivory JP, Ross AC. Children and the law. In: *Key Topics in Orthopaedics*, Oxford: BIOS Scientific Publishers, 1995; 65–67.

Worlock P, Stower M, Barbor P. Patterns of fractures in accidental and non-accidental injury in children: a comparative study. *British Medical Journal*, 1986; **293**: 100–102.

Related topic of interest

Paediatric fracture principles, p. 165

PAEDIATRIC SPINE TRAUMA

The paediatric spine differs anatomically from the adult, and consequently presenting patterns of injury differ.

Paediatric spinal injuries are uncommon, making up <2% of all spinal injuries and <1% of all paediatric injuries. The true incidence may be underestimated. Neurological deficit is rare and the prognosis better than in adult injuries. The commonest site of injury involves the upper three cervical vertebrae. The paediatric pattern of injury persists until about the age of 10 years, when patterns change to the adult type.

Anatomy and radiography

At birth, each vertebra is composed of three ossification centres – one for the body and one for each half of the neural arch. The axis has an extra ossification centre – the odontoid peg. Thus, through an open mouth view the physes appear as a capital 'H' (*Figure 1*). The vertical limbs are formed between the lateral neural arches. The horizontal line, or physis, lies between the dens and body. The 'H' fuses by the age of 6 years.

The vertebral apophyses are secondary ossification centres and form in the vertebral end-plates between 8 and 12 years, fusing with the body in the early 20s.

The paediatric spine is more mobile than the adult, thus the upper limit of normal for the atlanto-dens interval is 4.5 mm, compared with 3 mm in the adult. The body of C2 can appear anteriorly subluxed upon C3 – such 'pseudo-subluxation' is a normal variant. In pseudosubluxation however, the spinolaminar line of Swischuck should remain aligned (this is the radiodense line formed at the spinolaminar junction, seen posteriorly on a lateral radiograph).

The upper limit of normal prevertebral soft tissue thickness is 5 mm at the inferior border of C2, and 8 mm at the lower border of C6.

Clinical examination

The possibility of spinal injury should be considered after traumatic delivery in the flaccid neonate and in all children with head or facial injuries. Neck pain after trauma is an indication for X-ray.

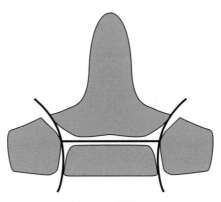

Figure 1. The open physes of the axis form an 'H', as seen on the open mouth view.

The child's large head causes flexion of the neck when immobilized on a standard spine board. The child's body should therefore be raised, or a cavity made for the occiput.

C1/C2 injuries

1. *Occipito-atlantal dislocation.* This is often fatal and those who survive require immediate immobilization in a halo. Traction should be avoided. Later posterior fusion should be considered.

2. *Atlas fractures.* These are rare.

3. *Atlanto-axial instability.* There are three principal patterns:

- Transverse ligament rupture can be acute or chronic. The chronic rupture is associated with Down's syndrome, Klippel–Feil syndrome and some skeletal dysplasias. In these cases, posterior fusion should be considered if the atlanto-dens interval is >10 mm, or if there is neurological compromise. The acute case is surgically stabilized.
- Odontoid peg fractures typically occur through the basal physis and the diagnosis is recognized on the lateral X-ray. Treatment consists of either a Minerva cast or a halo for 6 weeks. An *os odontoideum* is most probably an old undiagnosed peg fracture and if unstable or associated with neurological impairment, a C1/C2 fusion can be performed.
- Atlanto-axial rotatory instability classically presents with a torticollis, the 'cock robin' deformity, after an upper respiratory tract infection. Plain radiographs are difficult to interpret and the diagnosis is most easily made on CT. The condition should be treated seriously as cases of neurological deficit and even death are reported. Fielding and Hawkins classify four types:

Type 1: no AP shift.
Type 2: <4 mm anterior shift.
Type 3: >4 mm anterior shift.
Type 4: posterior shift of the atlas on the axis.
Treatment is usually a soft cervical collar and NSAIDs. In the more resistant cases, halter traction or even open reduction and posterior fusion, may be required.

4. *C2 spondylolisthesis.* The 'Hangman's fracture' is rare in children and treated by immobilization in a Minerva cast or halo.

C3-C7 injuries

These occur in older children at the cartilage/bone junction and may be difficult to diagnose on plain X-ray. Treatment is similar to that in the adult, although anterior fusion should be avoided, as this predisposes to growth arrest and kyphosis.

Thoraco-lumbar spine injuries

1. *Three-column model of Denis.* This is applicable to children and the most common pattern of injury is compression. Burst fractures, flexion distraction fractures (Chance) and fracture-dislocations all occur. Treatment is similar to that in the adult and in children of <10 years the vertebral height often reconstitutes.

2. *Vertebral apophysis.* This can fracture and displace into the spinal canal, with associated disc protrusion. This usually occurs in the lower lumbar spine and is often misdiagnosed as a prolapsed intervertebral disc. Laminotomy and removal of fragments from the spinal canal are required.

Spinal cord injury without radiological abnormality (SCIWORA)

SCIWORA is seen in 5–55% of children with spinal cord injury and is most common in the cervical and thoracic spine. Aetiology is excessive stretching of the spinal column in relation to the cord. The infantile column can be stretched by 5 cm, as opposed to the cord which stretches only 0.5 cm. In 25–50% the onset of symptoms is delayed. Evaluation is by X-ray, CT to exclude bony instability and MRI for soft tissue swelling or impingement.

Complications

Spinal fractures in children need follow-up into adulthood. There is a risk of spinal deformity, which can be secondary to bony deformity, or more commonly to neuromuscular imbalance. Late neurological deterioration should be considered, and if present, evaluated by MRI to exclude a syrinx.

Further reading

Jones ET, Loder RT, Hensinger RN. Fractures of the spine. In: Rockwood CA, Green DP, Bucholz RW, Heckman JD, eds. *Rockwood and Green's Fractures in Adults*. Philadelphia: Lippincott-Raven, 1996; 1023–1105.

Related topics of interest

Spine – C3 to C7, p. 269; Spine – occiput to C2, p. 272; Spine – thoracic and lumbar fractures, p. 275; Spine – whiplash and associated disorders, p. 278

PAEDIATRIC TIBIAL FRACTURES

The most common fractures of the lower limb in children are of the tibia and fibula, classified by site and pattern.

Tibial eminence fractures

Avulsion of the ACL tibial insertion is more common than cruciate rupture in the immature skeleton and not infrequent in adolescents playing sport. Haemarthrosis is the usual presentation with a fracture on X-ray.

1. Classification. 'Meyers and McKeever' (lateral X-ray).

- Type I: minimal displacement.
- Type II: hinged anteriorly, attached posteriorly.
- Type III: detached +/– rotated.

2. Management. Type I and II may be treated in a knee extension cast for 6 weeks. A check X-ray should be obtained to ensure reduction, as the intermeniscal ligament may be trapped under the anterior lip, preventing reduction. Type III and unreduced type II fractures require surgical reduction – open, arthroscopic-assisted or totally arthroscopic. Anatomical reduction and fixation with either a postero-inferiorly directed lag screw within the epiphysis, or tie over sutures passed out through the proximal tibia, is required. A cast brace is used for 6 weeks.

Proximal tibial epiphyseal fractures

These are rare injuries, as the collateral ligaments insert below the epiphysis, but may follow a direct valgus blow in adolescents. This is occasionally 'mis-diagnosed' as collateral ligament sprain. Vascular injury occurs in 10%, and peroneal palsy in 3%.

1. Classification. Salter–Harris II is the most common (43%), but S–H III (22%) and S–H IV (27%) also occur.

2. Management. Immobilization following reduction in an above knee cast for 6 weeks. Operative fixation is required for the unstable S–H II and to reduce the intra-articular extension of the S–H III and S–H IV fractures.

Proximal tibial apophysis and tubercle fractures

Chronic apophyseal problems such as Osgood–Schlatter's disease are common, but acute fractures are rare. However, as with eminence fractures, these are increasing in frequency and associated with adolescent sport. Fractures follow sudden resistance to quadriceps contraction, such as kicking the ground.

1. Classification (Ogden).

- Type 1
  A: distal tuberosity fracture with minimal hinged displacement.
  B: distal tuberosity fracture hinged up and separated from epi/metaphysis.
- Type 2
  A: all tuberosity hinged up.
  B: all tuberosity hinged up and fragmented.

- Type 3

    A: fracture line through epiphysis.

    B: fracture line through epiphysis plus comminution.

2. Management. Type 1A (undisplaced) are immobilized for 4 weeks in plaster. All displaced fractures require ORIF with sutures or lag screws avoiding the physis if possible, and cast immobilization. Growth arrest may lead to recurvatum and reduced quadriceps power.

Proximal tibial metaphyseal fractures

These occur in the younger age group – 3–7 years. A greenstick fracture follows indirect trauma. Direct high-energy trauma leads to significant displacement and associated risk of vascular injury.

1. Classification. Greenstick, buckle, displaced. A medial opening greenstick is the most common fracture.

2. Management. Undisplaced fractures require immobilization for 6 weeks. Displaced fractures require careful reduction, and exclusion or treatment of any vascular injury. Valgus angulated greenstick fractures are difficult to reduce and require immobilization in a moulded long leg cast in extension, with close follow-up, as re-angulation is common. Complications include a vascular injury and valgus deformity. The latter usually develops at 5–6 months and typically spontaneously resolves within 3–4 years. Rarely, varus osteotomy is required.

Shaft fractures

Certain characteristics of children's tibial shaft fractures differentiate the injury from the adult fracture. There is a thicker periosteum and the fibula is more likely to deform than fracture, generally leading to less displacement and fewer healing problems.

Most fractures follow low-energy indirect twisting injuries, resulting in long spiral fractures. Occasionally, these occur without significant obvious trauma; in 1–6 year olds, the fracture may present with reluctance to weight-bear and local inflammation similar to infection. X-rays may be unhelpful, but an isotope bone scan is usually positive. Direct 'bumper' injuries cause more complex fracture patterns.

1. Classification. Descriptive.

2. Management. Most isolated fractures are managed by closed reduction in a long leg cast. Close follow-up and cast changing or wedging is required to prevent loss of reduction. Wedging may be required in the first 3 weeks. Operative management is indicated in open fractures, compartment syndrome, neurovascular injuries, failure of closed management, and possibly in polytrauma victims.

Operative techniques differ slightly from adults, as consideration must be given to the growth plate. ORIF with plates or lag screws is tolerated well, with lower non-union and infection rates than in adults. External fixation is useful in polytrauma or open fractures. Locked, semi-rigid nails are avoided because of injury to the apophysis. Flexible nails inserted in a retrograde fashion are becoming popular as the growth plates are avoided, as are the disadvantages of plating or external fixation.

3. Complications
- Malunion. There is similar remodelling potential to adults. Five degrees varus-valgus and 10° anteroposterior angulation is acceptable.
- Length discrepancy. Overgrowth is not significant, so reduction should be anatomical.
- Compartment syndrome is occasionally recognized.

Distal tibial metaphyseal fractures

The soft metaphyseal bone is susceptible to buckle or greenstick fractures, similar to the proximal end. There is less tendency to coronal angulation, but anterior collapse and recurvatum may occur, which is overcome by casting the foot in plantar flexion. 15° saggital angulation and 30% translocation will remodel.

The 'bicycle spoke' distal tibial fracture is a specific injury occurring in young children. The foot is caught in the spokes and forced internal rotation results in an open, short-oblique metaphyseal fracture. There may be significant skin degloving.

Distal tibial epiphyseal fractures

An important variant is the *triplane fracture*, which occurs in children nearing skeletal maturity, as the physis closes in an asymmetrical fashion. These are generally two or three-part fractures, difficult to recognize on X-ray, which require careful reduction and fixation. The principle fragments are (i) the tibial metaphysis, (ii) the medial and posterior fragment of the distal epiphysis with a metaphyseal spike posteriorly, and (iii) the antero-lateral corner of the distal epiphysis. Evaluation is better with CT or plain tomography.

Treatment is in a cast, when displacement is minimal. Where displacement exceeds 2 mm, open reduction and internal fixation is required, sometimes through a generous exposure, depending on the nature of the fracture and degree of displacement.

Further reading

Heinrich S. Fractures of the shaft of the tibia and fibula. In: Rockwood CA, Wilkins KE, Beaty JH, eds. *Fractures in Children*. Philadelphia: Lippincott-Raven, 1996; 1331–1376.

Sponseller P, Beaty JH. Fractures and dislocations about the knee. In: Rockwood CA, Wilkins KE, Beaty JH eds. *Fractures in Children*. Philadelphia: Lippincott-Raven, 1996; 1231–1330.

Related topics of interest

Paediatric fracture principles, p. 165; Tibial shaft fractures, p. 291

PATHOLOGICAL FRACTURES

Pathological fractures occur in diseased, weakened bone following minimal trauma or, occasionally, spontaneously. Pre-existing disease includes metabolic bone disease, metastatic malignant disease, primary benign or malignant bone tumours and infection. Osteoporosis is the most common cause. Primary malignant bone tumours require specialist management and are beyond the scope of this chapter. The term 'insufficiency fracture' is used for fractures through bone weakened by a process other than neoplasia. Repeated loading may cause a 'stress fracture', most commonly in the athlete or military recruit's foot or tibia (this term is a misnomer and a stress fracture is not really a pathological fracture).

Any primary malignancy may metastasize to bone, but spread most commonly follows breast, bronchus, thyroid, kidney or prostate tumours. Multiple deposits are common, with solitary metastases in only 9% of cases. A solitary metastasis may be the presenting feature of undiagnosed malignancy.

Metabolic disease

Pathological fractures occur in bone affected by metabolic bone disease such as osteoporosis or osteomalacia, and in other systemic disease states such as osteogenesis imperfecta, Paget's disease, polyostotic fibrous dysplasia and osteopetrosis. The most common sites of osteoporotic fractures are the distal radius and femoral neck. Femoral neck fractures may occur without trauma and some patients report an acute event around their hip before their fall.

Treatment of fractures in metabolically diseased bone is by conservative or operative means, aiming for early mobilization. The underlying disease should be investigated and treated as appropriate. Future preventative measures are essential to reduce the ever rising number of fractures, in particular femoral neck fractures, related to osteoporosis. Increasing awareness of HRT, which to be effective should be started within 6 years of the menopause, may be an essential preventative measure.

Primary benign bone tumours

Presentation is either after a coincidental finding on X-ray, or with an acute fracture. There may be a recent history of pain. Displaced fractures need to be reduced and stabilized, undisplaced fractures often unite spontaneously. The underlying condition will need treatment, by curettage and bone grafting, cryosurgery, polymethylmethacrylate cement, or endoprosthetic replacement, either acutely, or later when the fracture has healed. Conditions such as unicameral bone cysts may resolve spontaneously after a fracture.

Secondary deposits

Presentation is either with increasing bone pain following a fracture, or rarely from a tertiary effect such as hypercalcaemia. The lower vertebral column, femur and humerus are most commonly involved, although metastasis may occur in any bone. Metastasis to the vertebral column from pelvic malignancy is explained by Batson's plexus, a valveless system of veins linking pelvic viscera to the vertebral veins.

Where appropriate, fractures through metastatic deposits should be treated aggressively, with internal fixation or joint replacement, to achieve early mobilization and discharge of the patient, who will usually, but not always, have a short life-expectancy. Liver function, blood clotting and the bleeding time may be deranged. Reaming causes embolization of tumour, as well as marrow products, and this may cause death during surgery. Where fixation is tenuous because of diseased bone, polymethylmethacrylate bone cement may be used to improve implant fixation. Tissue must be sent for histological confirmation. The development of further deposits, locally or systemically, following surgery has not been proven.

Following surgery, adjunct radiotherapy or chemotherapy should be considered.

Before surgery, the entire affected bone must be X-rayed, to exclude another deposit in the bone. Preferably before surgery, and certainly before mobilizing the patient, a technetium bone scintigram should be obtained to exclude other deposits, or a skeletal survey performed. Deposits from myeloma are not always identified by bone scintigraphy.

Consideration should be given to prophylactic fixation of painful secondary deposits, especially if >50% of the cortical circumference, or >2.5 cm of cortical length is involved. Prophylactic fixation is relatively easy and less technically demanding than reducing a displaced fracture, with less blood loss, less morbidity for the patient and a better outcome.

Spinal fractures require special consideration and even without a fracture, pain may be excruciating. A pathological deposit or fracture may be associated with spinal cord compromise. Spinal decompression and fixation is often required.

Stress fractures

This term is probably a misnomer, as it is *strain* that usually causes a fracture and not *stress*. With a steady increase in exercise, bone hypertrophies and strengthens according to Wolfe's law. A stress or fatigue fracture occurs in normal bone, with abnormal loading, as the strain and increased exercise has been too great to give the bone time to hypertrophy. There is typically a 4-week interval between an increased exercise load and the onset of pain, which is usually relieved by rest.

Tibial shaft fractures may occur around Looser's zones in osteomalacia.

Further reading

Galasko CSB. Pathological fractures. In: Gregg PJ, Stevens J, Worlock PH, eds. *Fractures and Dislocations.* Oxford: Blackwell Science Ltd, 1996; 889–908.

Nugent IM, Ivory JP, Ross AC. Bone tumours – benign. In: *Key Topics in Orthopaedic Surgery.* Oxford: BIOS Scientific Publishers, 1995; 63–67.

Nugent IM, Ivory JP, Ross AC. Bone tumours – malignant. In: *Key Topics in Orthopaedic Surgery.* Oxford: BIOS Scientific Publishers, 1995; 68–73.

Nugent IM, Ivory JP, Ross AC. Metabolic bone disease. In: *Key Topics in Orthopaedic Surgery.* Oxford: BIOS Scientific Publishers, 1995; 183–186.

PELVIS – ACETABULAR FRACTURES

Fractures of the acetabulum are significant skeletal injuries. Seventy-five per cent follow RTAs. Fifty per cent are associated with other major fractures or injuries. The fracture may be associated with dislocation of the hip and impaired sciatic nerve function. Femoral head dislocation should be reduced as an emergency and traction maintained until a definitive management plan for the fracture is devised – occasionally the femoral head may be incarcerated in the fracture or peri-acetabular muscles. The most important prognostic factors are the velocity of the injury, the restoration of congruity of the weight-bearing surface of the dome of the acetabulum and the stability of the femoral head.

This topic is concerned with the management of major acetabular fractures; lesser isolated rim fractures following dislocation are discussed in 'Hip dislocation', p. 104.

Classification

The acetabulum lies between the anterior column, the posterior column and the superomedial iliac root (quadrilateral element). Judet and Letournel have been instrumental in the understanding of acetabular fractures, with extensive cadaveric work. The Letournel and Judet classification considers fractures in five elemental and five associated, or more complex, configurations. The five elemental patterns include: posterior wall (25%), posterior column, anterior wall (20%), anterior column and transverse fractures. The five associated patterns include: T-shaped, posterior column and wall, transverse and posterior wall, anterior wall or column with posterior hemitransverse and, finally, both column fractures.

A detailed alpha-numeric classification has recently been proposed, using the traditional A,B,C approach and incorporating the Letournel classification. This will improve comparison and long-term outcome assessment.

Imaging

An AP pelvis X-ray will confirm clinical suspicion of an injury. More detailed assessment, including Judet views (AP views with the pelvis tilted 45° internally and 45° externally) (*Figure 1*), pelvic inlet and pelvic outlet views, is required to demonstrate the injury pattern and plan surgical reconstruction. The use of CT to delineate the intra-articular extent of the fracture is essential and the increasing availability of spiral CT with three-dimensional (3D) reconstruction will improve the understanding and surgical reconstruction of acetabular fractures.

Treatment

*1. **Conservative.*** Fractures with less than 4 mm displacement of the acetabular dome, and low column fractures, can be treated conservatively, with a period of 8 weeks traction and bed rest prior to mobilization when sufficient hip movement has been regained. Where displacement is greater, ORIF should be considered, with reference to the patient's age and functional demands. In elderly and low-demand patients, conservative treatment with a view to early total hip replacement may be preferable.

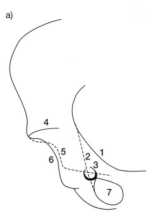

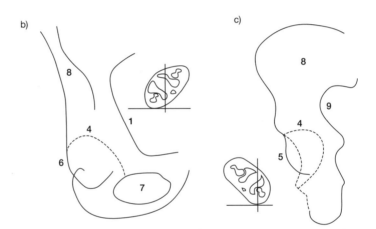

Figure 1. Bony outlines on the (a) AP, (b) obturator oblique and (c) iliac oblique views of the pelvis. The obturator oblique view profiles the anterior column and the posterior rim. The iliac oblique profiles the greater and lesser sciatic notches (posterior column) and the anterior rim. 1, ileopectinial line; 2, ilioischial line; 3, teardrop; 4, roof of acetabulum; 5, anterior lip of acetabulum; 6, posterior lip of acetabulum; 7, obturator foramen; 8, iliac wing; 9, greater sciatic notch.

2. Surgical reconstruction. While acetabular reconstruction should be undertaken promptly, within 1 week of the injury, appropriate investigations, facilities and expertise are imperative, as operative fixation represents a formidable surgical challenge.

Anterior column fractures are exposed through an anterior ilio-inguinal approach, exposing the hemi-pelvis medial and lateral to the ilio-psoas and the neurovascular bundle – this may also be appropriate for a two-column fracture. Posterior injury patterns should be exposed through an extended Kocher–Langenbeck approach. Some two column and transverse fractures, which are difficult to expose and reduce, may require a sequential anterior and posterior approach. An extensile approach, such as a tri-radiate transtrochanteric or an extended ilio-femoral incision, is also used.

The general principle of surgery is to achieve anatomical reduction and fixation with a combination of lag screws and contoured pelvic reconstruction plates. Patients should be mobilized early, with minimal weight-bearing for the first 8 weeks.

Where there is significant destruction of the articular cartilage, total hip replacement may be appropriate. This is undertaken either after the fracture has healed, or on occasion acutely, using bone graft and the multiple screw holes of an uncemented acetabular cup to stabilize the fracture and act as supplementary plate fixation.

3. Ipsilateral femoral shaft and acetabular fracture. This is one of the few indications for compression plate fixation of the femoral shaft. A retrograde femoral IM nail is another option. The shaft fracture should be stabilized acutely, keeping the wound away from the pelvis and the acetabular fracture addressed a few days later, after appropriate investigation.

Complications

1. Sciatic nerve injury occurs in up to 30% of acetabular fractures; femoral and superior gluteal nerve injuries are occasionally encountered. A subclinical traumatic injury to the sciatic nerve at the time of the accident may be dramatically aggravated by surgery and per-operative EMG monitoring of the calf should be available. Post-operative sciatic nerve palsies tend to recover; traumatic nerve injuries are permanent in 10% of fractures.

2. Thromboembolism occurs in a significant proportion of cases and anticoagulation should be routine.

3. Infection is reported to occur in 3–5% of cases.

4. Heterotopic ossification with an incidence varying from 5 to 15% (may be as high as 70%) is reported in the literature, yet only a minority of patients have significantly impaired movement. The prophylactic roles of indomethacin and radiotherapy are yet to be defined for this type of surgery.

5. Avascular necrosis, chondrolysis and post-traumatic degenerative arthritis are recognized late complications – the incidence is dependent on the severity of the initial injury, damage to the femoral head, other pelvic injuries, restoration of congruity of the weight-bearing dome of the acetabulum and stability of the femoral head. The incidence of avascular necrosis of the femoral head is 10% in posterior injuries. Post-traumatic degenerative change is more common in patients over the age of 40 and in those patients with residual displacement of the fracture. Where reduction is good, 90% will have a favourable result; where reduction is poor, 50–70% will achieve a satisfactory result.

Further reading

Judet R, Judet J and Letournel E. Fractures of the acetabulum: classification and surgical approaches for open reduction. Preliminary report. *Journal of Bone and Joint Surgery*, 1964; **46A**: 1615–1646.

Letournel E, Judet R. *Fractures of the Acetabulum*. New York: Springer-Verlag, 1993.
Tile M. *Fractures of the Pelvis and Acetabulum*, 2nd Edn. Baltimore: Williams and Wilkins, 1995.

Related topics of interest

Hip dislocation, p. 104; Pelvis – ring fractures, p. 189

PELVIS – RING FRACTURES

Fractures of the pelvis follow high-energy trauma, frequently in association with other major skeletal, thoracic, abdominal and pelvic trauma. Stability of the fracture depends upon the integrity of the pelvic ring. Blood loss may be dramatic, requiring swift intervention. Twenty to twenty five per cent of fatal accidents have associated pelvic fractures and the mortality rate following pelvic fractures is 9–19%. Less severe fractures occur in the elderly osteoporotic patient following low-energy trauma.

Anatomy and classification

An understanding of the anatomy and ligamentous structures of the pelvis is essential in order to appreciate the classification system. Fractures are classified according to the deforming force and stability depends upon the integrity of supporting ligaments. The closed ring of the pelvis is chiefly stabilized posteriorly by the congruity of the sacroiliac joints, interosseous sacroiliac, anterior sacroiliac, posterior sacroiliac, sacrotuberous, sacrospinous and ilio-lumbar ligaments. Anteriorly, the symphysis pubis plays a lesser role in supporting the closed ring.

The classification of Burgess and Young is commonly used, with four injury patterns including lateral compression (LC), antero-posterior compression (APC), vertical shear (VS) and combined mechanism (CM) injuries.

- **LC injuries** with a deforming force from the side are of three subtypes (LC-I, LC-II and LC-III), differentiated by disruption of the posterior sacroiliac structures. Pubic rami fractures are generally transverse, may buckle or overlap and are best seen on the pelvic inlet view. In LC-I injuries, the pubic rami are fractured, but there is no posterior instability. A crush fracture of the sacrum is common. In LC-II injuries, medial displacement of the anterior hemi-pelvis is associated with rupture of the posterior sacroiliac ligament complex or a fracture of the sacroiliac joint/wing, producing posterior instability. In LC-III injuries, the pelvis opens on the contralateral side as the deforming force is transmitted through the pelvis, resulting in a windswept pelvis. LC injuries are associated with acetabular fractures.

- **APC injuries** follow direct anterior or posterior trauma and are divided into subtypes (APC-I, APC-II or APC-III), depending on the degree of displacement. APC-I injuries have minimally displaced, usually vertical, pubic rami fractures or mild symphysis pubis diastasis (<2 cm). The anterior sacroiliac, sacrospinous and sacrotuberous ligaments are violated in APC-II injuries, as the pelvis splays open like a book. In APC-III injuries, all the sacroiliac structures, including the posterior ligaments, are disrupted. APC-II and APC-III fractures have the highest risk of haemorrhage.

- **VS injuries** typically follow a fall from a height, with a fracture pattern through the pubic rami and posterior pelvis, displacing the hemi-pelvis vertically.

- **CM injuries** result in a combined fracture pattern – most frequently LC and APC.

Tile classifies fractures as: A, stable; B, rotationally unstable, but vertically stable; and C, rotationally and vertically unstable. Isolated fractures of the sacrum, pubic rami, iliac wing or crest and avulsion fractures may occur.

Imaging

Plain X-rays may confirm a suspected injury, and should be included in the initial radiographic evaluation of all major trauma. Further assessment is with Judet views (see p. 186), and pelvic inlet and outlet views (X-ray beam angled 40° caudad and 40° cephalad). Where the state of the acetabulum is in doubt, a CT scan should be obtained. While CT has traditionally not been part of the investigation for assessment and planning of surgery, the advent of spiral CT with rapid 3D reconstruction may change the approach to radiological investigation.

Associated soft tissue injuries

1. Vascular. Haemorrhage from a pelvic fracture is often dramatic, either from the sacral venous plexus and other great veins, or an artery in close proximity to bone. The superior gluteal artery is the most frequently damaged, as it passes through the sciatic notch. Significant haemorrhage may also occur from exposed bony surfaces.

2. Urological. Urethral injury, more common in males, occurs in 15% and bladder rupture occurs in 5% of pelvic fractures. Injuries to the ureter are rare. Urethral injuries manifest as blood at the meatus, penile bruising, a high riding prostate on PR examination, or haematuria. Urological advice is required before attempted catheterization. Suprapubic catheterization is often preferable and further investigation includes a retrograde urethrogram, cystogram, intravenous pyelogram (IVP) or CT scan.

3. Neurological. Sacral fractures through neural foramina may compromise the lumbosacral plexus. The sciatic and other nerves may be damaged, depending on the injury pattern.

Treatment

1. Emergency management. Pelvic fractures may present with major haemorrhage. A widely displaced fracture, in a haemodynamically unstable patient despite fluid replacement, needs the pelvis closed and stabilized as a resuscitative measure in the emergency room, using an external fixator to tamponade blood loss. Two or three 5 mm pins should be passed into the anterior iliac crest and the fixator applied. An external fixator may be suitable for definitive management and should be retained for 8–12 weeks. A Ganz clamp can be applied to close the pelvis posteriorly.

When pelvic haemorrhage is uncontrollable despite the compression and tamponade effects of an external fixator, angiography and embolisation may be indicated. With a pelvic fracture, laparotomy is ill-advised without an external fixator applied.

2. Conservative treatment. Stable fractures, where displacement is minimal, may be treated conservatively. Minimally displaced pelvic ring fractures should be mobilized with protected weight-bearing after a period of 6 to 8 weeks bed rest. 'Stable' injuries can displace and radiological review is advisable. Simple pubic rami fractures can be mobilized early, to the tolerance of pain.

3.   Operative stabilization. Occasionally the pubic symphysis needs to be stabilized anteriorly, using a two or four-hole plate through a Pfannenstiel incision. Double plating is more stable. Displaced posterior injuries need fixation, either by a direct posterior, or anterior (extended ilio-inguinal) approach to the sacroiliac joints. Methods of fixation include reconstruction plates, trans-iliac rods or carefully placed ilio-sacral screws. Such surgery is complex, prone to hazard and should be undertaken by experienced surgeons in adequately equipped centres. In skilled hands, screws may be inserted percutaneously with image intensifier control.

Complications

1.   Infection and thromboembolism. There are few accurate figures available for these complications.

2.   Malunion. This can result in substantial disability, with abnormal gait, leg length inequality and attendant complications. The incidence is around 5%.

Further reading

Tile M. *Fractures of the Pelvis and Acetabulum*. Baltimore: Williams & Wilkins, 1995.

Young JWR, Burgess AR, Brumbach RJ, Poka A. Pelvic fractures: value of plain radiography in early assessment and management. *Radiology*, 1986; **160** :445–451.

Young JWR, Smith RM, Kellam JF. Mini-symposium: pelvic fractures. *Current Orthopaedics*, 1996; **10:** 1–23.

Related topics of interest

Pelvis – acetabular fractures, p. 185; Polytrauma – management and complications, p. 200

PERIPHERAL NERVE INJURIES AND REPAIR

Each peripheral nerve contains many nerve fascicles. The fascicles and intervening connective tissue are bound by a sheath of epineurium. Fascicles contain many individual nerve fibres surrounded by perineurium. A nerve fibre consists of an axon with a Schwann cell covering, bound by endoneurium.

Nerve fibres may be myelinated (A and B) or unmyelinated (C). The myelin sheath is produced by the Schwann cell. Sequential Schwann cells surround myelinated fibres, separated at the nodes of Ranvier. Each Schwann cell supports only one axon. In unmyelinated fibres, one Schwann cell may support several axons.

Myelinated fibres are larger (1–10 μm) than unmyelinated fibres (0.2–2 μm) and the conduction velocity is much faster (10–70 m/s compared with 2 m/s). Conduction velocity is faster due to the saltatory or skip conduction effect of the myelin sheath. Loss of the myelin sheath results in absent or delayed conduction.

Classification of nerve injury

Seddon (1943) described the most widely used classification of nerve injury:

1. *Neurapraxia.* A physiological block to conduction associated with either temporary ischaemia or focal demyelination.

2. *Axonotmesis.* Axon disruption, but the nerve covering or 'tube' remains intact.

3. *Neurotmesis.* Transection of both axon and nerve sheath/covering.

Sunderland (1951) expanded axonotmesis into three grades, differentiating whether the endo-, peri-, or epineurium were intact.

Mechanisms of injury

A peripheral nerve may be compressed acutely or chronically, stretched, transected, burnt or irradiated. Acute or chronic compression may cause neurapraxia or axonotmesis. Severe compression may cause axonal death. Stretching may cause any type of injury, but typically axonotmesis (>15% elongation). Transection usually follows a penetrating injury, causing neurotmesis.

Pathophysiological response to injury

1. *Neurapraxia.* Temporary ischaemia is reversed and function recovers. Focal demyelination is followed by remyelination over a period of 2 to 6 weeks.

2. *Axonotmesis and neurotmesis.* Axonal (Wallerian) degeneration occurs in the whole distal axon and the proximal stump up to the nearest node. Wallerian degeneration consists of enzymatic degradation and ingestion of the axon and myelin by macrophages and Schwann cells. This takes 1 to 3 months, leaving an empty neural tube, continuous or divided.

Nerve regeneration is governed by neurotrophism (growth stimulating factors) and contact guidance (Schwann cells). Regeneration occurs after a delay of 1 month, by axonal budding from the proximal stump and proceeds at a rate of

1 mm/day (1 inch/month) in adults. The bud is directed down the Schwann cell tube, but the regenerate fibre is smaller and less myelinated, with slower conduction.

The lack of an intact Schwann cell tube (neurotmesis) severely interferes with effective regeneration. The axonal buds lack direction, resulting in a functionless mass.

Clinical findings

Nerve dysfunction is usually immediately apparent, by either altered or absent sensory or motor function. Occasionally signs may evolve after the acute event, so repeated examination is important.

Electrophysiology

Nerve conduction studies (NCS) and EMG are used to assess the type of injury, recovery and prognosis. Timing of studies is important, as the type of injury cannot be identified before 2–3 weeks. Prior to this, axonal degeneration may not have occurred, leading to false results. At 3–6 months, repeat studies can assess the mode and degree of recovery.

In a neurapraxia, there is normal nerve conduction above and below, but not across the site of injury, where nerve conduction is slowed. In axonotmesis and neurotmesis, both EMG and NCS are abnormal. There is no conduction distal to the injury, and muscle exhibits denervation fibrillation within 3 weeks. Later EMG studies may predict both the mode (collateral sprouting or regeneration – see below) and degree of recovery in the case of axonotmesis, but not neurotmesis.

Recovery

- Most neurapraxias recover fully within 2 to 6 weeks, but occasionally take 3 months.
- Functional recovery from axonotmesis has two mechanisms. Firstly, by *collateral sprouting* from other axons at the nerves' destination, which effects fast functional recovery (3–6 months), but requires at least 30% of axons to be intact. Secondly, by *nerve regeneration* as above. This is slower and often incomplete. If nerve lesions are very proximal, the distal Schwann cell tubes may become obliterated prior to the fibre reaching the end plate (18 months) and recovery is incomplete. Prognosis is poor.
- Spontaneous recovery from neurotmesis is poor, with no collateral sprouting or effective regeneration.

Management

1. **Closed injury.** Observation, with baseline NCS/EMG documentation at 3 weeks and follow-up studies at 3 months is required. Joint and muscle contracture should be prevented by physiotherapy. Surgical exploration is considered after 6 months and neurolysis, co-aptation (repair) or resection and grafting may be required. The final outcome is assessed at 2 years. Evidence of nerve injury following manipulation of a closed fracture may require early exploration.

2. **Open injuries.** These should be explored, and acute co-aptation undertaken within 2 weeks. Clean, guillotine divisions are best co-aptated without delay. How-

ever, dirty, crushed or avulsed lesions should be debrided, allowed to heal and secondarily repaired.

Nerve co-aptation

Direct repair is undertaken if there is <2.5 cm nerve gap. Scarred portions should be excised. Both epineurial and group fascicular repairs have been advocated. No studies have shown any advantage of fascicular repair.

Recovery is hampered by intraneural oedema and scarring. The future may see the use of bioabsorbable tubes, into each end of which the cut nerve ends are placed. The proximal axons will grow to the distal Schwann cell tube, guided by intrinsic factors. This will avoid the use of sutures and may improve topography and subsequent functional outcome.

Grafting for segmental defects

Following exploration and mobilization of the nerve, intervals of >2.5 cm should be grafted to avoid tension and failure of repair. Nerve, muscle, vein conduit and synthetic materials have all been used. Nerve grafts are the most common, but have the disadvantage of donor site morbidity. The grafts are usually non-vascularized, but vascularized grafts can be used if the graft site is very scarred. The sural, medial and lateral cutaneous nerves of the forearm are commonly used.

Current research is investigating the use of frozen/thawed muscle grafts and synthetic tubes as conduits for nerve growth and repair. Results of muscle grafts have so far been disappointing.

Recovery: phases and prognosis

There are three phases of recovery:

- Axon growth.
- Simple protective function.
- Useful motor and sensory function.

Best outcomes are achieved in distal guillotine divisions of young, pure nerves rather than proximal crush or avulsion type injuries in old, mixed nerves.

Further reading

Bonney GLW. Iatropathic lesions of peripheral nerves. *Current Orthopaedics*, 1997; **11**: 255–66.

Hems TEJ, Glasby MA. Prospeccts for the treatment of spinal cord and peripheral nerve injury. *Journal of Bone and Joint Surgery*, 1996; **78B**: 176–77.

Nugent IM, Ivory JP, Ross AC. Paralysed hand. In: *Key Topics in Orthopaedic Trauma Surgery*. Oxford: BIOS Scientific Publishers, 1995; 214–217.

Related topic of interest

Shoulder – brachial plexus injuries, p. 243

PERI-PROSTHETIC FRACTURES (HIP AND KNEE)

Fractures around prosthetic implants most commonly affect the hip and knee, although fractures around shoulder and elbow prostheses occur. Fractures occur as an acute event following a fall, or as an acute on chronic process with established implant loosening and osteolysis, resulting in a fracture after minimal trauma. Management is best within a specialist revision arthroplasty unit.

Classification

It is essential to determine whether the fracture has occurred around a loose or well-fixed implant, as this has implications for definitive treatment and pre-operative planning. Sixty per cent of peri-prosthetic femoral shaft fractures occur around a loose stem and 25% occur around a loose stem in the presence of advanced loss of bone stock.

Several classifications exist for fractures around a total hip replacement (THR). The important factors are the degree of displacement and where the fracture occurs. The fracture can occur around the upper femur leaving a soundly fixed prosthesis below, around the tip of the prosthesis, or below the prosthesis. Johansson proposed a type I, II and III classification on this basis. The six-part American Academy of Orthopedic Surgeons (AAOS) classification of fractures integrates with the AAOS classification for femoral bone stock loss. Peri-prosthetic acetabular fractures without established lysis are rare.

Distal femoral fractures in relation to a total knee replacement (TKR) occur at the upper margin or above the level of the prosthesis. Fractures of the proximal tibia are rare.

Management

Treatment depends upon the level of the fracture, whether the prosthesis is well-fixed or loose and, if loose, the extent of osteolysis. Loose prostheses generally require revision surgery.

With the exception of very proximal and distal femoral fractures, conservative treatment is rarely successful as it is difficult to control alignment of the femur accurately. There is also a high incidence of subsequent prosthetic loosening. Should a patient require revision at a later date, malunion compromises surgery and an osteotomy through the previous fracture may be required.

When plate fixation is chosen, a specially designed plate can be fixed to the femur with cerclage cables at the level of the prosthesis and with large fragment screws below the prosthesis – four cables above a fracture are required for adequate fixation. Long stem prostheses for peri-prosthetic fractures should pass two femoral shaft diameters below the fracture site. Prostheses with distal cross locking bolts may be useful to control rotation.

1. ***Fractures around a loose THR*** should be treated with a revision THR, removing the implant and reconstructing the femur, unless medical conditions or age dictate otherwise. The femur may need reconstruction with a plate and cables, strut allograft

or morsellized impaction grafting. Soft tissue attachments to bone fragments should be carefully preserved. Sometimes bone loss is so severe that a combination of techniques is used, but it is important to restore bone stock and implant stability. Stable fixation of the stem into intact host bone is essential. Distal fixation is therefore required after reconstructing the femur. A cemented or uncemented implant may be used. It is important to ensure that cement does not interdigitate with the fracture site as this may prevent fracture union. An uncemented implant should have a porous coated stem or distal grooves. With advanced osteolysis, a massive allograft or femoral replacement prosthesis may be required.

2.   Fractures of the proximal femur around a well-fixed THR can be treated conservatively if there is minimal displacement. A period of bed rest and traction is followed by mobilization and partial weight-bearing when the patient regains leg control.

3.   Fractures around the lower end of a well-fixed THR require open reduction, fixation and bone grafting. Generally, a cemented prosthesis should be removed and the femur reconstructed before inserting a long stemmed prosthesis. Where there is minimal comminution, reconstruction of the femur with cables or wires alone may suffice before cementing a long stem prosthesis. Alternatively, an uncemented prosthesis may be favoured. With extensive comminution, allograft struts, plate and cables, augmented with morsellized autograft or allograft will be required.

A soundly fixed uncemented prosthesis may not need exchange, if the femur can be adequately reconstructed around the stem of the prosthesis.

4.   Fractures of the femur below a well-fixed THR require open reduction and internal fixation with a plate and cables, augmented with strut allograft, morsellized autograft or allograft.

5.   Undisplaced fractures of the distal femur around a TKR can be treated conservatively in traction and subsequently in a plaster or cast brace. Regular radiological assessment is required to check alignment is maintained.

6.   Displaced fractures of the distal femur around a TKR require open reduction and internal fixation with a contoured large fragment plate, or similar fixation device. Sometimes a blade plate or condylar screw plate may be used, depending on the presence of stems or pegs on the prosthesis. When plate fixation is employed, bone grafting is required.

An alternative to extramedullary fixation is supracondylar IM nailing. Provided a small diameter nail passes through the centre of the condylar prosthesis, adequate fixation can be achieved and additional bone grafting is rarely required. Good results are reported using this technique, with the advantage of minimal soft tissue disturbance.

In some circumstances a stemmed revision is required as definitive treatment. Controlling alignment of the distal femur is crucial, as varus or valgus malunion accelerates failure of the prosthesis.

7.   Fractures of the proximal tibia are rare. A stress fracture at the tip of a tibial stem may occur and often heals with conservative treatment. Occasionally, revision with a long stemmed prosthesis is required.

8. The principles of treating fractures around shoulder and elbow prostheses are similar. Fractures around a total shoulder replacement can generally be treated conservatively with early mobilization – prolonged immobilization leads to poor function. Fractures around a total elbow replacement (TER) are a more common complication, affecting around 5% of all reported TER series; treatment may be conservative or operative, with internal fixation or revision. The specific management of these problems is beyond the scope of this chapter.

Complications

- With good operative techniques non-union is rare, although revision arthroplasty surgery is prone to major complications and these are increased in the presence of a fracture.
- Malunion compromises subsequent surgery and may promote loosening.
- A large proportion of solid implants treated without revision become loose within a few years.

Further reading

Callaghan JJ. Peri-prosthetic fractures of the acetabulum during and following total hip arthroplasty. *Journal of Bone and Joint Surgery*, 1997; **79A**: 1416–1421.

Chandler HP, Tigges RG. The role of allografts in the treatment of peri-prosthetic femoral fractures. *Journal of Bone and Joint Surgery*, 1997; **79A**: 1422–1432.

Duncan CP, Masri BA. Fractures of the femur after hip replacement. In: *Instructional Course Lectures, The Academy of Orthopaedic Surgeons*. Rosemount, Illinois: The Academy of Orthopaedic Surgeons, 1995; **44**: 293–404.

Engh GA, Ammeen DJ. Peri-prosthetic fractures adjacent to total knee implants. *Journal of Bone and Joint Surgery*, 1997; **79A**: 1100–1113.

Lewallen DG, Berry DJ. Peri-prosthetic fracture of the femur after total hip arthroplasty. *Journal of Bone and Joint Surgery*, 1997; **79A**: 1881–1890.

Related topics of interest

Femoral fractures – shaft, p. 49; Pathological fractures, p. 183

POLYTRAUMA – FAT EMBOLISM AND RESPIRATORY DISTRESS

Fat embolism is the systemic release of bone marrow fat, or other fat, into the circulation. As the peripheral arterial circulation is affected, the term 'embolism' is a misnomer. Fat embolism syndrome (FES) is the systemic response to this phenomenon. Although FES is an infrequently recognized complication of trauma, the effects can be dramatic, a major cause of mortality, and an important cause of adult respiratory distress syndrome (ARDS). FES is really part of the spectrum of trauma-related insults which can lead to ARDS and treatment is aimed at reversing respiratory compromise.

The early stabilization of fractures and early patient mobilization may account for the falling incidence of FES.

Incidence

FES follows 0.5 to 2% of long bone fractures and 10% of polytrauma cases. The incidence is higher during treatment of metastatic deposits. Subclinical fat embolism follows 50% of long bone fractures, and occurs after instrumentation of the medullary canal in both trauma and joint replacement surgery.

Pathophysiology

The pathogenesis of FES remains unclear. After trauma there is probably a change in lipid solubility and membrane stability. There is also a change in micro-circulatory flow, causing increased tissue permeability and tissue hypoxia. Fat in the circulation is not purely from bone marrow. The volume released is not a critical factor either, but the size of the globules may be important. Agglutination may occur, resulting in larger fat globules.

Globules larger than 8–10 μm cause local irritation, damaging the pulmonary microvasculature and increasing pulmonary capillary permeability. These larger globules provoke an acute inflammatory response and become coated with platelets and leukocytes.

The release of thromboplastin after a fracture activates both the complement and extrinsic coagulation cascade, and may alter the binding of free fatty acids to albumin. This changes the permeability of vascular linings, especially in the pulmonary circulation, which can progress to disseminated intravascular coagulation (DIC).

The release of marrow fat may only be a part of, or even a catalyst for, a sequence of immune system events, altering the permeability of the pulmonary vascular endothelium, producing the pulmonary sequelae of FES.

Presentation

Features classically develop 24 to 72 hours after a long bone fracture, typically the femur, with confusion, restlessness, disorientation, tachycardia, tachypnoea, pyrexia and hypoxia. FES may follow non long bone fractures, even a skull fracture. The changes in mental state can progress to coma, and are a consequence of hypoxia and diminished perfusion. There is diminished urine output. Other features are conjunctival and upper trunk petechial haemorrhages, fat in the urine, or fat in the sputum. The diagnosis is made by clinical awareness and blood gas analysis, with a PaO_2 <50 mmHg.

There may be a thrombocytopenia, progressing to DIC and often the haemoglobin level falls.

Physiological effects

The pulmonary changes cause increased airway resistance and diminished compliance, leading to atrioventricular (AV) shunting and a metabolic alkalosis initially, which subsequently becomes a respiratory acidosis. AV shunting may explain why fat globules are found outside the pulmonary circulation. The corrected serum calcium may fall, due to increased calcium binding.

Treatment

Treatment of the life-threatening systemic and pulmonary effects is supportive, reversing the hypoxia with high flow oxygen and in some cases ventilation for 2 to 3 days, but occasionally 2 to 3 weeks. Blood gas analysis is the most sensitive method of determining severity, deterioration and response to treatment. The aim is to maintain a PaO_2 >70 mmHg. The chest X-ray demonstrates scattered infiltration and shadowing, progressing to a 'white-out' in fulminant ARDS. The platelet count may fall. Judicious fluid therapy should be maintained, to prevent overload. Diuretics are sometimes required.

Some centres and various clinical studies support the use of high-dose steroids once a diagnosis of respiratory compromise is established.

Recovery can be prolonged and there may be permanent neurological features. Long-term respiratory compromise is rare. Mortality is 10 to 50%, most commonly after multiple fractures.

Fracture stabilization

Early fracture stabilization is thought to diminish the risk of FES and the current aggressive approach to long bone fracture management is probably responsible for the decreasing incidence of FES. With both isolated femoral fractures and polytrauma, there is a strong association between early stabilization and decreased FES and ARDS, from around 35% to 5% when stabilization is undertaken within 24 hours of injury. Equally, intramedullary instrumentation should be avoided in the 24 to 96 hour interval after a fracture, as this may precipitate FES and ARDS.

Further reading

Ayres DC, Murray DG. Fat embolism syndrome and respiratory distress. In: Epps CH, ed. *Complications in Orthopaedic Surgery*. Philadelphia: Lippincott, 1994: 11–16.

Related topics of interest

Polytrauma – management and complications, p. 200; Polytrauma – metabolic response, p. 203

POLYTRAUMA – MANAGEMENT AND COMPLICATIONS

The management of the polytrauma patient is considered in four phases:

- Acute resuscitation: the first 4 hours.
- Primary definitive management: 1–72 hours.
- Secondary management: 3–8 days.
- Tertiary rehabilitation: >1 week.

Phase 1. Acute resuscitation and stabilization

The first phase follows the resuscitation principles of advanced trauma life support (ATLS), with airway, breathing, circulation and haemorrhage control, 'saving life before limb'. These principles are addressed in detail in the topic 'Polytrauma – resuscitation and ATLS', p. 209. The source of haemorrhage must be swiftly identified, as massive haemorrhage in the chest, abdomen or pelvis requires rapid surgical intervention.

The pelvis is a common site for massive haemorrhage after trauma. If pelvic haemorrhage is suspected, concurrent intra-abdominal or thoracic bleeding should be excluded, whilst rapid fluid resuscitation is started. Failure to respond within 10–20 min requires immediate intervention, with pelvic stabilization by external fixation, to achieve stability and reduce the potential space, to tamponade the haemorrhage. External fixation is usually applied anteriorly, but additional posterior stabilization using the 'C clamp' device may be required.

If external fixation does not bring the situation under control, continuing haemorrhage may become life threatening. Controversy surrounds subsequent management. Pelvic angiography and attempted embolization of pelvic vessels is advocated by some. However, the bleeding is usually from venous plexuses and is not identifiable by angiography or amenable to embolization. Furthermore, time may not allow such intervention. Many European trauma surgeons consider open surgical packing to be the next best option at this stage. The mortality from this is extremely high, but it may be the only opportunity to control haemorrhage, while the acute situation is allowed to stabilize.

Phase 2. Primary definitive management

1. The order of priority for the first 24 hours of surgical intervention is for injuries to:

- Head.
- Eye and face.
- Spinal cord.
- Viscera (non-haemorrhagic).
- Musculoskeletal system.

The severely traumatized patient requires a multidisciplinary approach to management, involving intensive therapy staff, appropriate surgical teams, specialist nursing care and physiotherapy. It is important to consider nutrition at an early stage, commencing early TPN or enteral feeding, for the hypercatabolic patient.

2. **Further investigations and imaging**, with special X-rays, CT and MRI should be undertaken early in this phase, as directed by signs and surgical planning.

3. **Intracranial collections** require urgent evacuation. Further trauma surgery should not be undertaken while the neurological condition remains unstable.

4. **Penetrating maxillofacial and eye injury** requires urgent surgery to preserve airway and sight. Treatment of lesser injuries may be delayed until swelling has settled or be undertaken simultaneously with skeletal surgery.

5. **Spinal cord compression,** with progressive neurological deterioration, is an indication for urgent decompression following appropriate imaging (MRI). Early steroid administration may be considered. Spinal stabilization protects the cord and allows earlier mobilization.

6. **Visceral and urological injuries** require attention at this stage and include diaphragmatic rupture, bowel perforation, duodenal or pancreatic injury.

7. **Early stabilization of all long bone fractures** in polytrauma patients is generally supported. However, there are certain situations in which the risks outweigh the benefits. Careful decisions have to be made with respect to salvage versus amputation, temporary versus definitive stabilization, and internal versus external fixation. Relative contraindications to early fracture surgery are:

- High intracranial pressures.
- Major pulmonary contusion/shunting.
- Clotting disorders.
- Hypothermia.

8. **Musculoskeletal injury priorities are:**

- Associated vascular injury.
- Compartment syndrome.
- Open fractures and wound management.
- Long bone fractures.
- Intra-articular fractures.

Multiple fracture stabilization requires thoughtful planning. Two surgical teams, ongoing re-evaluation and alteration to plans may all be required. In general, stabilization of the lower limb is undertaken before stabilization of the upper limb. Definitive pelvic or spinal surgery is usually delayed until phase 3. Most closed long bone fractures should be stabilized with IM nails. The management of femoral fractures in the place of severe pulmonary injury is controversial. Reamed IM nailing may precipitate a further pulmonary insult – ARDS. Unreamed nails, external fixation with or without conversion to an IM nail within 2 weeks, or plate fixation, are all alternatives to reduce this problem.

Phase 3. Secondary management: days 3 to 8

The first 5 days is the period of maximal systemic and metabolic response to trauma, and major surgical interventions should be avoided during this period if possible. Further wound management is undertaken (debridement, closure, flap formation) during phase 3. Pelvic, complex joint and spinal stabilization is usually undertaken after the fifth day following detailed imaging and planning.

Phase 4. Rehabilitation

The fate of the polytrauma patient is apparent at this stage. Those recovering require intensive and prolonged rehabilitative care, best supervised in dedicated rehabilitation units. Further surgical interventions and reconstruction may be required, as dictated by particular injuries and complications.

Further reading

Browner BD, Jupiter JB, Levine AM, Trafton PG, eds. *Skeletal Trauma*. Philadelphia: WB Saunders, 1998: 287–348.

Tscherne H, Regel G. Care of the polytraumatised patient. *Journal of Bone and Joint Surgery*, 1996; **78B**: 840–852.

Related topics of interest

Polytrauma – fat embolism and respiratory distress, p. 198; Polytrauma – metabolic response, p. 203; Polytrauma – outcome scores, p. 205; Polytrauma – resuscitation and ATLS, p. 209

POLYTRAUMA – METABOLIC RESPONSE

The metabolic response to injury is a physiological 'systemic inflammatory' reaction to tissue damage. It is a hormone-mediated defence response that establishes the optimum environment for wound control, debridement and subsequent repair. In some circumstances it may become prolonged or exaggerated. If control is lost, this may lead to a pathological systemic inflammatory response known 'host defence failure disease' or 'multi-organ failure'. This accounts for the third peak of the ATLS trimodal distribution of death following major trauma.

Metabolic response phases

The metabolic response is characterized by four phases:

- Injury.
- Turning point.
- Protein anabolism.
- Fat anabolism.

1. **The injury phase.** This lasts 5 to 7 days. During the first 2 days, there are large hormonal changes with an increase in catecholamine and corticosteroid levels, and an initial decrease in the level of insulin. These hormonal changes are thought to be stimulated by the release of numerous cytokines such as interleukin. The result is muscle, fat, and glycogen store catabolism, liberating substrates such as glucose, lactose, proteins and free fatty acids (FFA). These are important for energy, plasma protein formation, immune response and wound repair. The nitrogen balance is negative and albumin levels fall, while cardiac output, oxygen usage and energy consumption are high in proportion to the severity of the trauma. Energy consumption is increased by 20% in a single long bone fracture and by >50% in a burns victim. Water and sodium are in positive balance and potassium in negative balance, due to changes in antidiuretic hormone (ADH) and aldosterone levels.

    In the next 5 days (the flow phase), catecholamine levels continue to be high, but the insulin level increases and protein breakdown slows, with glucose directed at wound healing.

2. **The turning point phase.** This occurs from approximately the fifth to the tenth day, with a reversal of hormonal influences, a change to an anabolic state with positive nitrogen and potassium balance, and negative water and sodium balance.

3. **Protein anabolism phase.** This phase may last 4 to 5 weeks, as corticosteroid levels normalize and growth hormone levels increase. Plasma protein (such as albumin) levels rise and muscle is restored.

4. **Fat anabolism phase.** The final phase is slower and prolonged over several months. Insulin stimulates lipogenesis, as fat stores and body weight are regained.

Prolongation of the injury phase

The essential metabolic response may become exaggerated and detrimental, with 'failure to exit' leading to prolongation of the injury phase. This is called the *systemic inflammatory response syndrome* (SIRS). This is more likely to become established with the presence of pre-injury factors such as poor nutritional state, young adult males, severe injury, pain, fear, and the complications of trauma: sepsis, hypoxia, hypovolaemia, starvation, and acid/base disturbance.

SIRS is characterized by endothelial breakdown in multiple organs, particularly the lung and gut. This leads to ARDS and subsequently to multi-organ failure. The mechanism is thought to be related to cytokine-mediated free radical release. Once initiated, the outcome is poor, so preventing prolongation of the injury phase is vital. The polytrauma patient is especially at risk. Preventative measures should be taken from the outset, with particular attention paid to optimal oxygenation, fluid balance, nutrition, decontamination and analgesia.

Fat embolism syndrome is one of the trauma-related insults which also leads to ARDS. This can contribute to prolonging the injury phase.

Timing of surgery

Surgical 'insults' can prolong the injury phase, such as undertaking major operations at a time when the body is least able to cope (e.g. low acute phase proteins and immunocompetent cells).

Operative intervention should avoid the maximal catabolic phase, to reduce the risk of decompensation. Major operations should ideally be scheduled before day 2 or after day 5. Fracture stabilization should be undertaken on day one, with only dressing changes between day 2 and 5. Further major definitive fracture surgery is delayed until after this period.

Further reading

Hobsley M, Imms F. *Physiology in Surgical Practice.* London: E Arnold, 1993.
Tscherne H, Regel G. Care of the polytraumatised patient. *Journal of Bone and Joint Surgery,* 1996; **78B**: 840–852.

Related topics of interest

Polytrauma – fat embolism and respiratory distress, p. 198; Polytrauma – management and complications, p. 200; Polytrauma – resuscitation and ATLS, p. 209

POLYTRAUMA – OUTCOME SCORES

Scoring systems generate a measure of the severity of a patient's, or a group of patients' trauma, and provide a prediction of survivorship or mortality. Scoring systems can be applied to develop preventative measures, audit a region's trauma load, plan service delivery, audit the level of care and compare outcomes in different regions or countries. These latter functions are important as trauma is the leading cause of mortality and morbidity during the first four decades of life. Scoring systems are applied clinically to triage patients in major disasters and are used to monitor patient progress.

Scores either measure physiological parameters, anatomical injuries, or a combination of both. Some systems are applied at presentation and others at a later stage of injury documentation, even after autopsy. It is important to remember that some patients compensate better for trauma and potential physiological disturbance, which may mask a patient's condition and true level of injury. Therefore, weighting for age rather than absolute trauma scores is important.

Various systems have evolved by merging existing scoring systems, and with the benefit of analysing previous trauma cases, tables have been calculated to predict mortality. Although scoring systems measure the severity of an accident and predict mortality, these scores do not correlate well with the level of recovery and long-term morbidity. The SF-36 item questionnaire may be of more use in the future for long-term morbidity assessment.

In the acute phase, scoring systems are only of value if they assist with patient care. While it is possible to predict the chance of survival, or the need for amputation, the score must be carefully interpreted according to the individual clinical setting. In the longer term, when used to predict delivery of services, measure outcome, or develop preventative measures, the data is very much dependent on the accuracy of data collection and input skills.

Physiological scoring systems

1. **The Glasgow Coma Scale (GCS).** This is used as a quantitative measure of the conscious level following a head injury (*Table 1*). The maximum point score is 15, and is the combined total score for visual (max. 4 points), verbal (max. 5 points) and motor (max. 6 points) responses. Some units CT scan patients with a GCS of ≤13. A GCS of <8 represents a major head injury and a patient with a GCS of 3 points may be brain dead.

2. **Trauma Score (TS).** A modification of the Triage Index, the Trauma Score ascribes points to the parameters of systolic blood pressure, capillary return, respiratory rate, respiratory effort and GCS, with a maximum score of 16 (*Table 2*). A TS of ≤13 indicates major trauma with a 10% risk of mortality.

3. **Revised Trauma Score (RTS).** This is a more consistent predictor of outcome. The three parameters of respiratory rate, systolic blood pressure and GCS each score up to four points, with each score multiplied by a weighting factor (*Table 3*). The RTS is derived from the TS, but places greater emphasis on head injury status.

4. **Acute Physiology and Chronic Health Evaluation III (APACHE III) score.** This can be used as a predictor of mortality. The score is derived from 12 physiological and biochemical indices, and is used mainly in North America to plan delivery and audit the outcome of intensive care unit (ICU) services.

Table 1. Glasgow Coma Scale*

Best visual response (eye opening)	Score	Best verbal response	Score	Best motor response (to painful stimuli)	Score
Spontaneously	4	Orientated	5	Obeys commands	6
To verbal command	3	Confused	4	Localizes	5
To painful stimuli	2	Inappropriate words	3	Withdraws	4
No response	1	Incomprehensible sounds	2	Flexes	3
		No response	1	Extends	2
				No response	1

*Maximum score 15 points.

Table 2. Trauma Score*

Systolic BP (mmHg)	Score	Resp. rate (per min)	Score	Resp. effort	Score	Capillary return	Score	GCS	Score
>90	4	10–24	4	Normal	1	<2 sec	2	15–14	5
90–70	3	25–35	3	Shallow/	0	>2 sec	1	13–11	4
69–50	2	>35	2	reactive		Nil	0	10–8	3
<50	1	<10	1					7–5	2
Nil	0	Nil	0					4–3	1

*Maximum score 16 points.

Table 3. Revised Trauma Score

Resp rate	Score[a]	Systolic BP (mmHg)	Score[b]	GCS	Score[c]
10–29	4	>89	4	15–13	4
>29	3	89–76	3	12–9	3
9–6	2	75–50	2	8–6	2
5–1	1	49–1	1	5–4	1
Nil	0	Nil	0	3	0

[a]Multiply score by a weighting factor of 0.2908.
[b]Multiply score by a weighting factor of 0.7326.
[c]Multiply score by a weighting factor of 0.9368.

Anatomical scoring systems

1. *Abbreviated Injury Scale (AIS).* A complicated and detailed scoring system, the AIS measures the severity of injuries, based on the anatomical location, extent and importance of the injury. A code book lists and scores over 1000 penetrating and blunt injuries, ascribing scores from 1 point for a minor injury to 6 points for a fatal injury.

2. *Injury Severity Score (ISS).* This is an application of the AIS to predict outcome, by using the highest AIS identified in each of six different body areas – head and neck, abdomen and pelvic viscera, bony pelvis and limbs, face, chest and finally, body surface. From these six areas, the ISS is generated by adding together the sum of the square of the three highest AISs. An AIS of 6 in any body area will be fatal and scores the maximum of 75. If there are no fatal injuries, the highest score could still be 75, if the highest scores in three different areas are all 5 points ($5^2 + 5^2 + 5^2 = 75$). The next highest score would be 66 ($5^2 + 5^2 + 4^2 = 66$) and the lowest score 3 ($1^2 + 1^2 + 1^2 = 3$).

A score of 16 corresponds to a TS of $\leqslant$13 and 10% mortality, a score between 29–32 with 50% mortality, and a score of >40 with very low probability of survival. The ISS is not weighted for age, but lethal dose scores associated with 50% mortality (LD_{50}) for different ages have been reported.

Combined scoring systems

1. TRISS. This combines the RTS and ISS as a predictor of survival. A complex formula is used to derive the probability of survival, with weighting coefficients derived by regressional analysis of many thousands of North American trauma victims. There is additional weighting for age and blunt or penetrating trauma. Special charts, TRISSCAN tables, have been prepared from which the probability of survival is derived when the RTS and ISS are calculated.

Analysis can be taken further to produce a 'z statistic' for comparison of institutions, with a standard level of outcome and care.

2. Mangled Extremity Severity Score (MESS). This score ascribes points for soft tissue injury, ischaemia, blood pressure and age, with a maximum score of 14 points (*Table 4*). A score of $\leqslant$6 is a good predictor of a salvageable limb. This system was originally designed for lower limb injury, but is now being applied to the upper limb.

Comparison of data and outcome

The Major Trauma Outcome Study (MTOS) is an international retrospective study of injury and outcome, with a data base of almost 150 000 cases. Based on the RTS and ISS, the MTOS predicts outcomes and compares the performance of different institutions. This analysis started in North America and new weighting coefficients are being determined for UK trauma case mix populations.

Table 4. Mangled Extremity Score

Energy of injury	Score	Limb ischaemia*	Score	Systolic BP (mmHg)	Score	Age (years)	Score
Low energy	1	Diminished pulse,	1	Always >90	0	<30	0
Medium energy	2	Pulseless, paraesthetic, slow capillary refill	2	Transient hypotension	1	30–50	1
High energy	3	Cool, paralysed, insensate	3	Persistent hypotension	2	>50	2
Massive crush	4						

*Double points if ischaemia time exceeds 6 hours.

Further reading

McGowan A. Scoring systems. *Current Orthopaedics*, 1993; 7: 4–8.
Pailthorpe CA. Trauma scores. In: Pynsent PB, Fairbank JCT, Carr AJ, eds. *Outcome Measures in Trauma*. Oxford: Butterworth-Heinemann, 1994; 1–16.

Related topics of interest

Classification of fractures, p. 37; Polytrauma – management and complications, p. 200

POLYTRAUMA – RESUSCITATION AND ATLS

Immediate and effective resuscitation is paramount to the outcome of major and minor trauma. Trauma victims require rapid assessment, structured resuscitation, reassessment, appropriate observation and definitive management. The concept of advanced trauma life support (ATLS) is an effective, structured, safe, reliable, and increasingly well recognized method for the resuscitation of trauma victims.

Trauma is the most common cause of death in the first four decades of life.

Trimodal death distribution

There are three peaks of death following trauma:

- *The first peak* occurs within minutes, due to untreatable, catastrophic neurological or vascular events.
- *The second peak* occurs within an hour or two, due to reversible and treatable injuries.
- *The third peak* occurs after several days or weeks, due to multi-organ failure or infection.

ATLS concept

ATLS started in Nebraska, North America, after an orthopaedic surgeon crashed his plane, injuring his family. He found the delivery of emergency care to be inadequate. The aim of ATLS and resuscitation is to treat reversible, potentially life-threatening injuries, which become evident during the first 'golden' hour after trauma. ATLS provides a simple, structured system for the rapid assessment, treatment, re-evaluation, stabilization and possible transfer of the critically injured, enabling a physician to single-handedly and safely resuscitate a trauma victim, without specialist expertise.

ATLS emphasizes the need to treat trauma victims in a logical sequence, addressing resuscitation of life-threatening injuries in order of potential fatality, under the ABCDE mnemonic:

- Airway and cervical spine protection.
- Breathing and ventilation.
- Circulation and haemorrhage control.
- Disability and neurological status.
- Exposure and environment.

This forms the basis of the primary survey, interrupted only by regular re-assessment and simultaneous treatment of injuries, followed by the secondary survey.

Primary survey

1. Airway and cervical spine protection means rapidly assessing and securing a patent airway, while stabilizing a presumed cervical spine injury. The airway may respond to removal of debris, vomit and secretions alone, or elevation of the soft tissues of the palate with a chin lift or jaw thrust. A nasopharyngeal or oropharyngeal airway, or establishment of a definitive airway by endotracheal intubation, may be required. Oxygen should be delivered with a flow of 10–12 l/min.

Protection of the cervical spine and cord is initially by manual in-line immobilization, followed by a rigid cervical collar, sand bags, tape and a full spine board.

2. Breathing and ventilation are essential for adequate gas exchange, once the airway is secured. The chest should be exposed and examined. Examination may reveal an open chest wound, flail segment, tension pneumothorax or haemothorax, requiring immediate treatment.

A circulatory injury, such as massive haemorrhage or cardiac tamponade, may manifest as, and is easily confused with, a ventilatory problem. A haemothorax should not be drained until venous access is established. A simple pneumothorax, demonstrated on X-ray, may be treated by close observation unless ventilation or transfer are required, when a tube thoracostomy is indicated.

3. Circulation and haemorrhage control can be rapidly addressed. Haemorrhage is the main preventable cause of death in the 'golden' hour. Visible haemorrhage should be controlled by local pressure. Venous access should be established with two wide bore (16 gauge) cannulae, placed peripherally, in the femoral vein, or by venous cutdown. Blood is sent for analysis and cross-match. Fluid replacement may be with warmed crystalloid, but blood may be required. The blood may be fully cross-matched, type-specific or O negative, depending on the urgency.

Young or athletic patients have a large physiological reserve, but the elderly may only have a limited ability to respond following blood loss. Massive blood loss affects the level of consciousness. Immediate surgical intervention may be required for uncontrolled internal haemorrhage. Cardiac output may be reduced by cardiac tamponade – pericardiocentesis of a small amount of blood can have a dramatic effect.

4. Disability and neurological status should be assessed with the AVPU scale and measurement of pupillary size and reaction. This gives an indication of the neurological status of the patient. The Glasgow Coma Scale score is recorded during the secondary survey. AVPU denotes:

- Alert.
- Verbal stimulus response.
- Painful stimulus response.
- Unresponsive.

Breathing, circulatory problems and drugs may cause a diminished level of consciousness.

5. Exposure and environment is a reminder to expose and examine a victim, while keeping them warm and protecting medical personnel form risk and danger.

Resuscitation

Resuscitation is undertaken in tandem with the primary survey, addressing life-threatening injuries as they are identified.

Monitoring

Regular observations are essential and should be accurately recorded. Monitoring includes using an ECG monitor and pulse oximeter. A nasogastric tube and urinary catheter, which is a good monitor of perfusion, should be inserted.

Secondary survey

The secondary survey includes obtaining a history, thorough examination, appropriate X-rays and specialist investigations.

Specialist treatment and transfer

When a particular injury is identified, assistance from the relevant discipline should be requested, or the patient transferred to a suitable centre if local assistance is not available. Urgent transfer may be appropriate, or need arranging, before the secondary survey.

Re-assessment

Constant re-assessment of a patient is vital during the resuscitation period. If there are signs of deterioration, or failure to respond, the safest course of action is to return to the start of the primary survey, re-evaluate and request assistance.

X-rays

Chest and pelvic X-rays are mandatory requirements during initial resuscitation. A lateral cervical spine X-ray is required if there are any indicators of a neck injury.

Further reading

Advanced Trauma and Life Support Programme For Doctors – The Student Manual. Chicago: The American College of Surgeons, 1997; 125–141.

Related topic of interest

Polytrauma – management and complications, p. 200

PRE-OPERATIVE PLANNING

The aim of pre-operative planning is to ensure optimal patient selection, appropriate timing of surgical intervention and utilization of the appropriate technique of surgical stabilization. This optimizes the end result. A full understanding of the complications associated with these techniques is mandatory.

Adequate pre-operative planning will assist the other theatre staff, especially the scrub team, providing them with a greater understanding of the procedure and making preparation of the necessary equipment easier.

Considerations

Appropriate care of the injured patient does not start at the time of the operation. It is imperative that patients are prepared properly for surgery and that the timing of surgery does not cause any further unnecessary harm. Rapid stabilization of skeletal injuries is frequently encouraged, but can lead to further unnecessary or prolonged trauma to an already injured patient.

Non-operative treatment of musculoskeletal injuries is still appropriate for some types of injury. Surgical stabilization, while frequently possible can often be unnecessary, although opinion varies between surgeons. A clear indication for surgery is required and the complications and other harmful effects that could arise from the operation should be borne in mind before proceeding.

Planning

Once the decision to operate has been made, simple decisions regarding timing, type of anaesthesia, patient positioning and surgical approach should be made. Methods of surgical stabilization should be well thought out pre-operatively.

When planning the type of operative procedure required, the character of the fracture, degree of soft tissue injury, biology of fracture healing, and the patient's age and activity levels should all be considered. The surgeon must be fully conversant with the operative methods to be employed and, together with the theatre staff, should ensure that the appropriate instruments and implants are readily available.

A careful review of the radiographs should be undertaken prior to surgical intervention, as a clear understanding of the fracture pattern is essential. Proximal and distal extensions into joints, multiple fragments and the fracture pattern should be considered. This, together with a clear knowledge of the actual and possible soft tissue injuries, should help the surgeon to decide on the method of stabilization.

Pre-operative drawings

From an X-ray of the uninjured side, an outline drawing of the bone is traced and the fracture fragments drawn onto this in a different colour. A tracing of the chosen implant and screws is then made using a third colour. This helps to plan the operative approach, the implant required, and the number/type of screws or other implants that may be required.

While pre-operative templating is not always required with increasing experience, in difficult or complex fractures with extensive comminution, displacement or angulation, this can be an invaluable technique. However, if the surgeon is unfamiliar with this form of pre-operative planning, planning can be difficult. It is therefore recommended that surgeons practice templating procedures on relatively simple fractures, to gain the experience and skill for more complex procedures.

Further reading

Mast J. Preoperative planning and principles of reduction. In: Müller ME, Allgöwer M, Schneider R, Willenegger H, eds. *Manual of Internal Fixation*, 3rd Edn. Berlin: Springer-Verlag, 1991; 159–177.

Related topics of interest

Biomaterials – implants in trauma, p. 15; Biomechanics of fracture implants and implant removal, p. 19; Principles of operative fracture management, p. 220

PRINCIPLES OF EXTERNAL FIXATION

There are certain advantages and indications for skeletal stabilization by external rather than internal fixation. External fixation has unique characteristics, which differ from those of internal fixation. These include:

- Rapid skeletal stabilization by percutaneous pins and connecting frames, remote from the site of injury.
- Versatility to accommodate different injuries and anatomy.
- Soft tissue access.
- Adjustment of alignment and fixation during fracture healing.
- Indirect closed reduction by ligamentotaxis.

Indications for external fixation in trauma

- Grade III long bone fractures, especially the tibia.
- Closed fractures, with degloving skin injuries.
- 'Open book' pelvic fractures.
- Polytrauma.
- Paediatric femoral fractures.
- Peri-articular and metaphyseal fractures.

Types of fixator

1. **Simple fixators** may be of the clamp or pin type and may be uni-planar or multi-planar. Pin types (AO, Orthofix, Wagner) permit little adjustment to the reduction once applied. Clamp types (Hoffmann) allow reduction after application.

2. **Ring fixators** (Ilizarov, Monticelli–Spinelli, Sequoi) have components that surround the limb and allow considerable adjustment during treatment.

3. **Hybrid fixators** are a combination of simple and ring fixators.

Frame components and mechanics

Frames consist of pins or wires for fixation to bone, with a series of external bodies and connecting rods or rings.

1. **Pins.** The pin–bone interface is crucial to frame stability. Half pins pass through one side of the limb, whereas transfixion pins or wires pass all the way through the limb. Most are stainless steel with a threaded portion of variable length. The following pin characteristics are important:

- Pin stiffness $\propto$ radius^4.
- Pin diameter depends on the size of the particular bone.
- Pin diameter greater than one-third of the bone diameter risks fatigue fracture of the bone.

Tapered pins reduce screw deformation at the interface between the large shank and the threaded portion. Tapered pins can be tightened, should loosening occur. Two or three pins widely spaced in one plane, optimize stability.

2. Transfixion wires. Wires of 1.5–1.8 mm are unthreaded. When fixed and tensioned at 90–120 kg, deforming forces are resisted. Bone purchase is by tension and friction. Some wires have enlargements (olives) on one end to prevent movement of bone or to apply a deforming force.

Frame stability

Frame stability is increased by:

1. Multi-planar fixation with good frame/pin linkage.
2. Increasing the diameter and number of pins.
3. Reducing the distance between the frame and the bone.
4. Reduction of the fracture with bony apposition.

Fixation modes

The final construction and properties of the frame depend upon the indication for external fixation and the need for bone transport.

- *Static axial compression* is suitable for simple fractures.
- *Dynamic axial compression* allows the application of controlled reciprocal micro-movement or elastic deformation called 'dynamization'.
- *Neutralization* maintains alignment where the bone is multifragmented.
- *Distraction by ligamentotaxis* reduces peri-articular fractures.

Application considerations

1. Anatomy. Pins or wires must be placed in positions that minimize injury. It is especially important not to impale neurovascular structures. If possible, muscle penetration should be avoided to prevent tethering. Zones of safety are described with respect to a 360° arc based on cross-sectional anatomy studies.

- Half pins are generally safe in the subcutaneous border of the tibia and ulna, or around the lateral intermuscular septum of the humerus and thigh.
- In the distal tibia an oblique wire may safely be passed through the fibula and anteriorly through the tibia, with another perpendicular wire passing through the subcutaneous border of the tibia.
- In the proximal tibia, transverse wires are safe in an anterior arc of 220°.

2. Technical aspects. The following should be considered:

- Relaxed skin incisions should be made to prevent tension necrosis and infection.
- The pin–bone interface is vital for stability of the construct. Thermal injury should be prevented by cooled predrilling. Predrilling to a diameter slightly smaller than the pin, radially preloads the pin, and is recommended for half pins. Schanz pins are tapered for this purpose.
- Avoid bending to preload the pins.
- Wires are best placed at 90° (minimum 30°) to each other for stability.
- Rings should have a 3 cm gap from the skin circumferentially.
- A strict pin care regime is important to reduce infection frequency and severity.

Complications

Complications are often considered to be high, but this may reflect the severity of the presenting injury, for which the external fixator has been employed.

Pin tract infection occurs in 50%, ranging from minor inflammation to severe osteomyelitis.

Other complications can be classified as follows:

- Osteomyelitis.
- Joint stiffness.
- Non-union 5–10%.
- Malunion 5%.
- Frame failure (rare).
- Pin loosening.

Further reading

Behrens F, Searls K. External fixation of the tibia. Basic concepts and prospective evaluation. *Journal of Bone and Joint Surgery*, 1986; **68B**: 246–254.

Pollak AN, Ziran BH. Principles of external fixation. In: Browner BD, Jupiter JB, Levine AM, Trafton PG, eds. *Skeletal Trauma*. Philadelphia: WB Saunders, 1998; 67–86.

Related topics of interest

Bone defects, transport and late reconstruction, p. 25; Non-union and delayed union, p. 153; Open fracture management, p. 156; Principles of operative fracture management, p. 220

PRINCIPLES OF NON-OPERATIVE FRACTURE MANAGEMENT

The closed treatment of fractures follows the standard algorithm of reduce, immobilize and rehabilitate. The three principal forms of immobilization are casting, functional bracing and traction. Operative fracture treatment has advantages in many cases; however, there are patients for whom non-operative treatment is preferable and others for whom non-operative treatment augments operative methods.

Reduction

The principles of adequate closed reduction are:

1. *Anaesthesia* to provide analgesia and in some cases muscle relaxation.

2. *Planning*, with a rehearsal of reduction and cast application.

3. *Reduction* to re-align the fracture. When skeletal stability is lost, the soft tissues may provide some stability. Charnley described utilization of the soft tissue hinge or 'ligamentotaxis', on the concavity of a fracture (dorsally in a Colles' fracture). In high-energy injuries the soft tissue envelope is disrupted to a greater extent than in low-energy injuries – consequently reduction will be less stable.

4. *The reduction manoeuvre* consists of the following (Colles' fracture procedure described in parentheses):

- Disimpaction: traction, followed by increasing the deformity (dorsiflexing the distal fragment).
- Reduction: the mechanism of injury is reversed (pronation and palmar flexion).
- Locking the reduction: the distal fragment is brought into rotational alignment with the proximal; rotation is then exaggerated to lock reduction (further pronation).

5. *Splint application* with a moulded cast, to achieve three-point fixation, placing the soft tissue hinge under tension. (In a Colles' fracture the three points are dorsal, proximal and distal to the fracture, and volar just proximal to the fracture.)

6. *Clinical and radiological assessment* of the result and, if inadequate, repetition of the process.

7. *Excessive swelling, haematoma or soft tissue interposition* make the reduction more difficult. Interposed soft tissue requires open removal.

Casts

Undisplaced fractures require splintage for analgesia and to prevent displacement. Displaced fractures, which have been reduced, require a moulded cast, as outlined above. Fractures without a soft tissue hinge are inappropriate for cast management.

Traditionally, casts are applied without padding (Bohler), or more commonly with padding (Bologna). Application and moulding of the unpadded cast is easier, but associated with pressure complications. Application of the padded cast is more difficult, as excess padding in the absence of correct moulding produces a poor fit. Current preference is to use an intermediate amount of padding.

Traditional plaster of Paris relies on calcium sulphate taking up its water of crystallization ($CaSO_4 \cdot H_2O + H_2O \longleftrightarrow CaSO_4 \cdot 2H_2O$ + heat). Fibreglass casts are made of fibreglass impregnated with polyurethane prepolymer, which cures in ultraviolet light to form a light, durable cast.

Functional bracing

Functional bracing aims to improve function in the limb by allowing early joint movement. The patient's soft tissues and the external brace control alignment of the fracture. The patient controls the weight-bearing status, as pain indicates excessive fracture mobility. Clinical union precedes radiological union.

Sarmiento describes five stages of fracture healing:

- Stage 1: no healing has yet taken place.
- Stage 2: the callus is rubbery and allows bending.
- Stage 3: hard callus, starting to ossify.
- Stage 4: structural callus.
- Stage 5: remodelling callus.

In stage 1, the soft tissues are the only factors controlling alignment in two ways:

1. The extent of soft tissue stripping at the time of injury determines the maximum possible displacement of the fragments. With time, the soft tissues heal, reducing the potential for displacement. It is necessary to hold the limb out to length in the short-term (e.g. with traction) during stage 1.

2. The rigid brace encloses an essentially fluid limb segment (the soft tissues with a fractured bone approximately correspond to a fluid filled tube). If the fluid is surrounded by a tight fitting, rigid cast, the cast will act as an exoskeleton so that loading will not cause deformation.

This implies that the traditional dictum of 'the joint above and below should be immobilized' can be ignored to some degree, allowing the bracing to be more functional. Thus, a humeral shaft fracture can be treated without immobilizing the shoulder or elbow, while a tibial fracture requires at least 1 week in an above-knee cast. A humeral fracture heals in 8–10 weeks, a tibial fixture in 12–16 weeks. A femoral fracture reaches stage 2 at 3–5 weeks and stage 4 at 8–10 weeks.

Traction

1. Traction needs an opposing force, so is either *fixed* (consider a femoral fracture braced between the ring of a Thomas' splint on the perineum and the tapes attaching the limb to the distal end of the splint), or *balanced* (a weight attached to the splint and hung over the end of the bed 'balances' the body weight). Finally, the limb must be *suspended*, allowing care around the limb and avoiding pressure.

2. Traction can be applied by a hanging plaster (as in humeral fractures), or by using a pin above and below the fracture incorporated in plaster.

3. *Skin (Buck's) traction* can be used to a maximum of 4 kg, before causing skin damage.

4. *Skeletal traction* can be used with larger weights. A threaded Denham pin is preferred and prevents the migration seen with a smooth Steinmann pin.

The Thomas' splint is used for femoral fractures, with calico slings and padding behind the thigh to re-establish the femoral bow. After initial manipulative reduction the fracture position is usually maintained by *suspended, balanced skeletal* traction through a proximal tibial pin. Many varieties are described, including Hamilton–Russell, Perkins, and Fisk.

Contraindications to non-operative treatment

1. *Patient:* Obese, neuropathic, arteriopathic, non-compliant.

2. *Fracture:* Interposed soft tissue, excessive soft tissue damage.

3. *Surgeon:* Poor cast or reduction technique, improper supervision of technique, inadequate clinical and radiological follow-up.

Further reading

Charnley J. *The Closed Treatment of Common Fractures*, 3rd Edn. London: Churchill Livingstone, 1961.
Latta LL, Sarmiento A, Zych GA. Principles of non-operative fracture treatment. In: Browner BD, Jupiter JB, Levine AM, Trafton PG, eds. *Skeletal Trauma*. Philadelphia: WB Saunders, 1998; 237–266.

Related topic of interest

Principles of operative fracture management, p. 220

PRINCIPLES OF OPERATIVE FRACTURE MANAGEMENT

Producing a comprehensive list of indications for operative treatment is difficult. In the majority of cases, the reason for operative intervention is the belief that the outcome will be 'better' than with conservative treatment.

Indications for operative treatment

1. Articular fractures. For optimum results, intra-articular fractures require anatomical reduction and early mobilization.

2. Open fractures. These require debridement, fracture stabilization to reduce dead space and maintain alignment, followed by soft tissue reconstruction.

3. Vascular injury. Vascular repair follows fracture stabilization. Stabilization protects the repair, if limb salvage is attempted.

4. Haemorrhage. Massive haemorrhage may require swift intervention and the most important example is an 'open book' pelvic fracture, which should be closed and stabilized.

5. Compartment syndrome. Following fasciotomy, the fracture is usually stabilized.

6. Pathological fractures. Internal fixation provides analgesia and makes nursing easier in disseminated disease. Specialist management is mandatory for primary bone tumours.

7. Nerve injury. Exploration should be undertaken if there is neurological injury in the presence of an open wound, or if neurological deficit occurs after closed reduction.

8. Polytrauma. Operative stabilization in polytrauma reduces the incidence of ARDS and FES. The mortality at 1 month is reduced from 29% to 5% with operative stabilization.

9. Early mobilization. Avoiding the complications of prolonged recumbency by fixation and early mobilization is well accepted with the fractured neck of femur. There is evidence that nailing femoral and tibial fractures leads to earlier rehabilitation, reduced union times and a lower incidence of malunion.

10. Late reconstruction. Internal fixation is used in late reconstruction.

11. Physeal injuries. The aim of treatment is anatomical reduction. This sometimes requires operative fixation.

Timing of surgery

Timing depends on the indication, but the majority of fracture surgery can be undertaken during daylight hours, with full backup available. A few conditions require immediate or emergency surgery, including:

- Open fractures, or compromised skin.
- Vascular compromise.
- Neurological compromise, with gross displacement.
- Polytrauma.
- Compartment syndrome.
- Massive haemorrhage.
- Hip dislocation.
- Displaced subcapital femoral neck fracture in a young patient.

Surgical procedure

If a decision to operate is made, the approach to reconstruction depends on:

- Nature of the injury.
- Condition of the patient.
- Surgeon's experience and personal preference.
- Operating theatre availability.
- The 'fitness' of the surgical team.
- Implant availability.

Principles of operative treatment

There are two possible modes of fracture healing: (i) **primary or direct bone healing**, in a fracture rigidly stabilized by internal fixation, when there is direct contact between the fragments; (ii) **healing with 'callus'**. Fortunately both types of healing give satisfactory results. Primary healing is seen after rigid compression plate fixation and healing with callus after IM nailing. This should not be confused with **'indirect bone healing'**, which follows closed treatment in a cast.

Compression

Interfragmentary compression during fixation has been advocated by the AO group. The postulated advantages are:

- The increased stability produced by contact between fragments.
- The absence of a gap, which prevents motion at the fracture site. A gap can lead to fatigue failure of the implant.
- Loading of the bone by compression, prevents bone resorption at the fracture site.

Compression is a means of increasing the stability of fixation, but not a method of accelerating union. Nevertheless, it has a major effect on the biology of bone healing. Bone can withstand 300 kPa/cm^2 of pressure before undergoing necrosis.

There are many ways of achieving compression, but the two principal types are *static* and *dynamic*. Static compression is applied at the time of surgery, for example with a DCP. Dynamic compression is dependent upon loading of the fracture/implant construct and is seen with tension band wiring of the olecranon.

Tension band

The use of an unyielding band (wire, plate) on the tension side of a bone converts tension to compression. The compression is dynamic, optimal compression only being achieved with functional activity. The most common application of a tension band technique is for fixation of olecranon and patellar fractures. However, a plate applied to the lateral femoral cortex (the tension side) also produces dynamic compression. Such a plate may also be acting as a static compression plate.

Biological fixation

With massive comminution it may not be possible to reduce a fracture anatomically and compress the fragments. Healing therefore relies on soft tissue viability and callus formation. The emphasis with comminuted fractures is to maintain the 'biological milieu' around the fracture to enhance healing. This can be achieved using a number of techniques:

- Indirect reduction methods, with traction and a guide wire.
- Using implants that minimize fracture exposure, including IM nails, external fixators, and 'wave' plates. The wave plate has a bowed section around the fracture, preventing the need for periosteal stripping and soft tissue exposure. This can be applied with limited exposure.
- Using materials with an elastic modulus close to that of bone (e.g. titanium, carbon fibre).
- Reducing implant/bone contact (unreamed nails, LC-DCP).
- Avoiding devascularization of fragments.

A major concern with rigid fixation is the reduction in bone density under the plate – there are two proposed causes for this. Some propose that loss of density follows stress protection of the bone by rigidity of the plate (the elastic modulus of stainless steel is 12× that of bone), while others propose that it is the disturbance of the periosteal blood supply by the plate.

The LC-DCP has been introduced to try to address both of these issues. It is made of titanium, which is less rigid, and has a low contact profile.

Further reading

Mazzoca AD, Caputo AE, Browner BD *et al.* Principles of internal fixation. In: Browner BD, Jupiter JB, Levine AM, Trafton PG, eds. *Skeletal Trauma*. Philadelphia: WB Saunders, 1998; 287–348.
Muller ME, Allgower M, Schneider R, Willenegger H, eds. *Manual of Internal Fixation*. Berlin: Springer-Verlag, 1991.

Related topics of interest

PRINCIPLES OF SOFT TISSUE MANAGEMENT

There are three stages in the management of soft tissue injuries associated with open fractures:

- Prevention of further injury.
- Debridement.
- Reconstruction.

The first two stages are often managed solely by the orthopaedic surgeon.

Prevention of further injury

During resuscitation, avoiding hypovolaemia helps maintain peripheral perfusion. Local hypoxic damage can be minimized by prompt reduction of any fracture or dislocation causing arterial occlusion, or obviously distorting the soft tissues. Arterial injury and compartment syndrome should be addressed early. Exposed tissues must not become desiccated.

Debridement

Formal debridement to remove foreign material, dead tissue and haematoma, should be performed in an operating theatre. The aim is to reduce the bacterial load, preventing increase above 100000 microorganisms per gram. The use of a tourniquet is controversial. A tourniquet should perhaps be applied and only inflated if blood loss is excessive.

The edges of the traumatic wound are excised and the wound extended if required. Visualization is paramount, as the 'zone of injury' extends beyond the traumatic wound. All dead fascia, tendon, bone and muscle are excised. The viability of muscle is assessed according to the four 'Cs' – contractility, colour, consistency and capacity to bleed. The wound is irrigated with 9 l of isotonic saline and the fracture stabilized. Re-establishing alignment and stability reduces the dead space and improves perfusion.

Principles of reconstruction

The wound is reinspected at 48-hour intervals until the tissues are stable and viable. At this stage, which should be within 4 days, the traumatic wound is closed.

Wound closure requires a variety of techniques, from delayed primary closure to free flaps, based on a sound understanding of the vascular anatomy of muscle and skin.

Vascular anatomy of muscle and skin

Skin blood flow is from a deep dermal plexus of vessels running parallel to the skin in the superficial fascia. This plexus is principally supplied from musculocutaneous perforators. These vessels are derived from the muscular pedicular vessels. The perforating vessels supply limited areas of overlying skin and form the basis of the 'random pattern' flap (*Figure 1a*).

Muscular blood supply is from one or more pedicular arteries. The muscle can be rotated on its pedicle, or the pedicle divided creating a 'free' flap (*Figure 1a*).

A second pattern of blood supply occurs in defined anatomical regions (such as

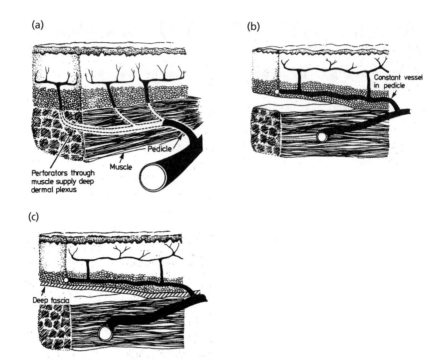

Figure 1. Blood supply to the skin. (a) Random pattern and myocutaneous flaps are based on perforating vessels from the muscle. The muscle can be rotated with or without the overlying skin. (b) An axial pattern flap. (c) A fasciocutaneous flap. This figure was first published in the BMJ (Davies DM Plastic and Reconstructive Surgery: Skin Cover, *BMJ* 1985, vol. 290, pp. 765–767) and is reproduced in modified form by permission of the BMJ.

the groin flap on the superficial circumflex iliac artery), where a specific cutaneous artery arising from a large artery, runs superficially to muscle in the subcutaneous fat. These vessels reinforce the musculocutaneous blood supply. The flap is raised so the vessels run axially, which allows the flap to be raised for a greater length than a random pattern flap. Such flaps are known as 'axial pattern' flaps (*Figure 1b*).

Random pattern flap size is limited, but can be increased by raising a flap with the deep fascia. This incorporates the superficial plexus of vessels into the random flap, forming a 'fasciocutaneous flap' (*Figure 1c*).

The reconstructive ladder

In order of increasing complexity, wound closure can be achieved in the following ways.

1. Delayed primary closure. This involves suturing the wound when the tissues are viable and not too tight.

2. Healing by secondary intention. Allowing a wound to granulate and epithelialize may be appropriate in certain cases. However, this leaves a portal of entry for microbes, allows drying of tissue and often an unsightly scar.

3. **Split skin grafting.** This is frequently employed, often in combination with other techniques. A vascularized bed is required, so split skin grafts cannot be applied to bone (in the absence of periosteum), cartilage, tendon or nerve. The graft relies on vascular in-growth and to improve 'take rates' the graft should be sutured to its bed. Haematoma should be avoided by attention to haemostasis of the bed, or by applying the graft after a delay of 48 hours. Split skin can be 'meshed' to increase the area of coverage. Skin can be stored in saline gauze at 4°C for 2 weeks.

4. **Full thickness skin or composite grafts**

5. **Local flaps.** These include:
- Cutaneous – random pattern, fasciocutaneous and axial pattern flaps. Random pattern flaps have a limited length, which is equal to the width of the base. Fasciocutaneous and axial pattern flaps can be raised to greater lengths.
- Muscle – a local muscle is rotated into the defect on a vascular pedicle.
- Myocutaneous – muscle, fascia and skin.

6. **Free flaps.** These include:
- Cutaneous – such as the groin flap.
- Muscular – commonly used muscles are latissimus dorsi, gracilis and the radial free forearm flap.
- Myocutaneous – free muscle with its overlying skin.
- Complex – including bone (free fibula or radius) and nerve. Nerve grafting can either give protective sensation (e.g. on the sole of the foot), or movement (e.g. gracilis to the forearm after Volkmann's).

Choice of cover

Choice of tissue cover depends on:
- The nature of the injury. Low-energy injuries can often be reconstructed with a cutaneous or fasciocutaneous flap. For high-energy injuries, reconstruction with muscle improves the local blood supply, which clears staphylococci better than a cutaneous flap. In a high-energy injury, local damage may preclude the use of local tissues, necessitating a free flap.
- Surgical experience.
- The location of the injury. A flap of a size and contour that does not interfere with function should be used. Local flaps have obvious restrictions in the area covered.

Skin flap failure rates

Failure rates can be reduced by avoiding:
- Systemic hypotension.
- Smoking.
- Infection.
- Haematoma.

- Tension in closure.
- Poor arterial inflow, which is more important than venous congestion.

  With good technique, failure rates are <10% and may be lower for free rather than local flaps.

Reconstruction techniques by location

Examples of these techniques are given below:

- Knee: one, or both heads of gastrocnemius.
- Tibia: proximal third – gastrocnemius.
  middle third – soleus.
  distal third – for low-energy wounds, a fasciocutaneous flap may suffice, but the majority require a free flap.
- Ankle: dorsalis pedis island pedicle flap, or a free flap, such as the radial free forearm. Both can be harvested as sensate flaps.
- Foot: plantar wounds require stable and sensate tissue. The medial plantar arch can be used as a sensate flap to cover the heel. For plantar wounds, innervated radial free forearm flaps have been used.

Further reading

McGregor IA. *Fundamental Techniques of Plastic Surgery*. Edinburgh: Churchill Livingstone, 1989; 45–118.

Sanders R, Swiontowski M, Nunley J *et al.* The management of fractures with soft-tissue disruptions. *Journal of Bone and Joint Surgery*, 1993; 75A: 778–788.

Related topic of interest

Amputation and replantation, p. 3

RADIATION EXPOSURE

It is accepted that there is no safe dose of radiation. While the average dose to the orthopaedic surgeon in a single year has been shown to fall within national guidelines, understanding of the principles of radiation protection is important.

Fundamentals of radiation biology

Ionizing radiation (e.g. X-rays, γ-rays) is defined as radiation with sufficient energy to release electrons from the atom. The electron release damages biological tissue, principally DNA. The unit of radiation absorbed is the Gray (Gy). The Gray is defined as 1 joule of ionizing radiation absorbed by 1 kg of matter; however, the Gray makes no allowance for the type of ionizing radiation. This is important as different types of ionizing radiation deliver their energy with differing spatial distribution and biological effect. Thus α-particles are $20\times$ more damaging than X- and γ-rays. This 'quality' factor (Q) is multiplied by the absorbed dose (D) to give the 'dose-equivalent' (H). H is measured in 'sieverts' (Sv).

As well as factors associated with radioactivity, different tissues have different sensitivities and the relative sensitivities are expressed as 'tissue weighting factors' (w_t). The organs most at risk are the gonads ($w_t = 0.25$), red bone marrow, lung, colon and stomach ($w_t = 0.12$). Gonadal irradiation causes both impairment of fertility and mutagenesis with resultant effects on offspring.

The effects of radiation

Ionizing radiation can:

- Kill cells.
- Cause long-term damage.
- Cause site-specific effects such as cataracts.

Long-term damage is mediated through damage to DNA. While cell killing is not significant in diagnostic imaging, long-term effects remain a concern. Animal studies have shown that 1 Gy non-specifically reduces life expectancy by 5%. This non-specific effect is unproven in man. However, there is no doubt that radiation can induce cancer; osteosarcomas are reported in radium-dial painters and excess malignancy is reported in patients with ankylosing spondylitis treated by radiation.

Environmental radiation

The average UK background radiation is 2.2 mSv per year (range 1.5–7.5 mSv), made up from various sources:

- 50% from radon gas, particularly in Devon and Cornwall.
- 14% from medical sources, such as X-rays, nuclear medicine scans and radiotherapy.
- 14% from γ-radiation in rocks and building materials.
- 11.5% from natural radionuclides ingested in food and drink.
- 10% from cosmic radiation.
- 0.5% from occupational sources, nuclear weapons testing, discharges and other sources.

Table 1. Dose from various common radiological procedures compared to a chest X-ray and background radiation levels

	Typical effective dose (mSv)	Equivalent number of chest X-rays	Equivalent period of background radiation
Limbs and joints (excl. hips)	<0.01	<0.05	<1.5 days
Hip	0.3	15	7 weeks
Pelvis	0.7	35	4 months
Lumbar spine	1.3	65	7 months
^{99m}Tc bone scan	4	200	1.8 years
CT pelvis	10	500	4.5 years

Table 1 summarizes the dose from various common radiological procedures, compared to a chest X-ray and background radiation levels.

Principles of radiation protection

Radiation protection is based on three principles:

- Justification – a proposed intervention should do more good than harm.
- Optimization – the magnitude of the dose should be kept as low as reasonably achievable (abbreviated as 'ALARA').
- Limitation – exposure of individuals should be subject to a dose limit.

1. Staff safety. Adequate training and local rules are paramount. New members of staff should be trained and copies of the rules should be available. There are three physical factors involved in protection:

- Time – reduction of the time of exposure to radiation.
- Distance – ionizing radiation obeys the inverse square law, such that the dose reduces as the square of the distance between the individual and source increases.
- Shielding – protective screens, lead aprons, etc.

The International Radiological Protection Board recommend an occupational limit on the effective dose of 20 mSv for an individual in a single year. This corresponds to an increased lifetime risk of an induced fatal cancer of 4% and compares to the population risk of dying from cancer of 20–25%.

Monitoring is important and local rules dictate that some, or all, staff should wear a personal dosimeter, which may either be of the film or thermoluminescent sort.

2. Patient safety. The number of radiological examinations should be minimized. CT imaging must be carefully justified, as CT contributes almost half of the collective dose from all radiological examinations. The additional risk of a lifetime cancer is 1:1000000 for a chest X-ray compared to 1:2000 for an abdominal CT scan. However, these figures are small in comparison to the overall risk of 1:4.

3. **Children.** Children are at increased risk for two reasons:

- Under the age of 10 years there is an increased risk of carcinogenesis.
- The dose equivalent depends on organ mass. The organ mass in children is smaller, thus the dose equivalent in a child will be greater for the same administered dose.

4. **Pregnancy and protection of the foetus.** There is evidence of leukaemia and mental retardation when the foetus *in utero* is exposed to ionizing radiation. The Royal College of Radiologists recommend the following:

- Irradiation of the foetus should be avoided whenever possible.
- Women of reproductive age should be asked if they are, or may be pregnant when the pelvic area is going to be irradiated. This in effect includes any X-ray between the diaphragm and knees.
- If pregnancy is a possibility, the radiologist and referring clinician need to decide whether to delay investigation until after the next menstrual period.
- If pregnancy cannot be excluded, but the menstrual period is NOT overdue and the procedure gives a relatively low dose to the uterus, the examination may proceed. Examinations giving high doses of irradiation (e.g. IVP, pelvic and abdominal CT) should be performed in the first 10 days of the cycle. If the examination is considered necessary, despite the possibility of pregnancy, the dose of irradiation should be minimized and the decision to proceed clearly recorded.

Even if the foetus has been irradiated the risk rarely merits either invasive foetal diagnostic studies (e.g. amniocentesis), or termination of pregnancy.

Further reading

Dendy PP, Palmer KE, Szaz KF. Radiation protection. In: Sharp PF, Gemmell HG, Smith FW, eds. *Practical Nuclear Medicine*. Oxford: IRL Press at Oxford University Press, 1989; 91–107.

Making the Best Use of a Department of Radiology, 4th Edn. London: The Royal College of Radiologists, 1998.

Radiation Exposure of the UK Population – 1993 Review. London: National Radiation Protection Board (HMSO), 1993.

RADIUS AND ULNA – DIAPHYSEAL FRACTURES

The bowed radius rotates around the ulna allowing supination and pronation. The aim of treatment is to restore bony anatomy and preserve movement.

Classification

The most commonly used classification is one which divides the bones into thirds. The AO classification has been shown to have a high degree of interobserver variability. Three eponyms are commonly used:

- Monteggia (ulna fracture with radial head dislocation).
- Nightstick (isolated ulna shaft fracture).
- Galeazzi (radial fracture and distal radio-ulnar joint (DRUJ) dislocation).

Clinical examination and imaging

1. Forearm fractures are the second most common open fracture. Clinical examination should include the elbow and wrist, and full neurovascular assessment. The earliest signs of compartment syndrome are palpable tension in the soft tissues and pain on passive finger movement.

2. AP and lateral radiographs of the forearm, including the wrist and elbow, are the minimum imaging requirement. A line through the centre of the radial head and neck should pass through the centre of the capitellum in all planes. Signs of DRUJ injury include fracture of the base of the ulnar styloid, widening of the joint on the AP radiograph, dislocation on a true lateral radiograph and radial shortening of >5 mm.

Treatment

Non-displaced fractures are rare. Angulation of <10° and translation of <50% is acceptable. Closed reduction is difficult to achieve and maintain, so ORIF is the mainstay of treatment.

1. An above elbow cast for 6 weeks, with weekly X-rays for the first 4 weeks is used in the non-displaced fracture.

2. Open reduction and internal fixation through a Henry approach is used in the distal two-thirds, and through a Henry or Thompson approach in the proximal third. Thompson's approach allows the plate to be placed on the tension side of the bone, but is technically more demanding. A 3.5 mm narrow DCP is used and should fix seven cortices on either side of the fracture. The use of primary supplementary bone grafting is controversial, but a reasonable guideline is to graft if cortical continuity is lost for more than one-third of the circumference. Union rates are >95%. Functionally good or excellent results are obtained in >90%.

3. Unlocked IM nails do not provide rotational or longitudinal stability. It is difficult to re-establish the radial bow and non-union rates of 10–20% are reported. Nailing is therefore not popular, although malleable locking nails are being developed and may gain popularity.

4. *External fixation* has a role in Gustilo IIIB and IIIC injuries. Ten per cent of patients require fixator adjustment and superficial infections are common. Only 2/3 of patients have good or excellent results. These poorer outcomes are probably related to the severity of the initial injury, rather than the method of fixation.

5. *Gustilo I, II and IIIA fractures* are treated with antibiotic prophylaxis, debridement and irrigation, before ORIF in the same manner as closed fractures. Bone grafting, if required, is performed at the time of final wound closure. IIIB and IIIC injuries can be treated by internal or external fixation. The decision is based on the soft tissue wound, bone loss and condition of the patient.

Monteggia fractures

These form <5% of forearm fractures. The injury is classified according to the direction of radial head dislocation (Bado classification):

- Type 1: anterior (commonest).
- Type 2: posterior.
- Type 3: lateral.
- Type 4: dislocation in association with both radius and ulna fracture.

Generally, a stable radial head reduction is achieved with ORIF of the ulna fracture. Occasionally open reduction is required, reduction being blocked by interposed capsule or annular ligament.

Nightstick fracture

This isolated ulna shaft fracture is usually not significantly displaced (angulation <10°, translation <50%) and can be treated in plaster. Displaced fractures require ORIF.

Galeazzi fracture

Treatment consists of ORIF of the radius (in some series 20% present with a fracture of both radius and ulna). Careful DRUJ assessment is essential. There are three possible situations:

- Stable DRUJ reduction (most common). Early mobilization is allowed.
- Reduced, but unstable DRUJ. A long-arm cast in supination usually holds the reduction. Occasionally K-wire fixation is required for 3 weeks.
- The DRUJ is irreducible, necessitating open reduction.

Complications – early

1. *Compartment syndrome* – vascular injury, coagulopathy and a crush injury predispose to this emergency.

2. *Nerve injuries* are rare, excepting a posterior interosseous nerve palsy which is seen in 20% of Monteggia fractures. This is usually a neurapraxia if occurring before reduction and most resolve spontaneously in 3 months.

3. *Vascular injuries* which involve both vessels require urgent repair. Single vessel repair is associated with higher non-patency rates, possibly due to back flow.

Complications – late

1. ***Stiffness*** depends upon the severity of the initial injury and precision of bony reduction. With ORIF, early mobilization is encouraged.

2. ***Fixation failure*** follows infection or poor surgical technique.

3. ***Infection rates*** are low, and should be treated by soft tissue debridement and maintenance of the plate fixation.

4. ***Synostosis*** occurs in 3%. The incidence is increased by: high-energy trauma, head injury, fracture of both bones at a single level, infection, a single surgical approach, surgery delayed more than 2 weeks, and screws or graft near the interosseous membrane. Synostosis is classified by Vince and Miller according to location:

- Type 1: at the DRUJ – responds poorly to resection.
- Type 2: middle two-thirds – amenable to resection.
- Type 3: proximal third – intermediate prognosis.

Resection is attempted after 1 year and before 3 years. These time intervals may be altered by the adjuvant use of single fraction radiotherapy.

5. ***Removal of metalwork*** should be performed with caution. Refracture rates are 4–20% and neurological injury 10–20%. Risk factors for refracture are removal of a 4.5 mm plate and early metalware removal. Bone density underneath a plate does not return to normal until a mean 21 months. Removal of symptomatic metalware is associated with worsening of symptoms in 9%.

Further reading

Bruckner JD, Alexander AH, Lichtman DM. Acute dislocations of the distal radio-ulnar joint. *Journal of Bone and Joint Surgery*, 1995; **77A**: 958–967.

Cullen JP, Pelligrini VD, Miller RJ *et al.* Treatment of traumatic radioulnar synostosis by excision and postoperative low-dose irradiation. *Journal of Hand Surgery*, 1994; **19A**: 394–401.

Hertel R, Pisan M, Lambert S *et al.* Plate osteosynthesis of diaphyseal fractures of the radius and ulna. *Injury*, 1996; 27: 545–548.

Related topics of interest

Radius and ulna – distal fractures, p. 233; Radius and ulna – fractures around the elbow, p. 236

RADIUS AND ULNA – DISTAL FRACTURES

Fractures of the distal radius and ulna represent one sixth of fractures presenting to the emergency department. Two characteristic fracture patterns present – the young patient with an intra-articular fracture following high-energy trauma, and the elderly osteoporotic patient who falls on the outstretched hand, suffering an extra-articular fracture.

Classification

There are many classifications and Frykman (1967) was the first to differentiate between intra- and extra-articular fractures (*Figure 1*). Melone's (1980) classification subdivided intra-articular radial fractures depending on involvement of the radio-scaphoid, or scapho-lunate articulation, describing four principal bone fragments – the shaft, radial styloid and lunate fossa, split into dorsal and volar fragments. The AO system is the most complete, with 27 classes, however, inter-observer reliability is poor.

Radiological imaging

On plain radiographs the most important normal values are:

- Volar tilt – 11°.
- Radial length – 11 mm between a transverse line across the radial styloid and across the distal ulna.
- Radial inclination – 22°.

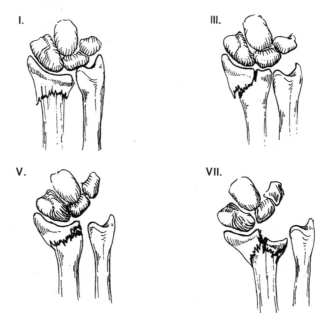

Figure 1. The Frykman classification of distal radial fractures. Type I is extra-articular, type III enters the radio-carpal joint, type V enters the radio-ulnar joint and type VII enters both the radio-carpal and radio-ulnar joints. The even numbers denote an associated ulnar styloid fracture (thus a type II fracture is an extra-articular fracture, associated with an ulnar styloid fracture, etc.). Modified from Kozin S.K. and Berlet A.C. *Handbook of Common Orthopaedic Fractures*, 1989, pp. 17, 19. Reprinted by permission of Medical Surveillance Inc.

These criteria determine treatment of extra-articular fractures. Less favourable results follow volar tilt changed >10°, radial inclination changed >5°, or >2 mm shortening. With intra-articular fractures, a step of >2 mm is significant. Articular disruption is better appreciated with CT or tomograms.

Treatment

It is difficult to predict which fracture configurations are unstable, or likely to redisplace, but the following factors are associated: dorsal angulation of >20°, shortening of >5 mm, dorsal/volar cortical comminution, marginal fractures (Barton's, Chauffeur), Smith's fracture and high-energy injuries. Many treatment modalities have been described:

1. Below elbow cast, in neutral or slight flexion, with ulnar deviation is the most common treatment. Three-point moulding is used. Above elbow casts are frequently used in North America, but there is no evidence that this give superior results. Excess flexion and ulnar deviation (the Cotton–Loder position) gives high carpal tunnel pressures.

2. Percutaneous wires supplementing a cast or external fixator, with K-wires inserted through the radial styloid and Lister's tubercle, may be used. Alternative techniques are those of Rayhack with multiple trans-ulnar pins, or Kapandji with dorsal pins transgressing the fracture. Percutaneous wires maintain length poorly in the presence of bi-cortical comminution.

3. External fixation can be used in distraction for ligamentotaxis or as a neutralization device to maintain position during union, perhaps after bone grafting. External fixators are associated with pin track problems, RSD, tendon and nerve transfixion, and stiffness. Dynamization after 3 weeks has been shown to help in some studies.

4. Open reduction is mandatory for most Smith's and Barton's fractures with carpal subluxation, but is more controversial in other fracture patterns.

5. Bone grafting is favoured to maintain anatomical reduction in intra-articular fractures, and angulation and length in extra-articular fractures. Either a dorsal approach between compartments 3 and 4 (between the tendons of EPL and EDC), or a volar approach between the radial artery and FCR can be used. Supplementary fixation is advised.

Complications

- Loss of reduction – remanipulation is usually possible at up to 3 weeks.
- Neurological complications occur in 10% (0.2 to 79%). Most common is median nerve palsy, which usually resolves spontaneously. Ulnar or radial nerve involvement is rare. Radial nerve involvement is usually secondary to cast pressure or wire transfixion.
- Compartment syndrome occurs in <1%.
- Acute tendon injury is rare in closed injuries, although the ECU trapped in the DRUJ can block reduction.
- Late tendon rupture classically affects EPL following a non-displaced fracture. Rupture occurs at the level of Lister's tubercle – a vascular watershed.

- Stiffness is caused by adhesions and prevented by early finger mobilization.
- Reflex sympathetic dystrophy occurs in up to 25%.
- Malunion. With intra-articular fractures, 2 mm of residual displacement leads to symptomatic degeneration in 50% at 30 years. The incidence can be reduced to 5–10% by anatomic reduction. With extra-articular fractures, dorsal angulation causes DISI, manifesting as wrist pain and instability. Correction is by opening dorsal osteotomy.

Prognosis

Ninety per cent of patients regain 90% of their movement by 1 year. Grip strength is usually reduced. Recent series imply that whatever method of treatment is chosen, the results at 1 year will be similar. In the longer term, there is evidence that anatomical reduction protects patients with intra-articular fractures from degenerative change. In extra-articular fractures the main predictor of a good result is the restoration of normal radio-carpal alignment.

Distal radio-ulnar joint

The DRUJ is formed between the ulna and the sigmoid notch of the radius. The flat distal end of the ulna is covered by the triangular fibrocartilage complex (TFCC) attaching to the fovea at the base of the styloid process.

DRUJ injury can be isolated (rare), or associated with other fractures. The classic is the Galeazzi fracture dislocation, but DRUJ injuries occur in association with fractures of both forearm bones and distal radial fractures.

The most helpful radiograph is a true lateral of the wrist – judged by the superimposition of the scaphoid, capitate and lunate. In this position the radius should overlie the distal ulna. Avulsion at the base of the ulnar styloid is indicative of a major TFCC injury. CT can be used to assess joint congruity. Isolated dislocations are reduced and treated by a long arm cast applied in supination for dorsal dislocation and pronation for volar dislocation.

A small avulsion fracture from the ulnar styloid, associated with a distal radial fracture can be ignored. When the fracture are at the base, some advocate internal fixation, using a screw or tension band wire. Chronic radio-ulnar instability, or arthritis, secondary to an old intra-articular fracture, are treated by the Sauve–Kapandji operation.

Further reading

Kozin H, Wood MB. Early soft tissue complications after fractures of the distal part of the radius. *Journal of Bone and Joint Surgery*, 1993; **75A**: 144–152.

McQueen MM, Hajducka C, Court-Brown CM. Redisplaced unstable fractures of the distal radius. *Journal of Bone and Joint Surgery*, 1996; **78B**: 404–409.

Nugent IM, Ivory JP, Ross AC. Carpal instability. In: *Key Topics in Orthopaedic Surgery*. Oxford: BIOS Scientific Publishers, 1995; 78–80.

Trumble TE, Culp R, Hanel DP *et al.* Intra-articular fractures of the distal aspect of the radius. *Journal of Bone and Joint Surgery*, 1998; **80A**: 582–600.

Related topics of interest

RADIUS AND ULNA – FRACTURES AROUND THE ELBOW

Simple fractures involving the radial head, coronoid process or olecranon, must be differentiated from fractures associated with ligamentous damage and elbow instability.

Radial head

There are two principal ligamentous injuries associated with radial head fractures; firstly, elbow dislocation, and secondly, disruption of the radio-ulnar interosseous ligament – acute longitudinal radio-ulnar dissociation (ALRUD). With dislocation the aim is to prevent valgus instability and with ALRUD to prevent longitudinal forearm collapse.

1. Classification of radial head fractures is based upon the 'Mason' classification:

- Type 1 – non/minimally displaced.
- Type 2 – displaced >2 mm or 30°.
- Type 3 – comminuted.
- Type 4 – associated with elbow dislocation.

2. Clinical examination reveals a swollen elbow, secondary to haemarthrosis. The haemarthrosis can be aspirated and local anaesthetic instilled into the joint. As well as providing analgesia, this allows the pronation and supination to be assessed.

3. Radiological evidence of a fracture may only amount to a 'fat pad' sign.

4. Treatment is determined according to Mason's type.

- Type 1. Early mobilization.
- Type 2. There is no universal consensus. A common approach is to examine the patient for a mechanical block to supination/pronation. In the absence of a block, the treatment is early mobilization. Where there is a block, ORIF is performed. In comparison to non-operative treatment, this reduces pain and increases motion and grip strength. If the head is non-reconstructable it should be excised.
- Type 3. The head is excised and early mobilization commenced. The optimum timing for radial head excision is controversial. While late excision reduces pain and improves function, early excision gives even better results in the majority. If the elbow is unstable following radial head excision, the treatment options are the same as following fracture dislocation – see below. Radial head excision reduces the movement by 15° and leads to a mean 2 mm of positive ulnar variance, but seldom leads to elbow or wrist pain.
- Type 4. With associated dislocation, an attempt must be made to preserve the radial head, as acute excision leads to recurrent dislocation and valgus instability. If the radial head is not salvageable, even temporarily, there are three options:

(a) The collateral ligaments should be repaired.

(b) If the elbow remains unstable a prosthetic radial head is implanted.

(c) The final option is a hinged external fixator to maintain mobility during healing.

5. ALRUD. Disruption of the interosseous ligament, or the Essex–Lopresti injury, can lead to progressive collapse of the radius on the ulna, if the radial head is excised. In these cases it is desirable to maintain radial length, by reconstructing the radial head, or using a metallic radial head prosthesis (silastic is inadequate). Temporary DRUJ stabilization with wires may also be helpful. Acutely, the problem is distinguishing this more serious pattern of injury from simple radial head fracture, but associated wrist and forearm pain may be indicative.

Coronoid process

The coronoid process forms an anterior buttress to the elbow. The anterior capsule and medial collateral ligament attach to the coronoid process and the brachialis inserts just distal. Two to ten per cent of elbow dislocations have associated coronoid fractures. A third of coronoid fractures are secondary to elbow dislocation. Malunion of large coronoid fragments can lead to elbow instability or cause a mechanical block to motion.

1. Classification. Regan and Morrey described three types:

- Type 1 – avulsion of the coronoid tip.
- Type 2 – <50% of the process.
- Type 3 – >50% of the process.

2. Treatment. Type 1 fractures are stable and treated with early mobilization. All type 3 and some type 2 injuries are unstable, requiring fixation. If ORIF does not stabilize the elbow, a hinged external fixator is added.

Olecranon

Olecranon fractures are most commonly caused by the pull of the triceps, or a fall onto the olecranon.

1. Classification. Numerous systems exist and that described by Colton is popular:

- Type 1. Non-displaced and stable.
- Type 2. Displaced.
  - A. Avulsion.
  - B. Transverse.
  - C. Comminuted.
  - D. Fracture/dislocation.

2. Non-displaced fractures. These are treated in a cast for 3 weeks, after which supervised mobilization is commenced.

3. Displaced fractures. Many techniques are described for displaced fractures, but tension band wiring, plating and olecranon excision are the principal options.

Transverse fractures are usually treated by tension band wiring, converting the tensile force into a compressive force. The tension band is supplemented by K-wires or a screw; 97% excellent or good results are reported. A screw reduces the irritation caused by prominent hardware. Oblique fractures can shorten with tension band wiring. Shortening is overcome by using a lag screw or a plate (pelvic reconstruction), which is preferable in the comminuted fracture.

Some authors prefer excision of the olecranon and reattachment of the triceps in the elderly. Up to 60% of the olecranon can be excised without destabilizing the joint.

4. *Elbow dislocation.* An olecranon fracture associated with elbow dislocation requires stable ORIF with a plate. Tension bands and wires do not have sufficient strength to resist the large AP forces.

5. *Complications.* Metalware prominence from backing out of wires, is probably the commonest complication. Non-union, reported in 5%, can be treated by grafting and refixation, or excision of the fragment and triceps repair. Limited range of motion occurs in 50%, but <5% of patients complain.

Further reading

Khalafyan EE, Culp RW, Alexander AH. Mason type II radial head fractures: operative versus non-operative treatment. *Journal of Orthopedic Trauma*, 1992; **6**: 283–289.
Morrey BF. Complex instability of the elbow. *Journal of Bone and Joint Surgery*, 1997; **79A**: 460–469.

Related topics of interest

Elbow dislocation, p. 43; Humeral fractures – distal, p. 107

SHOULDER – ACROMIOCLAVICULAR AND STERNOCLAVICULAR DISLOCATION

Acromioclavicular joint

Classification

Tossy classified injury of the ACJ into three types. This has been increased to six by Rockwood (*Figure 1*). Of these six types, 98% are type I, II or III (*Table 1*). Controversies regarding operative or non-operative management centre around type III which make up 40% of all ACJ injuries.

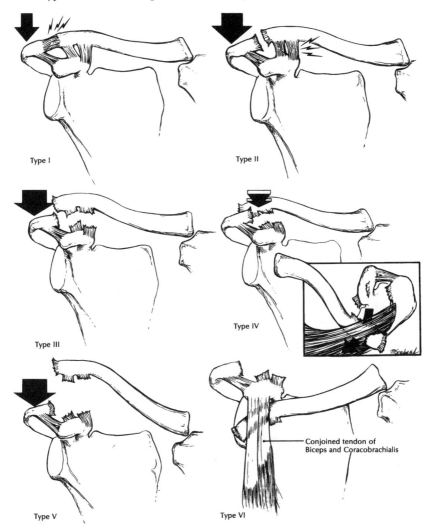

Type I

Type II

Type III

Type IV

Type V

Type VI

Conjoined tendon of Biceps and Coracobrachialis

Figure 1. Rockwood's classification of acromioclavicular joint injuries. Reprinted from Rockwood C.A., Williams G.R., Young D.C. Injuries to the acromioclavicular joint. In: *Rockwood and Green's Fractures in Adults*, Vol. 2, 4th Edn. Edited by Rockwood C.A., Green D.P., Bucholz R.W., Heckman J.D. © Lippincott Williams & Wilkins, 1996.

Table 1. Tossy/Rockwood classification of ACJ injuries

Type	ACJ	CCL	Deltoid and trapezius	Other
I	+	+	+	ACJ sprain
II	–	+	+	CCL sprain
III	–	–	+/–	Surgery controversial
IV	–	–	–	Clavicle in trapezius
V	–	–	–	Type III displaced 100–300%
VI	–	–	–	Clavicle subcoracoid

+: intact.
–: disrupted.

In type I and II injuries the coracoclavicular ligaments (CCLs) remain intact. In type III injuries the CCLs are ruptured and the ACJ is dislocated, but the deltoid and trapezius remain attached to the shoulder girdle. In the rare type IV to VI injuries, the soft tissue injury is greater.

Clinical examination and imaging

Type I, II and III injuries present with pain and tenderness over the ACJ. In type IV injuries the clavicle is displaced posteriorly (best seen by inspection from the side or above) into or through the trapezius muscle. Type V is a severe type II injury and type VI follows major trauma.

Specialist radiographs include:

- An AP with 10–15° cephalic tilt, outlining the joint and loose bodies.
- Stress radiographs, with 4 kg suspended from the patient's wrists. Comparative views of both sides are taken. This stress radiograph is most help in differentiating between type II and III injuries. In the type II injury there is partial overlap of the clavicle and acromion – this is not present in type III injury.

Treatment

1. Type I and II injuries. These are treated non-operatively, with a sling and early mobilization as tolerated.

2. Type IV, V and VI injuries. Such injuries are usually treated operatively.

3. Type III injuries. Treatment is controversial, with series in the literature justifying operative and non-operative management. Procedures described include:

- Transfixion of the ACJ with wires.
- Cerclage techniques between the coracoid and clavicle.
- Dynamic muscle transfers.

The current 'favourite' is a coracoclavicular screw (Bosworth), with repair of the CCLs and plication of the torn deltoid and trapezius. Screw removal is recommended.

Complications

- Cosmetic deformity of the distal clavicle – a 'bump'.
- Painful ACJ with degenerative change, treated by excision of the distal clavicle and reconstruction of the CCLs for instability.

- Surgery – migration of metalware, screw breakage and hypertrophic scarring.

Prognosis

Type I and II injuries do well, with reports of up to 100% good and excellent results. Patients with non-operatively treated type III injuries experience mild discomfort, but no reduction in strength or endurance compared to the non-injured side at 4 years. Return to work and rehabilitation are quicker with non-operative treatment.

Paediatrics

In children, ACJ injury is effectively a distal physeal fracture. The medial bony fragment herniates out of the periosteal sleeve. The CCL remains attached to the periosteum and does not rupture. Consequently, up to the age of 16 years these injuries are treated non-operatively, with remodelling of a new bone within the periosteal sleeve giving rise to normal anatomy.

Sternoclavicular joint

The SCJ is stabilized by three ligaments; the rhomboid-shaped costoclavicular ligament from the first rib, the interclavicular ligament and the capsular ligaments. The medial clavicular epiphysis closes at 25 years.

Classification

Classification is simply anterior and posterior dislocation of the clavicle, relative to the sternum. Anterior dislocation is less hazardous and more common.

Clinical examination and imaging

Dislocation typically follows an RTA or sporting injury – a blow to the shoulder drives the medial pole of the clavicle anteriorly or posteriorly. The diagnosis is made from the site of pain and deformity. Clinically, it can be difficult to determine the direction of the dislocation. Patients with hypermobility may exhibit voluntary joint subluxation.

Radiological diagnosis is difficult. A view with 40° cephalic tilt has been described, with anterior dislocation high riding and posterior low riding, in comparison to the normal clavicle. CT is the investigation of choice. Vascular studies should be considered in a posterior dislocation.

Associated injuries

The posteriorly dislocated clavicle can impinge upon any closely related structure – great vessels, trachea, oesophagus, heart or pleura. Anterior dislocation is relatively benign.

Treatment

1. Anterior. Closed reduction, under general anaesthesia, is performed. With a sandbag placed between the scapulae, the shoulder is abducted. Unfortunately, the reduction is often unstable, even with a figure-of-eight bandage and sling. In this case a decision should be taken to leave the joint dislocated with a cosmetic deformity, resect the medial clavicle trading a scar for a bump, or undertake open reduction and fixation – the least favoured option.

2. Posterior. After neurovascular assessment, closed reduction is by a manoeuvre similar to that described above. A percutaneous towel clip can be used to assist reduction. The reduction is usually stable and post-operatively a sling is worn for 3 months.

Open surgery in selected cases includes resection of the medial clavicle. Care should be taken not to resect the costoclavicular ligament, as this destabilizes the clavicle. If the ligament has ruptured, reconstruction is required.

Complications

Fixation of an unstable joint with K-wires, or similar, is not advised. There are several reports of fatalities secondary to pin migration.

Paediatrics

Dislocations up until 25 years are usually S–H I or II fractures. In the absence of pressure on vital structures, remodelling occurs within the split periosteal sleeve.

Further reading

Rockwood CA, Williams GR, Young DC. Injuries to the acromioclavicular joint. In: Rockwood CA, Green DP, Bucholz RW, Heckman JD, eds. *Rockwood and Green's Fractures in Adults*. Philadelphia: Lippincott-Raven, 1996; 1341–1413.

Rockwood CA, Wirth MA. Injuries to the sternoclavicular joint. In: Rockwood CA, Green DP, Bucholz RW, Heckman JD, eds. *Rockwood and Green's Fractures in Adults*. Philadelphia: Lippincott-Raven, 1996; 1415–1417.

Related topics of interest

Shoulder – clavicle fractures, p. 246; Shoulder – scapular fractures, p. 252

SHOULDER – BRACHIAL PLEXUS INJURIES

Injuries to the brachial plexus are uncommon, but are associated with considerable morbidity. Injuries most frequently follow motorcycle accidents or may occur during falls and sporting accidents. Open injuries are rare. The extent of the injury is related to the energy of the trauma – low-velocity injuries are generally neurapraxias with a better prognosis than high-velocity injuries, where an extensive or global defect is associated with a poor outcome.

A wide spectrum of injuries is seen, from neurapraxia and axonotmesis, to more extensive neurotmesis. The injuries are divided into infra- and supraclavicular, with supraclavicular being subdivided into pre-ganglionic (root avulsions) and post-ganglionic.

Neurapraxia and axonotmesis can recover spontaneously many months after the injury, whereas root avulsions are irreparable, and a salvage procedure (such as a nerve or tendon transfer) is required. In general supraclavicular lesions have a less favourable outcome than infraclavicular lesions.

Isolated nerve injuries are seen with fractures and dislocations around the shoulder. Vascular injuries occur in 15% of brachial plexus injuries and are more frequent with infraclavicular lesions.

Classification

Brachial plexus injuries are classified according to the aetiology and level of the lesion. The Leffert classification (*Table 1*) considers brachial plexus lesions in four types. Iatrogenic and tumour-related lesions can be added to this classification. Closed traction injuries account for >75% of lesions. Lesions may be at more than one level.

Table 1. Leffert classification of brachial plexus injuries

I	Open		
II	Closed	IIA	Supraclavicular
			Preganglionic – nerve root avulsion
			Postganglionic – traction injuries
		IIB	Infraclavicular
III	Radiotherapy induced		
IV	Obstetric	IVA	Upper root (Erb's palsy)
		IVB	Lower root (Klumpke's palsy)
		IVC	Mixed

The Sunderland classification is also popular, with five degrees of brachial plexus injury of increasing severity – neurapraxia is 1st degree, axonotmesis 2nd degree, lesions of increasing severity but in continuity 3rd and 4th degree, and complete transection is 5th degree.

Examination and investigation

A careful history and detailed examination, with a sound appreciation of the anatomy, will reveal the nature of the lesion in only 60% of cases. Associated vascular (15%) and musculoskeletal injuries are common.

Root avulsions occur proximal to the dorsal root ganglion, with loss of dorsal sensibility and denervation of dorsal neck muscles; plexus ruptures occur more distally. Mapping sensory and motor defects gives a good indication of the nature of the injury. Paralysis of the rhomboids or serratus anterior implies a proximal, usually preganglionic lesion, at the C5 or C6 level, respectively. Horner's sign (ptosis, miosis, anhidrosis, enophthalmos) implies a preganglionic C8/T1 lesion of the cervical sympathetic chain.

Chest, cervical spine and shoulder X-rays are mandatory. Further assessment with EMG studies may be necessary to localize the site of the injury. Supraclavicular injuries may need investigation with a CT myelogram or MRI, if surgery is contemplated. In cases of root avulsion pseudomeningoceles may be seen, which alter the prognosis and management. Investigation should be delayed a few weeks to allow CSF leaks to seal.

At a later stage, usually 3–4 weeks, the development of Tinel's sign implies recovery of a postganglionic injury – a favourable prognostic sign.

Treatment

Open, or penetrating injuries require primary surgical exploration and repair. Nerve roots cannot be reattached – although research is making some progress into this.

In the past, most closed injuries were treated by observation for 3 months, maintaining passive movement and using functional bracing if suitable. When there are no signs of recovery, or recovery ceases, surgical exploration with neurolysis and nerve grafting was undertaken.

The timing of surgery is controversial and now changing. Where the lesion is extensive there is now an increasingly strong argument in favour of early exploratory surgery, as both a diagnostic and therapeutic procedure. Surgery after 6 months has very poor results. When surgery is delayed, fibrous tissue encases the nerves, making the anatomy and pathology more difficult to define.

Surgical reconstruction

1. **Priorities of surgery** are to restore:

- Shoulder stability.
- Shoulder external rotation.
- Elbow flexion (some clinicians make this the priority).
- Wrist extension.

2. **Principles of surgery** are to perform:

- Neurolysis.
- Nerve repair.
- Nerve graft.
- Nerve transfer.

3. **A wide surgical exposure** from the mid-neck to the deltopectoral groove is required to define the anatomy and an osteotomy of the clavicle is sometimes used. Microsurgical neurolysis is required if scar tissue is dense, which may restore function and relieve intractable pain. Direct repair is rarely feasible. Nerve grafting is the most effective method of surgical reconstruction, using a sural nerve, or rapid

frozen/thawed muscle graft to reconstruct defects up to 4 cm in length. Reconstruction may also be achieved by nerve transfer (neurotization) or muscle/tendon transfer to restore basic shoulder, elbow or wrist function. Common examples of neurotization are: intercostal motor to musculocutaneous nerve and spinal accessory to suprascapular nerve. Recent evidence suggests intercostal nerve transfer may relieve intractable pain in preganglionic injuries.

4. **Late reconstruction.** Elbow flexion can be restored with a triceps to biceps transfer, which may cost the patient some loss of function, or by a Steindler flexorplasty. Latissimus dorsi to biceps can also be used, but is a rather lengthy and mutilating transfer. Pectoralis major transfer is no longer favoured as it has a poor result. Elbow extension can be restored by transferring part of deltoid to triceps. Free functioning muscle transfers may be appropriate, such as the transfer of gracilis to replace biceps and brachialis.

The use of orthotics and joint arthrodesis should be considered and are often essential. Amputation of a flail limb is occasionally requested.

Prognosis

The prognosis depends on the extent of the injury and early signs of recovery. However, the following are poor prognostic signs at initial presentation:

- Advancing age.
- High-velocity traction injury.
- Painful limb.
- Horner's sign.
- Flaccid limb.
- Root avulsions.

Further reading

Birch R. Advances in diagnosis and treatment in closed traction lesion of the supraclavicular brachial plexus. In: Catterall A, ed. *Recent Advances in Orthopaedics, No. 6.* Edinburgh: Churchill Livingstone, 1992; 65–76.

Kay SPJ and Scott MJL. Brachial plexus surgery – current indications. *Current Orthopaedics,* 1993; 7: 226–233.

Related topics of interest

Birth injuries, p. 23; Peripheral nerve injuries and repair, p. 192

SHOULDER – CLAVICLE FRACTURES

Fracture of the clavicle is usually treated non-operatively and seldom excites much interest. However, clavicle fractures represent 5% of all fractures and 44% of shoulder girdle fractures. Surgical fixation may be indicated.

Classification

The primary classification system divides fractures into those of the medial (5%), middle (85%) and distal (10%) thirds (Allman).

Fractures of the lateral third are subclassified into types I to V, based upon integrity of the coracoclavicular ligament (CCL) complex:

- Type I: non-displaced.
- Type IIA: fracture proximal to conoid and trapezoid ligaments.
- Type IIB: fracture between the conoid (proximal) and trapezoid ligaments.
- Type III: fracture into ACJ.
- Type IV: epiphyseal separation (children).
- Type V: three-part fracture, with intact ligaments connected to the middle fragment.

Examination and investigation

The clavicle is closely related to the brachial plexus, subclavian and axillary vessels, and the pleura. Open injury or compromise of the skin is important. Medial-third fractures, while uncommon, are associated with high-energy trauma and multiple injury.

As well as simple AP radiographs, 45° cephalic and 45° caudal views have been advocated. The cephalic view is valuable in medial-third fractures. Weight-bearing views of both shoulders are used to demonstrate ligament integrity in distal-third fractures. Tomograms and CT delineate intra-articular extension in medial and lateral-third fractures.

Management

1. Non-operative treatment with a broad arm sling is the mainstay of treatment, with or without devices attempting to hold a closed reduction (e.g. figure-of-eight bandage). The arm is mobilized when clinical union occurs (2 weeks in infants, 3 weeks in children, and 4–6 weeks in adults). Radiological union occurs after clinical union.

2. Operative treatment is reserved for:

- Open fractures.
- Polytrauma.
- Neurovascular compromise.
- Compromise of overlying skin.
- Floating shoulder.
- Type II distal-third fractures.
- Symptomatic non-union or degenerate ACJ.

3. Many techniques for operative fixation have been described. Intramedullary techniques allow closed fixation, but there is a significant risk of implant breakage or migration in this anatomically complex area. Plate fixation requires wide fracture exposure and raises the incidence of non-union. This is reduced by a low threshold for bone grafting.

4. Other techniques employed are coracoclavicular screw fixation for distal-third fractures with CCL disruption, and resection of the distal clavicle in cases of degenerative change following type III distal-third fractures.

5. A 'sensible' approach is to recommend non-operative treatment in the majority of middle-third fractures. In those cases requiring surgery, a plate and bone graft can be used. Distal third types I and III are treated conservatively, but type II and V fractures have higher non-union rates and the results of ORIF are superior.

Complications

1. Non-union is defined as the absence of clinical or radiological union at 6 months, occurring most frequently in distal-third fractures, although because middle-third fractures are more common, these patients present most frequently.

In the middle third, risk factors are severe trauma (with greater displacement and soft tissue disruption), primary ORIF, refracture, inadequate immobilization and patient age. Following non-operative treatment, the reported incidence varies from 0.1 to 4.0%. Neer reported a series with non-union of 0.1% after non-operative, and 4.4% after operative, treatment. Treatment of non-union is open reduction, bone grafting and fixation in the symptomatic patient.

In the distal third, non-union rates vary from 5% in type I fractures, to 30% non-union and 45% delayed union in non-operatively treated type II fractures.

2. Malunion with a 'bump' after conservative treatment is common. In children this usually remodels, but is persistent in adults. In the majority, treatment consists of advice, as surgical intervention is seldom required. However, osteotomy and refixation, or simple shaving of the bump, may be required. The patient should be warned that the scar may be less cosmetic than the bump and could also be painful (supraclavicular nerve injury).

3. Neurovascular compromise can be acute or chronic. Acute compromise relates to fracture displacement. Chronic compromise relates to excessive callus formation or mobile non-union. Typically the proximal part of the distal fragment in a middle-third fracture is pulled inferiorly and posteriorly against the neurovascular bundle.

4. Osteoarthritis may follow SCJ and ACJ injury.

Double disruptions of the superior shoulder complex

The 'superior shoulder complex' consists of the scapula, clavicle and soft tissues supporting the upper limb. If both the clavicle and scapula are fractured, a 'floating shoulder' results which should be stabilized. The clavicle should be plated and if the scapular fracture, usually of the glenoid neck, does not reduce spontaneously, fixation of this is also required.

Paediatrics

Childhood clavicular fractures may be obstetric or traumatic. Congenital pseudarthrosis is usually right-sided and asymptomatic. Treatment is non-operative. The early deformity remodels inevitably until the age of 10 years.

Further reading

Boyer MI, Axelrod TS. Atrophic nonunion of the clavicle: treatment by compression plate, lag-screw fixation and bone graft. *Journal of Bone and Joint Surgery*, 1997; **79B**: 301–303.

Hill JM, McGuire MH, Crosby LA. Closed treatment of displaced middle-third fractures of the clavicle gives poor results. *Journal of Bone and Joint Surgery*, 1997; **79B**: 537–539.

Related topics of interest

Shoulder – acromioclavicular and sternoclavicular dislocation, p. 239; Shoulder – brachial plexus injuries, p. 243

SHOULDER – DISLOCATION

Shoulder instability ranges from a post-traumatic unilateral Bankart lesion in which surgery is often indicated (TUBS), to atraumatic multidirectional instability, which is often bilateral, responding to rehabilitation and rarely requiring surgery with an inferior capsular shift (AMBRI). This topic deals with acute management of the dislocated shoulder, rather than chronic instability.

Classification

The direction of dislocation is the most useful system of classification for acute dislocation, as TUBS and AMBRI refer to non-acute situations. Thirty eight per cent of all joint dislocations involve the glenohumeral joint, of which 98% are anterior. Anterior dislocation is usually subcoaracoid, but can be subglenoid, subclavicular, or even intrathoracic. The remaining 2% are posterior, with the exceptional inferior 'luxatio erecta' and superior dislocation.

Clinical examination

Anterior dislocation occurs with the shoulder in extension, abduction and external rotation. Following dislocation the upper arm is held in slight abduction and external rotation. Characteristic emptiness is felt beneath the acromion.

More than 50% of posterior dislocations are missed at first presentation. The diagnosis should be suspected if the patient has a flat anterior contour of the shoulder, a prominent coracoid and difficulty abducting the arm. The most striking clinical finding is inability to externally rotate the shoulder.

Inferior dislocation presents with an arm fixed in abduction and the humeral head locked under the glenoid.

Radiological evaluation

Three views are recommended:

- AP in the plane of the shoulder (plate parallel to the scapula, not the body).
- Scapular lateral.
- Axillary.

A posterior dislocation classically gives a 'light-bulb' sign on the AP view.

Closed treatment

*1. **Anterior dislocation.*** Several eponyms are associated with closed reduction techniques. The essential principle is to apply gentle reduction with adequate muscle relaxation.

The Hippocratic technique is still recommended, using traction, with or without rotation. The foot is placed in the axilla as counter-traction; alternatively an assistant can provide counter-traction with a sheet looped through the axilla.

Kocher's method, which involves traction and abduction, followed by adduction and internal rotation, is no longer recommended. Kocher's method has been linked with fracture of the humeral neck and higher rates of recurrent dislocation (40% versus 12%).

2. *Posterior dislocation.* Traction is applied along the adducted arm. Forceful external rotation should be avoided, as it can cause fracture.

3. *Inferior dislocation.* This can usually be reduced by traction, but occasionally the head buttonholes through the capsule, necessitating open reduction.

Post-reduction care

Following reduction, neurovascular evaluation and radiographs should be repeated. Many surgeons use immobilization for 3 to 6 weeks following anterior dislocation. However, there is little evidence that the duration of post-reduction immobilization is related to the incidence of recurrent dislocation. Indeed there is evidence that an early rehabilitation programme reduces the incidence of recurrence, particularly in patients with an AMBRI lesion.

Early mobilization is particularly desirable in the patient over 40 years old. The emphasis should be on avoiding stiffness, strengthening the muscular stabilizers and avoiding positions provoking instability in this age group.

Posterior dislocation is often unstable after reduction. A shoulder spica in neutral rotation can be used (handshake cast).

Complications

1. *Recurrent dislocation.* The incidence of recurrent dislocation is inversely related to the age at first dislocation. In patients <20 years, 80% or more have a further dislocation within 2 years. Conversely, after 40 years, the rate is 10–15%. If the greater tuberosity is avulsed, recurrent dislocation is very rare. It is proposed that younger patients strip the labrum and capsule from the anterior glenoid (Bankart lesion), whereas older patients stretch the capsule or avulse the greater tuberosity.

Early repair of the Bankart lesion in a young active patient presenting with a first dislocation may be justifiable. Primary repair reduces recurrence from 80% to 14%.

2. *Rotator cuff tears.* Tears are common in the older patient with dislocation and should be suspected with excessive bruising and slow rehabilitation. Repair is usually required. The rotator cuff occasionally becomes interposed within the joint, blocking reduction.

3. *Fracture.* Dislocation is associated with two fracture types: intra-articular fractures of the head and extra-articular fractures.

The Hill–Sachs lesion (an impaction fracture of the postero-lateral head associated with anterior dislocation) is seen in 35% of acute and 60% of chronic dislocations.

Posterior dislocation can cause antero-medial impaction of the humeral head – the 'reverse Hill–Sachs'. If the impaction exceeds 20%, the subscapularis tendon is transferred into the defect (McLaughlin) and if it exceeds 45%, prosthetic replacement may be required.

Glenoid fractures should be fixed if displaced, or if there is persistent subluxation of the joint. Fractures of the greater tuberosity usually reduce after reduction of the shoulder. Persistent displacement of more than 1 cm requires

ORIF and repair of the cuff. Occasionally during reduction a non-displaced fracture can be displaced. For this reason, great care must be taken when reducing fracture dislocations.

*4. **Neurological injury*** occurs in 45% of dislocations when evaluated by electrophysiological testing. The incidence increases with age. The axillary, suprascapular and musculocutaneous nerves are most commonly injured, but the whole brachial plexus may be involved. The majority of lesions recover with conservative management. Nerve injury is rare with posterior dislocation, but almost all cases of luxatio erecta present with neurological compromise, which resolves after reduction.

*5. **Vascular injury*** can occur at the time of injury or reduction and manifests as vascular occlusion or haemorrhage. The second and third parts of the axillary artery are most commonly injured. The risk of bleeding is greatest in the elderly patient, where an attempt is made to reduce an old dislocation. This requires urgent treatment with open surgery. Arterial occlusion may occur in the presence of palpable distal pulses.

*6. **Irreducibility*** is usually secondary to biceps tendon or rotator cuff interposition. Open reduction is indicated.

Indications for acute operative treatment

These are rare, but include:

- Associated vascular injury.
- Open dislocation.
- Failure of closed reduction.
- Displaced greater tuberosity or glenoid fractures.
- Significant impaction of the humeral head.
- Gross instability following posterior dislocation.

Further reading

Arciero RA, Wheeler JH, Ryan JB *et al.* Arthroscopic Bankart repair versus non-operative treatment for acute, initial anterior shoulder dislocation. *American Journal of Sports Medicine*, 1994; **22**: 589–594.

Hovelius J, Augustini BG, Fredin H *et al.* Primary anterior dislocation of the shoulder in young patients. A ten-year prospective study. *Journal of Bone and Joint Surgery*, 1996; **78B**: 1677–1684.

Neviaser RJ, Neviaser TJ, Neviaser JS. Concurrent rupture of the rotator cuff and anterior dislocation of the shoulder in the older patient. *Journal of Bone and Joint Surgery*, 1988; **70A**: 1308–1311.

Nugent IM, Ivory JP, Ross AC. Rotator cuff injuries. In: *Key Topics in Orthopaedic Surgery*. Oxford: BIOS Scientific Publishers, 1995; 260–262.

Nugent IM, Ivory JP, Ross AC. Shoulder instability. In: *Key Topics in Orthopaedic Surgery*. Oxford: BIOS Scientific Publishers, 1995; 278–280.

Related topic of interest

Humeral fractures – proximal, p. 110

SHOULDER – SCAPULAR FRACTURES

Scapular fractures are in themselves a rarity (<1% of all fractures), but are often associated with other bony or soft tissue injuries to the shoulder girdle, neck or thoracic cage. The mean patient age is 35 to 45 years; motor car accidents account for 50% of all scapular fractures and motor cycle accidents 20%. Major trauma is required to fracture the scapula, so other injuries and complications are common (50 to 90% of cases).

Desault (1805), was most probably one of the first surgeons to describe injuries of the scapula, and since then a number of studies have suggested that the closed management of these fractures is the norm. Recent European studies have raised concerns about closed management of scapular fractures, especially those associated with fractures of the glenoid and resultant glenohumeral instability.

Fracture pattern and classification

Fractures of the scapula are classified on an anatomical basis:

- IA: acromion.
- IB: base of acromion.
- IC: coracoid.

- IIA: neck, lateral to the base of the acromion.
- IIB: neck, extending to base of acromion or spine.
- IIC: neck, transverse type.

- III: glenoid intra-articular.

- IV: body.

The most common fracture site is the body of the scapula (35%), followed by the neck (27%). Fractures of the spine, glenoid and acromion have similar occurrence rates.

Diagnosis

The diagnosis is often made as an incidental finding on plain radiographs in the skeletal survey of a multiply injured patient. AP and lateral scapular radiographs may suffice in most cases, but in more complex fractures, CT scans help to delineate the fracture pattern.

Treatment

As most fractures of the scapula occur in high-energy injuries it is important to recognize the high incidence of associated injuries. Pulmonary injuries are seen in 37% of cases, including a 30% incidence of haemopneumothorax. One third of patients have significant head injuries and ipsilateral clavicular fractures are seen in a quarter of cases.

Up to 10% of patients can have significant neurological impairment, due to injuries of the brachial plexus.

Simple fractures of the body of the scapula do well with closed treatment in a sling, followed by assisted mobilization. Even in the presence of significant displacement, the resultant disability from body fractures is small.

Fractures of the scapular neck can result in a high incidence of residual disability. Patients with a displaced neck fracture with >40° of angulation in either the transverse or coronal plane, or >1 cm of displacement, may require open reduction and internal fixation. Displaced fractures of the glenoid, especially when associated with glenohumeral instability, should be reduced and fixed in order to lessen the subsequent risk of glenohumeral osteoarthritic change or shoulder instability.

Fractures of the spine of the scapula can result in rotator cuff malfunction with pain and weakness on abduction. Scapular spine fractures at the base of the acromion and those with >5 mm of displacement may be at risk of non-union and should be considered for surgical treatment.

Surgical approach

The surgical approach is anterior for anterior glenoid rim and coracoid fractures. Posterior glenoid rim, neck and glenoid fossa fractures are best accessed through a posterior (Judet) approach.

Results

The reports of surgical fixation are few, but good or excellent results are reported in 79% of cases, in some series.

Further reading

Ada JR, Miller ME. Scapular fractures: analysis of 113 cases. *Clinical Orthopaedics*, 1991; **269**: 174–180.

Desault PJ. A treatise on fractures, luxations and other affections of the bone. Philadelphis, Fry and Kammerer, 1805; 57–67.

Hardegger FH, Simpson LA, Weber BG. Operative treatment of scapular fractures. *Journal of Bone and Joint Surgery*, 1984; **66B**: 725–731.

Neviaser J. Traumatic lesions: injuries in and about the shoulder joint. *Instructional Course Lecture XIII*. Rosemont: American Academy of Orthopaedic Surgeons, 1956; 187–216.

Related topics of interest

SPINAL CORD INJURY – ASSESSMENT AND MANAGEMENT

The management principles for the patient with spinal injuries are:

- Resuscitation.
- Assessment and investigation.
- Spinal immobilization.
- Prevention and management of complications.
- Rehabilitation.

Resuscitation

The priority in trauma management is, of course, resuscitation, following the principles of ATLS, with airway, breathing, circulation and haemorrhage control, 'saving life before limb'. Control of the spine is paramount during resuscitation and transfer. The spine is immobilized in the neutral supine position, on a long spinal backboard, with a hard neck collar, tape and sandbags.

Hypotension may be due to hypovolaemia or neurogenic shock. In most cases, particularly in multi-system trauma, hypovolaemia is the usual cause of shock. Treatment is initially volume replacement; failure to respond may indicate neurogenic shock. Typically with neurogenic shock there is a bradycardia. Treatment with leg elevation, atropine and occasionally vasopressors is required.

Assessment and investigation

1. History. A clear description of the accident is useful in determining whether there is an occult spinal injury, the extent and level of primary cord or root trauma, and any likely associated injuries. Polytrauma may result in delayed diagnosis of spinal injury, especially in the cervical spine.

2. Examination and special tests. A full examination of the spine and detailed peripheral neurological assessment is undertaken. The patient is log-rolled, by four experienced personnel, with the examiner observing for visual signs of head or spinal injury such as abrasions, tenderness, step off, interspinous widening, etc.

3. Neurology. Levels of motor and sensory function are summarized in *Table 1.* Reflex activity is indicative of the nature and level of cord injury (*Table 2*). Absent reflexes are indicative of spinal shock, or a lower motor neurone lesion. Brisk reflexes are indicative of an upper motor neurone lesion or intracranial event. The bulbocavernous reflex and anal wink test are indicators of spinal cord function. The return of these reflexes marks the cessation of spinal shock.

4. Investigations. Initially, plain X-rays are sufficient to establish spinal alignment and bony deformity. CT is useful to determine the extent of a fracture and plan operative intervention. MRI delineates cord injury, especially local haemorrhage or oedema. MRI is particularly useful where there is no obvious bony injury and in bifacet cervical dislocations where disc prolapse is suspected.

Table 1. Levels of motor and sensory function

Level	Motor function	Sensory function
C3,4,5	Diaphragm	
C4		Clavicle
C5	Elbow flexion	Lateral arm
C6	Wrist extension	Radial forearm/thumb
C7	Finger extension	Long finger
C8	Finger flexion	Ulnar hand
T1	Finger abduction	Ulnar forearm
T2		Medial arm/axilla
T4		Mid sternum
T7	Intercostals	Xiphoid
T10		Umbilicus
T12		Inguinal
L1	Hip adductors	Upper thigh
L2	Hip flexion	Mid thigh
L3	Knee extension	Knee
L4	Ankle dorsiflexion	Medial shin
L5	Great toe extension	Lateral calf, dorsum foot
S1	Ankle plantar flexion	Lateral foot, posterior leg
S2		Posterior thigh
S3,4,5		Peri-anal

Table 2. Reflexes levels

Reflex	Level
Biceps	C5
Supinator	C6
Triceps	C7
Knee	L4
Ankle	S1

Spinal immobilization

*1. **Immobilization*** of the 'unstable' spinal column is required to prevent secondary injury. This may be achieved by non-operative or operative means. Non-operative immobilization may be safely continued, with bed-rest, supervised nursing care, neck collar, tape and sandbags, etc. Skeletal traction via tongs or a halo is more secure and makes nursing easier in cervical spine injuries. Halo traction can be converted to halo-vest immobilization for early rehabilitation.

*2. **Operative immobilization*** of spinal fractures in the patient with a cord injury is controversial.

(a) Absolute indications for operative intervention:

- Severe malalignment.

- Progressive neurological deficit.
- Cauda equina syndrome.

(b) Relative indications for operative intervention:

- Incomplete deficit.
- Complete deficit with unstable fracture configuration.
- Polytrauma.
- To facilitate earlier transfer, nursing care and rehabilitation.
- Unacceptable alignment (angulation exceeding 30° in the saggital plane).

3. Surgical decompression. There is no clear evidence to support operative decompression except in the case of a progressive neurological deficit.

Prevention and management of complications

1. Complications. These include:

- Pressure sores.
- Infection – urinary, respiratory, skin.
- Gastrointestinal perforation or haemorrhage.
- Deep venous thrombosis (DVT) and pulmonary embolism.
- Shock.
- Autonomic dysreflexia.
- Joint contractures.
- Death.

Urinary retention or faecal impaction may precipitate autonomic dysreflexia, which manifests as headache, anxiety, sweating, nasal obstruction and blurred vision.

2. Prevention. The patient with a spinal cord injury is best managed in a specialized unit and early transfer after initial stabilization is advised. Most hospitals have a 'spinal protocol' for medical and nursing staff to follow. The protocol should include:

- Spinal immobilization control at all times on a spinal bed.
- Skin care with 2-hourly turning, logrolling, a well-padded mattress, etc.
- Gastric decompression by nasogastric tube if required.
- Intravenous fluid support.
- Bladder catheterization.
- Mechanical DVT prophylaxis.
- Monitoring for neurogenic shock and autonomic complications.
- Judicious antibiotic administration for infections.
- Adequate analgesia.
- Early physiotherapy.

3. Cord oedema control (steroids). The present evidence marginally favours early steroid administration in cord injury, in an attempt to reduce secondary cord injury and reduce the level of injury from oedema. However, such treatment has obvious risks and remains highly controversial. Methylprednisolone acts by membrane stabilization, decreasing inflammation and oedema; whether this leads to improved useful motor function is unclear. However, the gain of even minor grades of motor function at the cervical level may make a considerable difference.

The standard regime is a bolus dose of methylprednisolone (30 mg/kg) within 8 hours of presentation, followed by a continuous infusion of 5.4 mg/kg/hour for 23 hours, ideally with gastrointestinal protection. Ongoing trials suggest the time limit for the initial bolus dose may be extended to 24 hours from the time of injury and other agents such as gangliosides may be useful.

Rehabilitation

Following skeletal stabilization, by whatever chosen means, and the control of early complications, rehabilitation continues over a prolonged period during which the patient requires substantial support. A multidisciplinary team approach is required, involving physiotherapy, occupational therapy, orthoses, and social and welfare support. This is best co-ordinated by a Spinal Injuries Unit.

Further reading

Grundy D, Swain A. *Spinal Cord Injury*. London: British Medical Journal Publications, 1993; 4–18.

Related topics of interest

Polytrauma – resuscitation and ATLS, p. 209; Spinal cord injury – basic science, p. 258; Spinal fracture classification, p. 262

SPINAL CORD INJURY – BASIC SCIENCE

Spinal cord trauma is a catastrophic event, with a prevalence of 5 per 100 000 population. The mechanism of injury is RTA 50%, falls 20% and sport 20%, varying with age. Associated injuries include head injury 10%, chest injury 20% and multiple skeletal injuries 25%.

Anatomy

The cord occupies 35% of the spinal canal at C1 and about 50% elsewhere, being tightest in the upper thoracic region. The cord ends in the conus at the L1–2 disc level in adults, but is lower in children. Below the conus lies the cauda equina, which has more space in the spinal canal and hence is less susceptible to trauma than the cord. The dura ends at S2.

Table 1. Functional outcomes following injury at various levels

Level of injury	Transfer, ADL, dress and bowel function	Bladder control	Upper limb function	Trunk control	Lower limb function	Special aids
Above C3	Dependent	Dependent	–	–	–	Respiratory Elec. w/chair
C4	Dependent	Dependent	Some shoulder	–	–	Elec. w/chair
C5	Dependent	Dependent	Elbow flexion	–	–	Elec. w/chair
C6	? Independent	Dependent	Some grasp	–	–	Splints/ manual w/chair
C7	? Independent	Dependent	Grasp	–	–	Manual w/chair
C8	Independent	Assistance	Some hand	–	–	Manual w/chair
T1	Independent	Assistance	Good hand	Poor	–	Manual w/chair
T2–7	Independent	? Assistance	Normal	Fair	–	Manual w/chair
T8–9	Independent	Independent	Normal	Fair	–	Manual w/chair
T10–11	Independent	Independent	Normal	Good	Some pelvis	KAFO
T12–L2	Independent	Independent	Normal	Normal	Hip flexion	KAFO
L3–4	Independent	Independent	Normal	Normal	Knee extension	KAFO
L5	Independent	Independent	Normal	Normal	Ankle fair	AFO
S1–2	Independent	Independent	Normal	Normal	Ankle good	

ADL, activities of daily living; KAFO, knee ankle foot orthosis; AFO, ankle foot orthosis.

The cord blood supply is via the anterior and posterior spinal arteries, entering at segmental levels, with a vascular watershed in the mid-thoracic cord, where complete vascular lesions of the cord are most common.

Peripheral neurological function is related to cord levels and segments, so a sound knowledge of the myotomes and dermatomes is required. *Table 1* summarizes the effect of a cord injury at various levels on motor function, the level of independence achieved and the amount of support required. Similarly, different areas within the cord have specific functions (*Figure 1*). A partial cord injury may spare some cord function, while other areas are sacrificed.

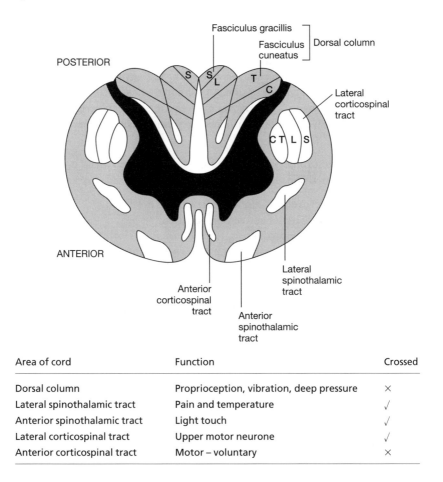

Area of cord	Function	Crossed
Dorsal column	Proprioception, vibration, deep pressure	×
Lateral spinothalamic tract	Pain and temperature	√
Anterior spinothalamic tract	Light touch	√
Lateral corticospinal tract	Upper motor neurone	√
Anterior corticospinal tract	Motor – voluntary	×

Figure 1. Transverse section of spinal cord in the cervical region. C, cervical structures; T, thoracic structures; L, lumbar structures; S, sacral structures. Reprinted from Browner BD, Jupiter JB, Levine AM, Trafton PG, *Skeletal Trauma*, 1998, p. 747, fig 26–2, by permission of W.B. Saunders Company.

Pathophysiology

Primary cord injury results from intrinsic flexion, stretching or rotation, or by extrinsic compression from bone or disc. Secondary cord injury follows ischaemia, hypoxia and metabolic disturbance. The timescale for cord damage is:

- 1 hour – petechial haemorrhage.
- 3 hours – necrosis.
- 6 hours – oedema.
- 1 week – cystic degeneration, syrinx.

Classifications

1. Complete versus incomplete cord lesions. Complete lesions are defined as absent motor or sensory function extending below the injury level. Incomplete lesions have some function spared, which indicates partial continuity of long tracts. Sacral sparing is typical and is assessed by testing peri-anal sensation, anal tone and squeeze, and great toe flexion. An incomplete deficit has a good prognosis for some functional motor recovery and may require urgent surgery, whereas true complete deficits have little hope of recovery if this persists beyond the period of spinal shock.

2. Level of injury. The lowest level with bilateral intact motor (MRC 3+) and sensory function, defines the level of injury.

3. Frankel grade. Classifies the severity of the deficit:

- A: Absent motor and sensory function.
- B: Sensation present.
- C: Sensation present, motor active not useful.
- D: Sensation present, motor active useful.
- E: Normal.

4. Cord syndromes, with incomplete cord lesions, are as follows:

- Central: The most common. Cervical hyperextension in the elderly, resulting in quadriplegia, classically flacidity (LMN lesion) in the arms, with spasticity (UMN lesion) in the legs. Bladder function may be preserved. There is a 75% recovery rate.
- Anterior: Dense motor/sensory loss (proprioception preserved). Poor prognosis. Ten per cent functional recovery.
- Posterior: Rare, usually following hyperextension injuries. Proprioception loss resulting in a foot slapping gait (syphilis).
- Brown–Séquard: Penetrating injuries. Ipsilateral motor and position/proprioception loss. Contralateral pain and temperature loss. Recovery is variable.
- Root: Recovery of one level is common and often important for function.

Spinal shock

Spinal shock is a transient condition, shortly after cord trauma, whereby cord function below and often above the level of injury is totally suspended. It is characterized by generalized flaccidity and the absence of local spinal reflexes, such as the bulbo-cavernosus reflex (S3–4). This is tested by looking for anal contracture after squeezing the glans penis or clitoris, or pulling on a catheter.

Spinal shock may prevent accurate assessment of the extent of a cord injury (complete or incomplete) and usually lasts for 24–48 hours. Recovery of spinal shock is marked by the return of reflex activity and UMN signs.

Neurogenic shock

Neurogenic shock is vascular hypotension with bradycardia, secondary to disruption of systemic sympathetic outflow and unopposed vagal tone. It is most commonly encountered with a high cord (above T7) lesion. Hypovolaemic shock with a tachycardia is more common, particularly in polytrauma, so management should first be directed at volume replacement and control of haemorrhage. Failure to respond is suggestive of neurogenic shock.

Treatment is with judicious volume replacement, leg elevation, atropine and occasionally vasopressors.

Further reading

Grundy D, Swain A. *Spinal Cord Injury*. London: British Medical Journal Publications, 1993; 4–18.

Related topics of interest

Spinal cord injury – assessment and management, p. 254; Spinal fracture classification, p. 262

SPINAL FRACTURE CLASSIFICATION

There is no universally accepted spinal fracture classification at present. Most classifications attempt to incorporate the three aspects of *mechanism, morphological appearance* and *stability.*

A. Mechanism

From the history, the *position* of the spine and the *force direction* at the time of injury are useful in understanding the extent of the disruption.

B. Morphological appearance

Radiological descriptions from plain X-ray, CT and MRI are used. The upper cervical spine, occiput, C1 and C2, are anatomically unique and hence there are a number of individual fracture classifications. The lower cervical spine, C3 to C7 and the thoracolumbar spine are similar and have generic classification systems.

Upper cervical fractures

See 'Spine – occiput to C2', p. 272.

Lower cervical fractures

Fractures may be classified purely on a morphological basis such as minor avulsions, teardrop, isolated posterior element, body compression or burst fractures and facet subluxations. This gives little information about the mechanism or stability. Several classifications which have attempted to expand on this are described.

1.   Allen and Ferguson classification. This is the only system specifically developed for this region, but is complicated. It is a mechanistic system based on the *presumed position* (flexion, extension, lateral flexion, or vertical) of the spine at failure and the initial dominant *direction of force* applied (compression or distraction).

2.   Denis 'three column spine' system or the AO system. Both systems, developed from analysis of thoracolumbar fractures, may be used, as the lower cervical region is broadly similar, allowing one comprehensive system.

Thoracolumbar spine fractures

1.   Holdsworth classification. Holdsworth divided the spine into two columns. Anterior body and posterior elements. The spine is unstable if both columns are injured.

2.   Denis classification. This describes fractures as four types: *compression, burst, flexion/distraction (Chance)* and *fracture-dislocation.* Denis divided the spine into three columns (*Figure 1*):

- Anterior: anterior longitudinal ligament and the anterior half of the vertebral body and disc.
- Middle: posterior half of the vertebral body and the posterior longitudinal ligament.

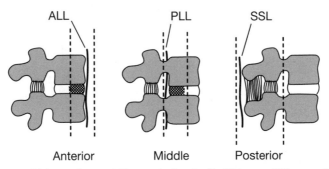

Figure 1. Denis' three columns. ALL, anterior longitudinal ligament; PLL, posterior longitudinal ligament; SSL, supraspinous ligament. Reprinted from Browner BD, Jupiter JB, Levine AM, Trapton PG, *Skeletal Trauma*, 1998, p. 967, fig 32–20, by permission of W.B. Saunders Company.

- Posterior: facet joints, ligamentum flavum, posterior arch, spinous process, and interspinous and supraspinous ligaments.

The principle of Denis' system is that if two columns are fractured then the spine is likely to be 'unstable'. Remember, however, that a column constitutes soft tissue as well as bone!

3. AO alphanumeric system. An accurate comprehensive, mechanistic system, incorporating the concepts of stability. While this system may prove to be predictive, it is not yet universally accepted as 'usable'. It is based upon Holdsworth's two-column model.

- Type A: vertebral body compression; 1: impaction, 2: split, 3: burst. Usually stable.
- Type B: anterior and posterior element injury with distraction; posterior disruption; 1: ligament, 2: bony, 3: + anterior disruption.
- Type C: anterior and posterior element injury with rotation; 1: type A + rotation, 2: type B + rotation, 3: rotational shear.

Sacral fractures

1. Vertical. These form part of a pelvic injury. Classified by Denis into ypes I to III; type I – lateral to neural foramen, type II – through foramen, and type III – medial to foramen.

2. Transverse. Fractures are undisplaced or displaced and are really spinal fractures which do not affect pelvic stability. Treatment is symptomatic.

C. Stability

Stability is defined as 'the ability of the spine under normal physiological loads to maintain a normal relationship between vertebrae, such that neurological structures are not injured and deformity or pain does not develop'. It is best to consider this with respect to the *acute* and *chronic* states.

*1. **Acute.*** If the patient is mobilized immediately, will one vertebra move with respect to its neighbour, putting the cord or nerve roots at risk?

*2. **Chronic.*** Will 'physiological loads', for example walking, in time lead to progressive unacceptable deformity and pain?

If the answer to either of these questions is 'yes', then the spine may be considered 'unstable' and management to control stability should be instigated. This may be non-operative or operative.

Further reading

Denis F. The three column spine and its significance in the classification of acute thoracolumbar spinal injuries. *Spine*, 1983; **8**: 817–831.

Magerl F, Aebi M, Gertzbein SD *et al*. A comprehensive classification of thoracic and lumbar injuries. *European Spine Journal*, 1994; **3**: 184–201.

O'Brien MF, Lenke LG. Fractures and dislocations of the spine. In: Dee R, Hurst LC, Gruber MA, Kottmeier SA, eds. *Principles of Orthopaedic Practice*, 2nd edn. New York: McGraw-Hill, 1997; 1237–1293.

Related topics of interest

Spinal cord injury – assessment and management, p. 254; Spine – C3 to C7, p. 269; Spine – occiput to C2, p. 272; Spine – thoracic and lumbar fractures, p. 275

SPINAL IMPLANTS

The range of commercial spinal implants continues to grow with new materials and designs. Implants are classified as internal or external fixation devices, including plates and screws, wires and rods, hooks and rods, lag screws, cages and external fixators.

Cervical spine implants – anterior devices

1. Anterior locking plates. Used in unstable anterior column compression/burst fractures. The low profile, smooth, titanium 'H' shaped-plates are applied to the anterior body and secured with unicortical locking screws. The screws are 'locked' by a short inner screw.

2. Lag screws. These include an odontoid peg screw (cannulated 3.5 mm cortical), inserted transorally, and transarticular screws for C1–C2 fusion.

3. Cages. Used to reconstruct the anterior column following vertebrectomy or fracture malunion. The cage provides support and the hollow structure is filled with bone graft.

Cervical spine implants – posterior devices

1. Wires and rods. Sublaminar, interspinous or interfacet wires may be used alone (Gallie and Brooke techniques) or with posterior metal rods, triangles or rectangles (Hartshill). Bone graft is added for posterior fusion and stabilization.

2. Plates and screws. Occipito-cervical plates extend stabilization of the upper cervical spine to the occiput, and are secured to the skull with short screws. Lateral mass plates are applied to the posterior aspect of the lateral masses, and require very precise (CT-guided) screw/hook placement (lateral angulation of 30°) to avoid the vertebral artery.
Transarticular 3.5 mm cortical screws (Magerl) may be used to stabilize C1–C2.

Thoracolumbar spine implants – anterior devices

1. Plates. Various plates, usually named after the designer (Thalgott, Kaneda, Zdeblick), may be applied to the lateral aspect of adjacent vertebrae to supplement an anterior decompression and bone graft reconstruction of the anterior column.

2. Cages. Hollow metal cages (e.g. Moss) packed with bone graft, are used to reconstruct the anterior column following trauma, tumour and degenerative spinal surgery. Cages include vertebral and disc-space types. Vertebral cages are used to replace the body after anterior vertebrectomy. Disc cages are inserted into the disc space following disc excision, to restore height and support bone graft. These may be inserted with an anterior or posterior approach. There are various complications associated with cages including incorrect placement and subsequent displacement. The use of these devices is increasing, as will their complications.

Thoracolumbar spine implants – posterior devices

Posterior 'tension band' stabilization may be achieved with sublaminar wires, screws and hooks, secured to posterior metal rods or rectangles. Hook-and-rod constructs are best suited to the thoracic spine, whereas pedicle screw-and-rod systems are favoured in the lower thoracic and lumbar spine. Rod systems may be classified as distraction, segmental or pedicle screw systems.

1. Distraction systems (Harrington). This system relies on three-point bending for mechanical fixation. Hooks secure the posterior rods to three vertebrae above and three below the injured segment. This system was very popular and is still used for thoracic injuries. The device is unsuitable for distraction injuries.

2. Segmental fixation systems (Cotrel–Dubousset or Luqué). These systems rely on the distribution of forces over multiple vertebral levels, with attachment of hooks, wires or screws. Compression and distraction may be used at different segmental levels within the same construct. The Cotrel–Dubousset system is widely used for trauma. The Luqué system was principally developed for deformity associated with paralytic disorders.

3. Pedicle screws. Inserted through the pedicles into the vertebral body, pedicle screws give very secure fixation. The screws (modified Schanz screw) are linked via clamps to plates or rods. Rod systems (AO, Colarado, Olerud, Vermont) are versatile and may extend over a few or many vertebral levels, allowing segmental compression or distraction. These systems are commonly used in the trauma setting to stabilize unstable fractures at the thoracolumbar junction and in the lumbar spine.

Screw entry point and direction of insertion is critical for safe use, and two-plane fluoroscopic guidance is essential. The entry point is best identified at the junction of the transverse process and the outer facet. An awl is used to carefully create a guide hole down the pedicle into the vertebral body. As the antero-medial direction of the pedicle varies with vertebral level (L1 – 10°, L5 – 25°) from the saggital plane, it is best to start laterally and aim medially. A pedicle 'feeler' and depth gauge are used to ensure that the pedicle walls have not been penetrated and the correct length screw is used. Complications include pedicle fracture, malposition, facet impingement, implant failure, nerve root and even cord injury. Computer-assisted techniques may help reduce complications.

Further reading

Bolesta MJ, Viere RG, Montesano PX, Benson DR. Fractures and dislocations of the thoracolumbar spine. In: Rockwood CA, Green DP, Bucholz RW, Heckman JD, eds. *Fractures in Adults*. Philadelphia: Lippincott-Raven, 1996; 1529–1571.

Stauffer ES, MacMillan M. Fractures and dislocations of the cervical spine. In: Rockwood CA, Green DP, Bucholz RW, Heckman JD, eds. *Fractures in Adults*. Philadelphia, Lippincott-Raven, 1996; 1473–1528.

Related topics of interest

SPINAL ORTHOSES

An orthosis is a device which provides external support to a body part and corrects or compensates for deformity or weakness. All orthoses are classified according to the joints crossed by the orthosis; the spine is no exception.

- CO: Cervical orthosis.
- CTO: Cervicothoracic orthosis.
- TLO: Thoracolumbar orthosis.
- TLSO: Thoracolumbosacral orthosis.
- LSO: Lumbosacral orthosis.

Most spinal orthoses act as static splints using the principle of three-point fixation. Orthoses are made from various materials, ranging from soft elasticated textiles to rigid thermoplastics, depending on the degree of support required.

Cervical orthoses

The degree of immobilization varies with vertebral level and depends on the material and design (*Table 1*). The range of devices is as follows:

1. Soft collars. These are constructed from foam, PVC or rubber and provide soft tissue support, but minimal skeletal support. Soft collars are used for 'whiplash type' injuries, stable fractures (such as clay shoveller's) and weaning from stiffer collars.

2. Semi-rigid collars. For example the 'Philadelphia' and 'Airflow' collars are for partial immobilization of stable flexion fractures. The Philadelphia collar is a two-piece plastazote collar, which provides good occipito-mandibular support, restricting flexion and extension. The Airflow collar is similar, but made of polyethylene with or without a chin extension.

3. Rigid trauma collars. These are stiff, foam-lined polyethylene collars. These immobilize the upper cervical spine very well, but are uncomfortable and only temporary.

4. Cervicothoracic braces. These two include two and four-poster braces, and the sterno-occipito-mandibular immobilizer (SOMI) brace. The SOMI specifically avoids a posterior thoracic pad which is uncomfortable. Cervicothoracic braces transfer load from the base of the skull to the thorax, immobilizing the neck very well and may be used for prolonged periods.

5. Halo vest system. The halo system may initially be used for cervical traction and later converted to static immobilization with shoulder struts to the chest jacket. The halo ring is attached to the skull by four skeletal pins equally spaced just below the widest part of the skull, avoiding contact with the ears. The anterior pins are placed above the outer aspect of the eyebrow. Care must be taken to avoid the supraorbital nerve and to ensure that the ring is equidistant from the skin all round.

The halo vest system allows general mobilization of the patient, while maintaining greater than 90% immobilization of the cervical spine, and is used for most unstable cervical injuries.

Table 1. Extent of immobilization achieved with cervical orthoses

Orthosis	Reduction in movement (%)		
	Flexion/extension	Rotation	Lateral flexion
Soft	20	15	10
Semi-rigid	70	20	40
Rigid	95	90	90
SOMI	70	70	40
Halo	95	95	95

Thoracolumbosacral orthoses

Many orthoses are available, ranging from simple elasticated canvas belts, to rigid plastic or plaster jackets with increasing degrees of immobilization. None is very effective in supporting above T8. In the trauma setting there are essentially two types:

- Hyperextension brace.
- TLSO.

Both utilize three-point fixation with anterior sternal, suprapubic/pelvic and posterior thoracolumbar pads to resist flexion. Hyperextension braces are used for stable flexion fractures. The TLSO extends to the pelvis, providing some rotation and lateral bending resistance.

Other 'corrective' rigid braces are used for non-traumatic conditions, such as scoliosis, and are beyond the scope of this topic.

Further reading

Johnson RM, Hart DL, Simmons EF *et al.* Cervical orthoses. *Journal of Bone and Joint Surgery*, 1977; **59A**: 332–339.

Related topics of interest

Spinal fracture classification, p. 262; Spine – C3 to C7, p. 269; Spine – occiput to C2, p. 272; Spine – thoracic and lumbar fractures, p. 275

SPINE – C3 TO C7

Sixty per cent of spinal cord injuries involve the cervical spine. The most commonly injured levels are C1, followed in order of frequency by C5, 6 and 7. Historically, 33% of patients with a significant cervical spinal injury were transported to hospital without immobilization. The factors predisposing to delayed diagnosis are altered consciousness, head injury and inadequate radiographic visualization of the cervical spine.

Classification

Unlike the lumbar spine, there is no universally agreed classification of cervical spine fractures. The three-column model of Denis has been extended to the cervical spine. The anterior column includes structures anterior to a line through the middle of the vertebral body. The middle column lies posterior to this line and extends posteriorly to include the posterior longitudinal ligament. The posterior column lies posterior to this ligament. An unstable injury is one with two-column, or middle-column failure.

Examination and investigation

1. **Examination.** After resuscitation and stabilization, the patient should be thoroughly examined.

2. **Radiological assessment.** This commences with a lateral radiograph, including the cervicothoracic junction (traction on arms/swimmer's view), which identifies 85% of injuries. AP and open mouth views should also be obtained. If plain radiological evaluation is inadequate, CT should be considered.

3. **Instability.** The criteria are:
- Angulation between vertebral bodies >11°.
- Translation of vertebral bodies >3.5 mm.
- Spinous process widening on lateral X-ray.
- Malalignment of the spinous processes on AP X-ray.
- Facet joint widening or rotation.
- Lateral tilting of the vertebral body on AP X-ray.
- Loss of >25% vertebral height.
- Pedicle widening.

4. **Ligamentous injuries.** The following may be associated with such injuries:
- Increased anterior soft-tissue interval; >3 mm to C3, >10 mm below C4.
- Minimal compression fractures of the anterior vertebral bodies.
- Avulsion fractures at the spinal ligament insertions.
- Non-displaced fractures through the vertebral body or posterior elements.

5. **Dynamic tests.** These can be used with normal radiological findings, where clinical suspicion remains. Flexion/extension views are obtained with the patient moving their head through a pain-free arc, under medical guidance. If these are normal, the patient is treated in a collar and reviewed with repeat dynamic radiographs at 3 weeks.

6. *Further imaging.* CT can be used for evaluation. The role of MRI to exclude a disc herniation is unclear. Cases of neurological deterioration due to disc retropulsion during reduction have been reported, but a risk/benefit assessment is required. If obtaining MRI causes unacceptable delay, especially in a conscious patient who is having the spine reduced under neurological and radiological monitoring, a scan is not obligatory.

Unilateral facet dislocation

Classical presentation is with the chin turned to the opposite side and the neck laterally flexed to the injured side. Seventy per cent have a radiculopathy, 20% are normal and 10% have spinal cord injury. The vertebral body is anteriorly subluxed 25% on plain lateral X-ray. The injury is often missed and is more easily demonstrated on oblique views. Reduction is by traction (often unsuccessful), or open reduction. Stabilization is either with a halo, or preferably posterior cervical fusion due to the incidence of non-union.

Bilateral facet dislocation

On lateral X-ray there is 50% anterior shift of the vertebral body. This is frequently associated with spinal cord injury and 9% of patients have disc material in the canal. In the absence of extruded disc material, reduction is usually achieved by traction. Immobilization using a halo has been associated with an unacceptably high incidence of non-union, and surgical fusion has been recommended.

Flexion injuries

If the anterior column is <25% compressed, the fracture is technically stable and can be treated with an orthosis. Fractures involving >25% anterior column compression, or the middle column, are unstable. Immobilization in a halo, or open reduction (usually anterior corpectomy) and stabilization, is required. The teardrop fracture (triangular fragment from the antero-inferior vertebral body) is associated with compression injury of the spine and instability. This can be treated by anterior decompression and fusion.

Extension injuries

Extension injuries are usually associated with compression. The most common pattern is fracture of the laminae, facets and pedicles. Laminar fracture is often associated with a facet or pedicle fracture. Bilateral laminar fractures are associated with major vertebral body injuries.

Ankylosing spondylitis

Fractures of the cervical spine in patients with ankylosing spondylitis are unstable, easily overlooked and associated with a high incidence of neurological injury. Immobilization in a halo or with surgical stabilization is required.

Clay shoveller's fracture

This is an isolated fracture of the spinous processes, most commonly C7, and is a stable injury in the absence of further ligamentous damage. Assessment is by flexion/extension views, and if the spine is stable, treatment is symptomatic in a collar.

Principles of treatment

1. *Traction.* The cervical spine can be stabilized using Gardner–Wells tongs and 5 kg of traction. After application, a lateral film should be obtained and neurological observations undertaken. Closed reduction should be attempted in all patients with malalignment. Reduction is performed under close radiological and neurological observation, after each weight addition. The initial weight is 10 kg, with 2.5 kg increments. A maximum weight of 30 kg is applied for the lower cervical spine and 10 kg for C1 and C2. Traction should be discontinued in the presence of:

- Neurological deterioration.
- Distraction >1 cm.
- Reduction.

After reduction, the traction is reduced to 10 kg or less, to maintain alignment.

2. *Surgery.* Timing is the major issue in surgery. Many authors consider that maximal damage occurs at the time of injury. However, there is evidence in dogs that decompression at 1 hour post-injury gives a better neurological outcome. Other studies also show that neurological deterioration is more common in patients operated on within 5 days than in patients who are operated on later. Thus the emphasis should be on resuscitation, closed immobilization and restoration of alignment. There is agreement that neurological deterioration in the presence of canal compromise is an indication for emergency surgery. Conversely, neurological deterioration without canal compromise is a contraindication to surgery.

Further reading

Beyer CA, Cabanela, Berquist TH. Unilateal facet dislocations and fracture-dislocations of the cervical spine. *Journal of Bone and Joint Surgery*, 1991; **73B**: 977–981.

Mahale YJ, Silver JR, Henderson NJ. Neurological complications of the reduction of cervical spine dislocations. *Journal of Bone and Joint Surgery*, 1993; **75B**: 403–409.

Slucky AV, Eismont FJ. Treatment of acute injury of the cervical spine. *Journal of Bone and Joint Surgery*, 1994; **76A**: 1882–1894.

Related topics of interest

Paediatric spine trauma, p. 177; Spinal fracture classification, p. 262; Spine – occiput to C2, p. 272

SPINE – OCCIPUT TO C2

The upper cervical spine is functionally and anatomically distinct to allow 'nodding' (occiput/ atlas) and 'shaking' (atlas/axis) of the head. This anatomical specialization leads to unique patterns of injury.

Anatomy

C1 (the atlas) is essentially a ring of bone, with articular facets for the occiput and axis. The body of C1 develops into the odontoid process of C2 (the axis). Ligamentous structures stabilizing the occiput to the spine include the apical and alar ligaments. The joint capsules provide additional stability. The most important stabilizer of the atlanto-axial joint is the transverse ligament passing between the lateral masses of the axis posterior to the dens, preventing anterior displacement of the atlas on the axis.

Occipital condylar fractures

These have been classified by Anderson and Montesano – the third type is potentially unstable:

- Type 1: impaction fracture of the occipital condyle.
- Type 2: fracture associated with a base of skull fracture.
- Type 3: rotation or lateral bending causing fractures secondary to ligamentous damage.

Occipital condylar fractures are rare and diagnosis requires a high index of suspicion. Types 1 and 2 are treated in a hard cervical collar, and type 3 in a halo.

Occipito-atlantal dislocation

Usually a fatal injury caused by a combination of hyperextension, rotation and distraction. X-rays can be dramatic, but less severe injuries may be overlooked. Injuries are of three types, with the occiput lying anterior, posterior, or distracted from its articulation with the atlas. Acute treatment is by application of a halo vest – traction is contraindicated. Definitive treatment is with occipito-cervical fusion.

C1 fractures

- Axial loading of C1 can cause the ring to fracture and the classic 'Jefferson' fracture is a four-part fracture in which the lateral masses are displaced laterally. Instability is determined according to the integrity of the transverse ligament, implied on the plain X-ray if the atlanto-dens interval is >3 mm, or if the measured sum of the overhang of the lateral masses is >8 mm. CT may show bony avulsion of the ligament and MRI images the ligament directly.
- Stable fractures are treated in a hard collar.
- Unstable fractures require 8 weeks in a halo, followed by 4 weeks in a Philadelphia collar.

- Some patients progress to stable fibrous union and, if asymptomatic, do not require treatment. If symptomatic (causing pain and torticollis), but stable, a C1–C2 fusion can be performed.
- If there is residual instability, an occipito-C2 fusion is necessary.

C1–C2 subluxation

Rupture of the transverse ligament is diagnosed when the atlanto-dens interval is >4 mm. If associated with bony avulsion confirmed on CT, a halo can be used; otherwise C1–C2 fusion is indicated.

Atlanto-axial rotatory subluxation

Rotation between C1 and C2 is typically seen in children, but also in adults, and occurs either spontaneously, or following trauma. The classification is based upon the paediatric spinal classification of Hawkins and Fielding. The only difference is that rupture of the transverse ligament should be suspected if the atlanto-dens interval is >3 mm (rather than 5 mm in children). Treatment with a short period of traction is followed by a cervical orthosis. Posterior fusion is rarely indicated.

Odontoid peg fractures

Peg fractures have been classified by Anderson and D'Alonzo (*Figure 1*).

- Type 1 fractures are at the tip, above the transverse ligament, and are caused by alar ligament avulsion. These fractures are stable and treated in a collar or brace.
- Type 2 fractures are level with the body of the axis, which is a watershed for the blood supply. Non-union rates of 67% have been reported. The risk of non-union increases with displacement of >4 mm, angulation of >10°, in patients who smoke and those over 40 years old. The results of treatment in a halo are better if the fracture is reduced. Surgical techniques include posterior C1/C2 fusion and transoral fixation with one or two screws into the peg.
- Type 3 fractures pass into the cancellous body of C2, with an 85–90% union rate after 12 weeks of halo treatment.

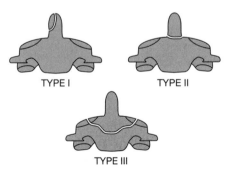

TYPE I   TYPE II

TYPE III

Figure 1. The Anderson and D'Alonzo classification of odontoid fractures. From Anderson LD, D'Alonzo RT (1974) Fractures of the odontoid process of the axis. *Journal of Bone and Joint Surgery*, vol. 56A, pp. 1663–1674. Redrawn by permission of the Journal of Bone and Joint Surgery, Inc.

Traumatic spondylolisthesis of the axis

This injury is caused by hyperextension and axial loading. Typically these injuries widen the spinal canal and therefore rarely produce neurological damage. The traditional 'Hangman's fracture' (extension in association with distraction) is seldom seen today. Spondylolisthesis of the axis was classified by Effendi and later modified by Levine:

- Type I: a stable injury with <3 mm displacement, treated in a collar for 6 weeks.
- Type II: an unstable injury, with >3 mm C2/3 displacement and angulation. Traction in slight extension usually achieves reduction, followed by application of a halo for 6 to 8 weeks.
- Type IIA: Levine proposed 5% of patients have this pattern of injury, from **flexion**-distraction and resultant C2/3 disc disruption. Angulation between C2 and C3 is more severe. These injuries mimic the traditional Hangman's fracture and with traction the cord can be distracted. A halo in slight compression and extension is required.
- Type III: a pars fracture, with uni- or bi-facet dislocation of C2/C3 and associated neurological injury. Treatment is again with traction, followed by halo immobilization. If the dislocation is irreducible, MRI is required to exclude disc herniation. A posterior fusion is performed between the inferior facet of C2 and the spinous process of C3. If the reduction of the body of C2 cannot be maintained, anterior fusion should be considered.

Further reading

Clark CR, White AA. Fractures of the dens: a multicenter study. *Journal of Bone and Joint Surgery*, 1985; **67A**: 1340–1348.

Fielding JW, Francis WR Jr, Hawkins RJ *et al.* Traumatic spondylolisthesis of the axis. *Clinical Orthopaedics*, 1989; **239**: 47–452.

Levine AM, Edwards CC. Fractures of the atlas. *Journal of Bone and Joint Surgery*, 1991; **73A**: 680–691.

Related topics of interest

Paediatric spine trauma, p. 177; Spine – C3 to C7, p. 269

SPINE – THORACIC AND LUMBAR FRACTURES

The objectives of spinal management are to prevent further displacement and neurological injury. Pre-hospital transport involves in-line immobilization on a long spinal board and a hard cervical collar. The initial management of the patient with a spinal injury in the Accident and Emergency Department follows ATLS guidelines, to identify and treat life-threatening conditions. Assessment, management and transfers should maintain in-line spinal control with log rolls and five-person lifts. Patients should be cared for in dedicated wards by personnel experienced in spinal injuries and many units have a spinal injury protocol.

Initial management

Early management is aimed at preventing and controlling complications.

1. *Skin.* The patient is kept on a well-padded mattress and turned, or log rolled, every 2 hours to reduce the risk of pressure sores.

2. *Bowels.* An ileus is common, particularly in fractures at the thoracolumbar junction. Intravenous fluids, restriction of oral intake and nasogastric intubation may be necessary.

3. *Bladder.* Urinary retention may occur secondary to recumbency, pain or neurological injury. Catheterization is required.

4. *DVT.* Mechanical prophylaxis with thigh-length compression stockings starts immediately. Subcutaenous heparin is started 48 hours after injury.

5. *Neurological injury.* See 'Spinal cord injury – assessment and management', p. 254.

Definitive management

Definitive management of thoracolumbar fractures depends on age, fracture level, fracture type, displacement and stability.

1. *Anterior wedge compression fractures* are common and management depends on the severity of the fracture.

- Less than 40% loss of anterior column height. The majority of these fractures are considered 'stable'. Management is directed at pain control, prevention of further deformity and obtaining the best position for healing. Spinal orthoses, such as a plaster jacket or a hyperextension brace, may be used at an early stage and maintained for 3 months.
- Greater than 40% loss of anterior column height. It is unusual for this degree of compression or wedging to occur without middle or posterior column injury. The fracture should therefore be considered 'unstable' and managed as a 'burst' fracture.
- Elderly. Multiple level compression fractures in osteopoenic bone may occur following minor, often unrecognized, trauma. Treatment is symptomatic, with early mobilization.

2. Burst fractures follow high-energy trauma with axial compression and flexion, causing an anterior body compression fracture and posterior ligamentous disruption. Burst fractures may be treated non-operatively or operatively.

(a) Non-operative. Treatment consists of bed rest followed by the application of a hyperextension brace, which reverses the deforming force, for 3 months. Most neurologically intact patients with <50% canal compromise and minimal segmental deformity may be managed in this manner.

(b) Operative. The indications for operative management are controversial.

- Absolute indication: progressive deterioration in neurological status.
- Relative indications:
  Kyphosis >30°.
  Subluxation at the fracture site.
  >40% loss of anterior height.
  >50% canal compromise.
  Neurological compromise.
  Pathological fracture – tumour, ankylosing spondylitis.
- Operative stabilization in cases of complete neurological compromise may reduce bed rest, facilitating nursing care and rehabilitation.

(c) Surgery by an anterior or posterior approach may be undertaken:

- Anterior approach. Canal decompression and anterior column reconstruction may be undertaken with strut graft of rib or iliac crest, or corporectomy and insertion of a graft-filled metal cage. Supplementary fixation with a plate or rod system may be used. Anterior approaches are as follows:
  T1 to T10 – thoracotomy, above the diaphragm.
  T11 to L1 – thoraco-abdominal, through the tenth rib and diaphragm.
  L2 to L5 – extraperitoneal approach below the diaphragm.
- Posterior approach. Correction of the sagittal alignment and re-establishment of the tension band effect of the posterior structures may be addressed posteriorly. Various systems are available, incorporating screws, rods and plates. Anterior grafting may also be accomplished posteriorly by trans-pedicular grafting.

3. Flexion–dislocation injuries are associated with a high incidence of neurological deficit due to severe vertebral malalignment. The management of these very unstable injuries is open reduction and fixation. Owing to the instability of the segment, posterior stabilization prior to anterior decompression is favoured.

4. Flexion–distraction (Chance) fractures are characterized by a line of disruption passing through bone or soft tissue (ligaments/disc). The latter are similar to facet subluxations in the cervical spine.

'Chance' fractures may be managed in a hyperextension brace and usually heal well.

Brace management of soft tissue disruptions may not heal and are better managed operatively with posterior reduction and stabilization.

A greater than 50% subluxation (bifacet type) may be associated with a traumatic disc herniation. Decompression prior to reduction is essential in these cases.

Complications

1. Non-operative
(a) Early
- The problems of prolonged bed rest and immobilization.
- Poor tolerance of, and cooperation with, bracing.

(b) Late
- Residual or progressive kyphotic deformity.
- Chronic pain.
- Instability/pseudoarthrosis.
- Spinal stenosis (central or root).

2. Operative
(a) Early
- Surgical complications; major vessel, lung, neurological trauma, wound healing, infection.

(b) Late
- Implant or graft failure.
- Loss of motion with fused segments and secondary degeration.
- Loss of correction and deformity.

Further reading

Bohlman HH. Treatment of fractures and dislocations of the thoracic and lumbar spine. *Journal of Bone and Joint Surgery*, 1985; **67**A: 165–169.

Kasser J. Spine: trauma. In: *Orthopaedic Knowledge Update 5*. Rosemont: American Academy of Orthopaedic Surgeons, 1996: 573–588.

Related topics of interest

Spinal cord injury – assessment and management, p. 254; Spinal cord injury – basic science, p. 258; Spinal fracture classification, p. 262; Spinal implants, p. 265; Spinal orthoses, p. 267

SPINE – WHIPLASH AND ASSOCIATED DISORDERS

Whiplash is a mechanism of injury, with acute neck flexion/extension, and is typically caused by a rear-end motor vehicle collision. The Quebec task force used the term '*whiplash-associated disorders*' (WAD) to describe the resulting clinical manifestations.

Classification

The Quebec task force graded WAD into:

- Grade I: complaint of neck pain, stiffness or tenderness.
- Grade II: neck complaints with musculoskeletal signs of point tenderness and decreased range of movement.
- Grade III: neck complaint and neurological signs.
- Grade IV: neck complaint and fracture or dislocation.

The first three grades are considered below.

Clinical presentation and imaging

The most common presenting symptoms are neck pain (88–100%) and occipital headaches (54–66%). Other complaints are stiffness, shoulder and arm pain, paraesthesiae, weakness, vertigo, memory loss, fatigue, dysphagia, and visual and auditory symptoms. A thorough clinical examination is mandatory to exclude significant bony or neurological abnormality requiring specific treatment.

At presentation, 44% of patients are grade I, 39% grade II, 16% grade III, and 1% grade IV.

A patient who is fully alert and oriented, with a grade I injury, does not routinely require radiographs. Patients with neurological abnormality or bony tenderness require radiographic evaluation. Only 35–50% of patients have normal radiographs – the most common abnormalities are loss of the lordosis and long-standing degenerative change. These factors are associated with a poorer outcome.

MRI and CT are not routinely indicated. MRI is abnormal in 19% of asymptomatic individuals and 28% of those over 40 years of age.

Pathology

The pathology is unclear. Injection studies demonstrate the zygoapophyseal joints are the most common sites of origin for chronic neck pain in WAD. Other possible causes are soft tissue damage, intramuscular bleeding and microinjury to the cord or brain. Intervertebral disc prolapse or end plate avulsion is rare.

The minimum speed involved is estimated between 6 and 10 km/hour, which generates forces of 4.5 G. Seatbelts may increase the incidence of WAD, whereas the preventative effect of headrests depends on design and adjustment.

Incidence

The estimated incidence varies greatly. A recent study from Lithuania, where there is little knowledge of the disability associated with WAD, showed no patient with persisting symptoms. Other studies show annual incidences of 16 (New Zealand),

39 (Australia) and 70 (Quebec) per 100 000. There are an estimated 250 000 cases per annum in the UK.

The most common age group involved is 20–24 years. Women are affected twice as often as men, and front seat passengers twice as often as those in the rear.

Treatment

1. Mobilization. Soft collars do not immobilize the neck. Immobilization, or 'rest', of the neck has been shown to slow recovery. The recommendation is that mobilization (Maitland manipulations encourage neck movement) is started within 72 hours – this may be supervised by a physiotherapist, or take the form of education and home exercise. In all cases the emphasis is on early return to normal activities, and reassurance that the injury is a benign and self-limiting condition for the majority.

2. Analgesia. The sparing use (1 week) of NSAIDs is sometimes necessary in grade II or III injury. The Quebec task force discouraged narcotics or benzo-diazepine therapy.

3. Reassessment. If the patient has not returned to their usual activities by 6 weeks (grade I), or 12 weeks (grade II and III), the task force recommended 'multidisciplinary team evaluation' The persistence of some pain or residual restriction of movement is not an indication for such assessment.

4. Surgery. Discectomy and anterior fusion has good results in the rare cases of disc protrusion and radicular symptoms.

Factors predicting a poor outcome

Many factors have been described which predict a less favourable outcome:

1. Patient factors
- Older age: it is unclear if this is an independent factor or related to the increased incidence of degenerative change in the elderly.
- Female.
- Multiple trauma.
- Referred upper limb pain.
- Abnormal neurological signs at presentation.

2. Radiological factors
- Pre-existing radiographic degenerative change.

3. Accident factors
- Severity of the accident.
- Single vehicle accidents where the collision involves a stationary object (e.g. a lamp-post).

4. Behavioural factors
It has been shown that patients with symptoms persisting at 2 years developed abnormalities shown by psychological testing (somatization, anxiety and depression) during the first 3 months after injury. The patients were not abnormal in the first week after injury. Compensation neurosis and secondary gain increase the

reported suffering; however, settlement of the litigation is not always associated with rapid recovery.

5. Long-term effect of WAD on the development of degenerative change.
This is unknown, although it has been shown that there is no radiological progression in the first 8 years.

Prognosis

The exact proportion of patients with persisting symptoms and the time after which no further resolution can be expected is difficult to determine from the literature. Nevertheless, the majority of patients do recover. In Quebec, 53%, 87% and 97% of patients had returned to their usual activities or work by 1, 6 and 12 months, respectively.

A larger number of patients have persistent symptoms, ranging from 0% in Lithuania, to 70% at 15 years in England. The consensus is that 6–18% of patients will have some persisting symptoms and disability.

Prevention

1. Prevention of accidents by improving road safety, and reduction of neck injury in each accident by the provision of proper head rests.

2. Early mobilization of the neck is useful, as is avoidance of advice to 'rest and wear a soft collar.' There may be merit in psychological intervention within the first 3 months.

3. Reducing the secondary gain and compensation neurosis by the provision of early positive reinforcement and reassurance that a good outcome can be expected.

Further reading

Freeman MD, Croft AC, Rossignol AM. 'Whiplash associated disorders: redefining whiplash and its management' by the Quebec Task Force. A critical evaluation. *Spine*, 1998; **23**: 1043–1049.
Ratliff AHC. Whiplash injuries. *Journal of Bone and Joint Surgery*, 1997; **79B**: 517–519.
Spitzer WO, Skovron ML, Salmi LR, *et al*. Scientific monograph of the Quebec Task Force on Whiplash-associated Disorders: redefining 'whiplash' and its management. *Spine*, 1995; **20**: 15–73S.

Related topics of interest

THORACIC TRAUMA

Thoracic trauma causes ventilatory or circulatory compromise and should be addressed in the resuscitation of all trauma victims after securing the airway and cervical spine. Initial measures include high flow oxygen, intubation and ventilation, and i.v. fluid therapy. Twenty five per cent of fatalities following major trauma are due to thoracic injuries, but only 10% of thoracic injuries present in time for, or require, surgical intervention. Continuous reassessment is mandatory.

Thoracic injuries are often manifest by external signs of thoracic cage injury with bruising or penetrating wounds. Internal deceleration injuries may occur without visible external trauma.

The function of the lungs and heart are closely interrelated and injury to either organ can result in ventilation/perfusion mismatch.

Injury patterns

*1. **Thoracic cage injuries*** often have visible external bruising, indicating damage to the ribs, lung parenchyma, small or great vessels. A fracture of the upper ribs indicates severe trauma and is often associated with spinal, brachial plexus or shoulder injuries. Fractures of the lower ribs can indicate injury to abdominal viscera. Fractures of the sternum are painful and can be associated with a flail segment and cardiac or pulmonary contusion.

*2. **A tension pneumothorax*** is diagnosed clinically and requires immediate decompression by needle thoracocentesis and a definitive tube thoracostomy. A tension pneumothorax may develop during assisted ventilation.

*3. **A simple pneumothorax*** is often diagnosed clinically, although may not be immediately evident and only seen on chest X-ray. Lung collapse should be treated by tube thoracostomy. Small pneumothoraces can be treated with close observation. However, if a patient is being transferred to another centre, or being ventilated, tube thoracostomy is essential. An untreated simple pneumothorax can progress to a tension pneumothorax.

*4. **Flail chest*** occurs with multiple rib fractures, disrupting chest wall movement, which may become paradoxical. The lung parenchyma may be damaged. Some patients require assisted ventilation and tube thoracostomy.

*5. **Open pneumothorax*** due to a defect in the chest wall, leaves a sucking wound. If the diameter exceeds two thirds of the trachea, the air enters preferentially by this route. The defect should be occluded, with a dressing taped on three sides and a definitive tube thoracostomy established.

*6. **Lung parenchymal damage or pulmonary contusion*** following a crush injury can cause early, rather than immediate, respiratory failure, sometimes progressing to ARDS requiring prolonged ventilation.

*7. **Tracheo-bronchial tree ruptures*** are uncommon, occurring in fewer than 10% of severe chest injuries. The diagnosis is suspected if widespread surgical emphysema or prolonged drainage through a thoracostomy tube are observed. Surgical closure is required.

8. *A haemothorax* occurs in isolation or with a pneumothorax. This can lead to ventilatory and circulatory collapse. Drainage of the blood is required after establishing venous access, as there may be sudden massive haemorrhage. Haemorrhage is usually self-limiting. If the initial drainage exceeds 1500 ml, or persistent drainage exceeds 200 ml/hour, surgical thoracotomy is required.

9. *Rupture of the diaphragm,* usually on the left, with herniation of abdominal viscera, impairs ventilation. Initial X-rays can be difficult to interpret. A nasogastric tube may help the diagnosis. Surgical repair is required. Late presentation occurs and 50% of hernias are diagnosed more than 1 year after injury.

10. *Penetrating cardiac injuries and cardiac tamponade* follow a sharp or penetrating injury. The diagnosis is often difficult in a noisy resuscitation room and a high index of suspicion is required. Draining 10 to 20 ml of blood from the pericardium can increase the cardiac output by 2 l/min.

11. *Great vessel disruption* usually results in sudden death. However, smaller defects in the great vessels are often repairable, if diagnosed promptly. Failure to respond to fluid resuscitation, or a widened mediastinum on chest X-ray are indicative of this injury.

12. *Myocardial contusion and valve damage* may follow a severe crush injury.

Investigation

In addition to clinical signs, a chest X-ray, ECG or CT scan may be required.

Resuscitation procedures

1. *Needle thoracocentesis* is performed as a life-saving procedure to relieve a tension pneumothorax in a rapidly deteriorating patient. An over-the-needle wide bore (14 gauge) cannula is passed over the second rib in the mid-clavicular line, after skin preparation and, ideally, local anaesthetic. Leaving the cannula in place, attached to a three-way tap, allows relief of any reaccumulation prior to establishing a definitive tube thoracostomy.

2. *Insertion of a thoracostomy tube* is a surgical procedure and should be undertaken by skilled personnel, with appropriate facilities. Ideally the insertion site is the fifth intercostal space in the anterior axillary line. After advising the patient of the procedure, the skin is cleaned and infiltrated with local anaesthetic. A transverse incision is made, followed by blunt dissection through the subcutaneous tissues and over the fifth rib, through the pleura. A finger is inserted into the thorax before introducing a clamped thoracostomy tube (26–30 French gauge). This is connected to an underwater sealed drain or a flutter valve. The thoracostomy tube is sutured in place and dressed.

3. *Needle pericardiocentesis* is performed with a 16 gauge, 15 cm over-the-needle catheter, with a three-way tap. Monitoring with ECG is essential. The needle is advanced at an angle of 45° to the skin, from an entry site 2 cm below the xiphoid, towards the tip of the left scapula. If the myocardium is penetrated, the ECG electrodes will show an injury pattern.

Further reading

Advanced Trauma and Life Support Programme For Doctors – The Student Manual. Chicago: American College of Surgeons, 1997; 125–141.

Watson DCT. Thoracic injury and sepsis. In: Ellis BW, Paterson-Brown S, eds. *Hamilton Bailey's Emergency Surgery.* Oxford: Butterworth-Heinemann, 1995; 281–286.

Watson DCT. Heart and great vessels. In: Ellis BW, Paterson-Brown S, eds. *Hamilton Bailey's Emergency Surgery.* Oxford: Butterworth-Heinemann, 1995; 287–294.

Related topics of interest

Polytrauma – management and complications, p. 200; Polytrauma – resuscitation and ATLS, p. 209

TIBIAL PILON FRACTURES

Tibial pilon or plafond fractures involve the weight-bearing intra-articular surface of the distal tibia. An uncommon but devastating injury, occurring most frequently in men of working age, which represents 1% of lower limb fractures.

Twenty per cent are open injuries with wounds of variable appearance, often antero-medial. Swelling and skin contusion may be severe at an early stage, worsening over the next few days. Associated injuries related to axial loading in the limb or axial skeleton should be excluded.

Mechanism

There are two mechanisms of injury – rotational and direct axial loading or compression.

1. Rotational forces cause low-energy fractures with relatively little associated soft tissue injury or fracture comminution.

2. Axial compression causes high-energy, 'explosive' fractures with extensive surrounding soft tissue disruption.

Imaging

Plain X-rays demonstrate the injury, but a CT scan is essential to determine the fracture configuration and to plan management. Spiral imaging with multiplanar reformatting identifies displacement and comminution.

Classification

Several classifications have been proposed, but the Ruedi and Allgower three-part classification (1969) is favoured. It both helps planning and is of prognostic value.

- Grade I: undisplaced articular fracture.
- Grade II: displaced articular fracture without comminution.
- Grade III: comminution of articular surface and metaphysis with impaction.

Low-energy rotational injuries tend to be grade I or II, and high-energy axial injuries grade III.

Initial management

Following resuscitation of a patient with life-threatening injuries, management objectives for the limb include:

- Protection of the soft tissue envelope.
- Correction of gross deformity.
- Initial stabilization.
- Fracture assessment.

Open fractures need debridement, lavage, antibiotics and delayed closure or skin cover. Closed fractures need attention to the soft tissues to reduce skin tension and minimize swelling. High elevation with or without cryo-cooling is used.

Correction of deformity and stabilization is by simple reduction, cast splintage or traction with a calcaneal pin or external fixator.

Further imaging is undertaken over the next few days while swelling subsides.

Definitive management

The objectives are:

- Anatomical reduction of the articular surface.
- Restoration of length.
- Bone union.
- Non-infected, viable soft-tissue envelope.
- Early movement and restoration of function.

1. *Grade I fractures* may be managed non-operatively, with cast immobilization for 6 weeks, followed by 6 weeks graduated weight-bearing. Surgical stabilization allows earlier movement.

2. *Grade II and III fractures* are difficult and unforgiving injuries. Various techniques have been advocated.

Open reduction with a fibular plate to restore length, a medial tibial buttress plate, with bone grafting and reconstruction of the plafond with interfragmentary screws, has >80% good or excellent results in low-energy grade I and II injuries. More than 50% of high-energy grade III injuries suffer major complications.

External fixation or traction alone provide ligamentotaxis and effect indirect joint reduction. Results are no better than ORIF in grade III injuries.

Combined fixation with a fibular plate to restore length and a medial external fixator crossing the ankle joint, with minimal open reduction, bone grafting and interfragmentary screw fixation, has similar results to ORIF for grade II injuries, but >70% good results for grade III injuries.

Newer techniques include Ilizarov circular frames in combination with minimal internal fixation, allowing early mobilization of the ankle. As yet, there is no substantiated evidence that these will improve previous results; however, any system allowing earlier joint movement is theoretically beneficial.

Early arthrodesis is a reasonable option for the non-reconstructable joint and facilitates rehabilitation.

Current recommendations

- Low-energy (Grade I/II): ORIF
- High-energy (Grade III): combined internal/external fixation with fine wire frames

Complications

Early complications are:

- Delayed wound healing.
- Infection of wound, pin tracks, or osteomyelitis.
- Loss of reduction.

Late complications include:

- Mal/non-union.
- Joint pain, stiffness and instability.
- Joint degeneration occurs despite optimal management and follows cartilage damage at the time of injury. Late arthrodesis is 50% in some series for grade III injuries.

Further reading

Ruedi T, Allgower M. The operative treatment of intra-articular fractures of the lower end of the tibia. *Clinical Orthopaedics*, 1979; **138**: 105–110.

Tornetta P, Weiner L, Bergman M *et al.* Pilon fractures: treatment with combined internal and external fixation. *Journal of Orthopaedic Trauma*, 1997; 7: 489–496.

Related topics of interest

Ankle fractures, p.6; Principles of external fixation, p. 214

TIBIAL PLATEAU FRACTURES

Tibial plateau fractures follow high-energy trauma in young adults. Cotton and Berg first described these as 'bumper' or 'fender' fractures in the late 1920s. RTAs account for 40–60% of tibial plateau fractures. In the elderly, with osteoporotic bone, tibial plateau fractures follow lesser trauma.

The degree of comminution, displacement and compression of the articular surface is variable. Management depends on the severity of the injury and the demands of the patient, but the aim of treatment is to restore alignment of the knee joint and congruity of the articular surface.

Classification

Hohl and Luck's classification of the 1950s has been superseded by Schatzker's classification (*Figure 1*) with six fracture patterns:

- Type 1 – vertical shear.
- Type 2 – vertical shear and compression.
- Type 3 – local compression.
- Type 4 – medial condyle fracture (a fracture/subluxation of the knee).
- Type 5 – bicondylar.
- Type 6 – tibial plateau and segmental fracture (separating metaphysis and diaphysis).

AO classify the fractures as: 41-B or 41-C.

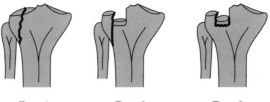

| Type 1 | Type 2 | Type 3 |

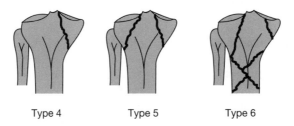

| Type 4 | Type 5 | Type 6 |

Figure 1. Schatzker classification of tibial plateau fractures. Modified from Schatzker, J., McBroom, R. and Bruce, D. The tibial plateau fracture. The Toronto experience 1968–1975. *Clinical Orthopaedics and Related Research*, vol. 138, 1979, pp. 94–104. With permission from Lippincott Williams & Wilkins.

Imaging

Plain AP and lateral X-rays are insufficient. Imaging with a plateau view (X-ray beam angled a few degrees off vertical), oblique views or tomograms give better evaluation of the injury. A CT scan with 3D reconstruction demonstrates the fracture pattern in considerably more detail and greatly assists surgical reconstruction.

Associated ligament injuries

Collateral ligament injuries occur in 4–25% of isolated fractures and are most common in compression fractures of the articular surface. Less than 10% of tibial plateau fractures are fracture/dislocations and ligament injuries occur in 60% of this group.

Management

1. Traction and early mobilization was advocated by Apley in the 1950s, who reported excellent or good results in 78% of patients. The current indication for conservative management is a depressed fracture of less than 4 mm. Conservative treatment consists of early mobilization in skeletal traction, followed by a cast brace for at least 6 weeks, touch-weight bearing initially. In the osteoporotic patient, pin loosening and infection on traction can be reduced with a double Steinmann pin technique.

Fractures with 4 to 8 mm of depression should be considered for elevation, bone grafting and internal fixation, depending on the age and physical demands of the patient. Where varus/valgus instability is >15°, or there is >8 mm depression, internal fixation is indicated.

Multifragmentary fractures in the elderly often benefit from manipulation and moulding with an Esmarch bandage, from distal to proximal.

2. Arthroscopically assisted reduction of a vertical shear fracture, without depression of the articular surface, can often be achieved with minimal exposure and large fragment transverse cancellous lag screws. Arthroscopy allows irrigation of the haemarthrosis, visualization of fracture reduction and confirms congruity of the articular surface. Type 1 fractures are more common in young people.

3. Surgical approach. A midline incision should be used, with dissection around the joint line and an arthrotomy beneath the meniscus. An extensive lateral approach jeopardizes the opportunity for late reconstructive surgery, but a small lateral incision may be used for type 1 fractures.

4. Elevation, bone graft and buttress plate fixation are required for depressed articular surface fractures. The antero-lateral (or antero-medial) aspect of the upper tibia is exposed and a cortical fenestration fashioned with a drill and osteotome. Using a punch, the articular surface can be elevated 'en masse' and graft from the ipsilateral iliac crest impacted, which is supported with two large fragment cancellous screws incorporating a contoured buttress plate. The joint surface must be visualized to ensure restoration of the articular surface, and in some instances to remove a meniscus displaced into the fracture. In skilled hands, arthroscopy is an alternative to arthrotomy. However, adequate visualization is difficult. After the procedure the joint surface should be slightly convex as there will be some collapse of the fracture and graft.

5. ***Post-operative management.*** Early movement is encouraged after surgery and the knee supported with a cast brace for 8 weeks, avoiding more than touch-weight bearing for the first 6 weeks. Even if the articular surface cannot be accurately reconstructed, realignment of the knee joint is important for subsequent reconstructive surgery.

6. ***External fixation*** may be required for bicondylar and segmental fractures, or cases where the skin and soft tissues are severely traumatized. Such injuries follow high-energy trauma, often with extensive comminution or soft tissue damage. Aggressive surgical intervention should be avoided, as extensive exposure with both medial and lateral plates is associated with wound breakdown and chronic infection. One series reports an 82% wound failure rate. These fractures may be stabilized with an external fixator across the knee for 6 to 8 weeks, followed by a hinged cast brace and intensive physiotherapy to regain movement. Alternatively a peri-articular ring can be used and knee movement started early. Stabilization of the articular surface may be augmented with percutaneous cancellous screws.

Pitfalls

- Type 4 (medial plateau) fractures tend to displace, with the knee assuming a varus deformity. Aggressive surgical treatment is required to prevent this.
- Type 4, 5 and 6 fractures are associated with neurovascular complications.

Complications

1. ***Wound healing.*** Primary skin contusion and substantial swelling follow these injuries. The upper tibia is poorly covered by soft tissue, especially on the medial side, and wound breakdown, which can be catastrophic, is common without a meticulous surgical approach.

2. ***Joint stiffness.*** Stiffness is not usually severe, with the majority of patients achieving full extension and flexion in excess of 90°.

3. ***Osteoarthritis.*** The incidence is variable and relates to the degree of comminution and the reduction achieved. Residual malalignment, medial and bicondylar fractures are poor prognostic factors. Symptoms may develop over a period of one to two decades following the injury. There is a poor correlation between radiological and functional results. Depending on the age, occupation and lifestyle of the patient, a knee replacement is appropriate. An osteotomy should be considered for varus malunion.

Further reading

Schatzker J, McBroom R, Bruce D. The tibial plateau fracture. The Toronto experience 1968–1975. *Clinical Orthopaedics*, 1979; **138**: 94–104.

Wiss DA, Watson JT. Fractures of the proximal tibia and fibula. In: Rockwood CA, Green DP, Bucholz RW, Heckman JD, eds. *Rockwood and Green's Fractures in Adults*. Philadelphia: Lippincott-Raven, 1996; 1919–1956.

Related topics of interest

Femoral fractures – distal, p. 46; Knee – dislocation, p. 137

TIBIAL SHAFT FRACTURES

Fracture of the tibial shaft is the most common long bone fracture. The numerous management approaches to closed fractures should be tailored to the morphology of the fracture and the patient. The advent of IM nailing has revolutionized the treatment of tibial shaft fractures. Management of the 20–25% of tibial fractures which are open injuries requires immediate input from plastic surgeons, and the method of stabilizing severely contaminated fractures remains controversial.

Classification

Shaft fractures are described by the anatomical site (mid-shaft, junction of upper and middle thirds, etc.), fracture configuration (transverse, short oblique, multi-fragmentary, etc.), and the extent of associated soft tissue damage. Fractures are most appropriately classified by the AO alphanumeric classification: 42-A, 42-B or 42-C for the tibia, with various subtypes to describe the morphological pattern.

Associated injuries

There is a high incidence of associated injuries accompanying closed tibial shaft fractures, including compartment syndrome, arterial and neurological injury. Twenty per cent of fractures have an associated knee ligament injury. A bifocal fracture may involve the tibial plateau or ankle in 5% of cases. In other cases the fracture may extend from the diaphysis to intra-articular regions. Pathological fractures due to metastatic spread are rare; however, metabolic bone disease may manifest as a tibial fracture. Stress fractures, even in the young, are recognized.

The popliteal artery and trifurcation are tethered by the anterior tibial artery passing through the interosseus membrane, and are more susceptible to injury with displaced fractures around the proximal diaphyseal–metaphyseal junction. The peroneal nerve is prone to injury from an associated fracture of the proximal fibula. Compartment syndrome is most common in the leg.

Treatment

Treatment includes closed manipulation and cast immobilization, functional bracing with graduated weight-bearing, plate fixation, IM nailing, external fixation and, for severe open fractures, amputation. Deformity of 10° in the saggital plane, 5° in the coronal plane and 10° of rotation, with up to 1 cm of shortening, are considered acceptable. Careful evaluation and documentation of any associated soft tissue injury is essential.

*1. **Closed treatment*** in a cast is ideal for low-energy, minimally displaced, isolated leg fractures. A long-leg cast is applied after closed reduction, with the knee flexed 20° and the ankle joint in neutral. Partial weight-bearing can be allowed if the fracture configuration is stable – if not, weight-bearing should be delayed until early signs of union. At around 4–6 weeks, the cast can be changed to a patellar tendon-bearing cast and weight-bearing increased. Later, a protective gaiter may be used. Regular clinical and radiological assessments should be made and residual angulation corrected by wedging the cast. The total period in plaster is usually 14–16 weeks.

With functional bracing applied 4 weeks after the injury and early weight-bearing, Sarmiento reports very successful union rates of 98.9% in 1000 selected fractures, with healing at 14–18 weeks and mean shortening of less than 5 mm. Functional bracing requires the patience of a skilled surgeon and orthotist, and a co-operative patient. The technique is unsuitable for major open fractures, poly-trauma, irreducible fractures, a segmental fracture configuration, angulated fractures with an intact fibula, and patients with an associated sensory deficit.

2.   *Plate and screw fixation* is seldom indicated with the advent of IM nails. Good results have been reported in only 85 to 90% of patients and complication rates are high – around 30%. In some series delayed union was as high as 48% and infection around 20%. Plate and screw fixation is suitable only for occasional bifocal fractures with metaphyseal involvement, when alternative means of treatment are contraindicated, and in some instances for the treatment of delayed or non-union. The complication rate is higher with open fractures where plate fixation is contraindicated.

3.   *IM nailing* is the treatment of choice for displaced diaphyseal fractures and for polytrauma, associated vascular injuries and pathological fractures. With conventional nails, fractures within 5 cm of the knee or ankle joint are difficult to control, and those within the proximal third of the tibia difficult to reduce. Union rates, functional outcome and residual deformity are all superior to closed treatment for displaced fractures. Interlocking bolts control rotation and length. Routine removal of interlocking bolts at 6 weeks to dynamize the fracture and promote union seems unnecessary.

The relative merits of reamed and unreamed IM nails remains unclear. The perceived benefits of not reaming, and avoiding disturbance of the endosteal blood supply, may be outweighed by slower union rates and higher rates of implant failure.

The rate of rehabilitation and post-hospitalization costs are lower after IM nailing than closed treatment and the outcome more predictable. However, the occasional complications of IM nailing, especially infection, may be catastrophic.

4.   *External fixation* is advocated for severe compound fractures and may be used for closed diaphyseal fractures with early weight bearing. However, delayed, non and malunion rates are higher. Pin tract infection or loosening occurs in up to 50% of patients. Dynamization of the frame may encourage healing. The use of circular frames, is now being extended for severe fractures with associated bone loss, restoring bone defects by early bone transport.

5.   *Traction* is rarely advocated for tibial fractures, unless co-morbidity prevents definitive treatment. A calcaneal traction pin and plaster backslab may be used for provisional control of a fracture when definitive treatment is delayed.

6.   *Paediatric tibial fractures* can usually be treated in plaster. Proximal tibial fractures (Cozen's fracture) have a tendency to malunite in valgus, requiring careful clinical and radiological assessment. Osteotomy is occasionally required. Following polytrauma, external fixation and plate fixation may be helpful.

Open fractures

Gustilo–Anderson type IIIB injuries are the most common, accounting for 35% of all open tibial fractures. IIIC fractures are the least common. Meticulous debridement and copious lavage of all open fractures are essential. Soft tissue cover should be achieved within 5 days of the injury, preferably sooner.

Type I, II and IIIA fractures may be treated by closed means or by IM nailing. Controversy surrounds the management of type IIIB and C fractures, which may be treated by IM nailing or external fixation. The latter may interfere with soft tissue reconstruction. Unreamed nails causing less damage to the endosteal blood supply are currently fashionable, but are associated with higher implant failure and non-union rates.

Union rates in I, II and IIIA injuries are almost comparable to closed fractures. Delayed bone union should be treated by exchange IM nailing and bone grafting, which is required in about 10% of all cases, but more commonly for IIIC injuries. The period to union is greater, and infection or non-union rates as high as 50% or more in IIIB and IIIC fractures. Compartment syndrome reportedly occurs in 20% of open injuries.

Consideration should be given to amputation in IIIC injuries with posterior tibial nerve damage, warm ischaemia time exceeding 6 hours or a severe ipsilateral foot injury. Overall amputation rates for IIIC injuries exceed 50%.

Delayed union, non-union and infection

Delayed union is defined as failure to progress to union by 16 weeks (20 weeks in some texts) and non-union is the absence of union at 8 months. Delayed union can be addressed by fibular osteotomy, IM nailing or exchange nailing. Additional bone grafting is recommended. Poor prognostic factors for union include the energy of the initial injury, the degree of initial displacement, comminution, infection and associated soft tissue damage.

Chronic infection is the worst prognostic factor and most frequent after high-velocity, open fractures. Management includes thorough debridement, soft tissue coverage, rigid fixation and antibiotic therapy. Stabilization with an external fixator may be required with extensive infection. Lesser infections may be treated by IM reaming and exchange nailing. Amputation is often the end result.

Complications

- Compartment syndrome: 3–20% (anterior compartment most common).
- Infection – closed fractures: 0.9-2% after IM nailing; 5–20% after plate fixation.
- Infection – open fractures: 7% after IM nailing.
- Delayed union: 16–30% after plate fixation; 8–10% after IM nailing.
- Non-union: 1.5% after closed treatment of stable fractures; 2–4% after IM nailing; 4–8% after plate fixation; 18% after external fixation of open fractures.
- Malunion: 2.5–11%.
- Ankle and subtalar joint stiffness: 30%.

Further reading

Russell TA. Fractures of the tibia and fibula. In: Rockwood CA, Green DP, Bucholz RW, Heckman JD, eds. *Rockwood and Green's Fractures in Adults*. Philadelphia: Lippincott–Raven, 1996; 2127–2200

Wiss DA, ed. Symposium: The treatment of tibial fractures. *Clinical Orthopaedics and Related Research*. Philadelphia: JB Lippincott, 1995; **315**: 1–198.

Wiss DA, Gibson T. IM nailing of the femur and tibia: indications and techniques. *Current Orthopaedics*, 1994; **8**: 245–254.

Related topics of interest

VASCULAR INJURIES

Arterial injury

Epidemiology and mechanism

Arterial injury may result from 'trauma' or 'surgery'. Most peripheral vascular injuries follow penetrating trauma – in Europe largely stab wounds and in North America low-velocity gunshot wounds. Blunt vascular trauma is less common. Certain fractures and dislocations predispose to arterial injury (*Table 1*).

In children, 1% of supracondylar elbow fractures have an associated vascular injury. In adults, 50% of fractures or dislocations about the knee have a vascular injury and 10% require surgical management. Open tibial fractures have a 10% incidence of vascular injury.

Some orthopaedic surgical procedures can have arterial complications. Presentation is typically intra-operative, but may be delayed with a pseudoaneurysm or arteriovenous fistula. Common sites are given in *Table 2*.

Table 1. Fracture/dislocation and the corresponding arteries predisposed to injury

Bone	Artery
1. Upper extremity	
Clavicle and first rib	Subclavian
Shoulder dislocation	Axillary
Distal humerus	Brachial
2. Lower extremity	
Femoral shaft	Superficial femoral
Supracondylar femur	Popliteal
Knee dislocation	Popliteal
Proximal tibia	Popliteal/tibial/peroneal
Distal tibia	Tibial/peroneal

Table 2. Surgical procedures and the arteries that can be affected

Procedure	Artery
Clavicle plating	Subclavian
THR/acetabulum	Iliac/gluteal/common femoral
TKR	Popliteal
Spine	Iliac/aorta

Classification of arterial injury

Five types of arterial injury are described:

- Spasm.
- Intimal flap tear or haematoma.

- Wall defect.
- Transection.
- Arteriovenous fistula.

Spasm and intimal flaps may be associated with blunt trauma. The remaining types follow penetrating trauma.

Presentation

The classic presentation of arterial insufficiency or injury are the five Ps (pallor, pulselessness, paraesthesiae, paralysis and pain), but the most acute and dramatic presentation is massive haemorrhage. Other hard signs are an expanding haematoma, a thrill or bruit. These signs usually indicate the need for urgent surgical intervention.

Subtle features in both the history and examination should raise suspicion of an arterial injury. These include penetrating trauma, location of the wound, associated nerve injury, non-pulsatile haematoma over an artery, tardy capillary refill (>2 sec) and clinical awareness in certain fracture or dislocation patterns.

Investigations

1. Doppler flow. In the absence of palpable pulses, the quickest test is with a hand-held Doppler flow probe. The ankle/brachial index may be calculated (<0.9 is indicative of arterial injury).

2. Duplex ultrasound. This more sophisticated technique is increasingly available and highly accurate.

3. Arteriography. This is the 'gold standard' technique to establish the presence and anatomical site of a lesion. This may be undertaken in the X-ray department or operating theatre, obtaining single or biplanar images following injection of contrast. Multiplanar images with or without digital subtraction taken in the angiography suite are superior, but time-consuming and can be difficult to arrange acutely.

Initial management

1. Acute massive haemorrhage needs immediate control and is best achieved by direct pressure. Tourniquet application is seldom indicated. Following temporary control and immediate life-saving measures, the patient is transferred to the operating theatre.

2. Deformity and absent peripheral pulse requires reduction and reassessment. This may be undertaken in the accident department or operating theatre.

Definitive management

1. Non-operative. In some injuries, such as single vessel occlusion (below the knee or elbow), the distal circulation may be adequate. This is usually determined by adequate capillary refill (<2 sec). In such cases, close monitoring is maintained and surgery may not be required. Some intimal flaps may heal spontaneously without occlusion.

2. Operative. Combined orthopaedic and vascular injuries usually require skeletal stabilization prior to vascular repair, to avoid disruption of the repair during fracture or joint reduction. Where surgery is delayed, with a warm ischaemia time >6 hours, immediate revascularization is required. This may be achieved by temporary shunting and subsequent definitive repair after skeletal stabilization.

3. Techniques. Knowledge of the principles of vascular repair is essential for all trauma surgeons. Positioning and draping should allow full access to the whole limb, with incisions directly over the artery concerned.

- In the upper limb, the clavicle may be divided to access the subclavian artery in the supraclavicular region. Extension of the deltopectoral incision allows access to the axillary and brachial artery. A lazy 'S' incision is used at the elbow.
- In the lower limb, the femoral artery in the groin is accessed anteriorly. In the thigh and around the knee vascular injuries are approached from the medial side.
- Surgical repair follows proximal control with vascular clamps and resection of the damaged vessel. Repair is achieved with a number of techniques (using 6/0 non-absorbable suture), including:

> Direct closure.
> End to end anastomosis.
> End to side anastomosis.
> Vein graft patch.
> Reversed vein graft.
> Prosthetic graft.

Proximal and distal embolectomy may be required to restore flow, in addition to local heparinization and flushing. Direct repairs under tension should be avoided as occlusion is common. Deficits >4 cm should be grafted. Vein graft is superior to prosthetic graft.

Venous injury

Damaged large veins above the knee or elbow should be repaired, although this is technically difficult and the vein may still occlude. Techniques are similar to arterial repair, but direct closure is the favoured method.

Complications
- Occlusion.
- Infection.
- Embolus.
- Ischaemia.
- False aneurysm.

Further reading

Feliciano D. Evaluation and treatment of vascular injuries. In: Browner BD, Jupiter JB, Levine AM, Trafton PG, eds. *Skeletal Trauma*. Philadelphia: WB Saunders, 1998; 349–364.

Related topics of interest

Compartment syndrome, p. 41; Peripheral nerve injuries and repair, p. 192

INDEX